Manual of Paediatric Intensive Care Nursing

Manual of Paediatric Intensive Care Nursing

Edited by

Bernadette Carter

Senior Lecturer
Department of Health Care Studies
Manchester Metropolitan University

CHAPMAN & HALL
London · Glasgow · New York · Tokyo · Melbourne · Madras

Published by Chapman & Hall, 2–6 Boundary Row, London SE1 8HN

Chapman & Hall, 2–6 Boundary Row, London SE1 8HN, UK

Blackie Academic & Professional, Wester Cleddens Road, Bishopbriggs, Glasgow G64 2NZ, UK

Chapman & Hall Inc., 29 West 35th Street, New York NY10001, USA

Chapman & Hall Japan, Thomson Publishing Japan, Hirakawacho Nemoto Building, 6F, 1–7–11 Hirakawa-cho, Chiyoda-ku, Tokyo 102, Japan

Chapman & Hall Australia, Thomas Nelson Australia, 102 Dodds Street, South Melbourne, Victoria 3205, Australia

Chapman & Hall India, R. Seshadri, 32 Second Main Road, CIT East, Madras 600 035, India

Distributed in the USA and Canada by Singular Publishing Group Inc., 4284 41st Street, San Diego, California 92105

First edition 1993

© 1993 Bernadette Carter

Typeset in 10/12 Times by Mews Photosetting, Beckenham, Kent
Printed in England by Clays Ltd, St. Ives plc

ISBN 0 412 44050 4   1 56593 042 8 (USA)

A catalogue record for this book is available from the British Library

Library of Congress Cataloging-in-Publication data available

∞ Printed on permanent acid-free text paper, manufactured in accordance with the proposed ANSI/NISO Z 39.48-199X and ANSI Z 39.48-1984

To Mum and Dad

Contents

Contributors

Julie Asquith RGN, RSCN, ENB 100, Diploma in Nursing
Senior Clinical Nurse
Paediatric Intensive Care Units
Guy's Hospital
London

Jackie Browne RSCN, RGN
Sister
Children's Intensive Care
Queens Medical Centre
Nottingham

Steve Campbell BNurs., RGN, RSCN, RHV, NDNCert., Cert. Ed.
Lecturer in Child Health Nursing
Nursing Studies, University of Southampton
Southampton General Hospital
Southampton

Bernadette Carter RSCN, RGN, BSc(Hons) Nursing Studies, PGCE, RNT
Senior Lecturer in Health Care Studies
Manchester Metropolitan University
Manchester

Margaret Clancy RGN, RSCN, ENB 160, ENB 998
In-service Education Manager (Paediatrics)
Royal Brompton National Heart and Lung Hospitals
London

Frances Clarke RGN, RSCN, RN, DPSN, ENB 603, ENB 927, ENB 998
Nurse Specialist Teacher (Paediatrics)
Newcastle College of Health
Newcastle

Dot Cooper NNEB, RGN, RSCN, DN (Lond), Cert Ed, RNT, BA(Hons) Psychology
Senior Lecturer
Liverpool John Moores University
Liverpool

Carolyn Davies RSCN, RGN, ENB 405, ENB 160
Nurse Manager,
Women and Children's Services
Hull Hospitals
Hull

Carmen Griffiths RGN, RSCN, ENB 136
Sister
Paediatric Haemodialysis Unit
Guy's Hospital
London

Margaret Hicklin RGN, RSCN, ENB 136
Senior Sister
Paediatric Nephrology Ward
Guys Hospital
London

Eiri Jones RGN, RSCN, ENB 100
Formerly Senior Nurse
Paediatric Intensive Care Unit
Royal Brompton National Heart and Lung Hospitals
London

John Lockwood BPharm, MRPharmS
Director of Pharmacy
Booth Hall Children's Hospital
Manchester

Susan Maxwell RSCN, RGN
Sister
Paediatric Intensive Therapy Unit
Royal Hospital for Sick Children
Glasgow

Cathy McCarthy RGN, RSCN
Clinical Nurse Manager
Neonatal and Paediatric Intensive Care
The Hospital for Sick Children
Great Ormond Street
London

Christine Oldfield RGN, RSCN, QDN, ENB 934
Sister
Paediatric Intensive Care Unit
Booth Hall Children's Hospital
Manchester

Adelaide Tunstill RGN, RSCN, BA
Clinical Nurse Manager
Cardiac Unit
The Hospital for Sick Children
Great Ormond Street
London

Pip Waddington RGN, RSCN
Sister
Children's Intensive Care Unit
Queens Medical Centre
Nottingham

Mary Wallis RGN, SCM, RSCN
Senior Sister
Neonatal Surgical Ward
The Hospital for Sick Children
Great Ormond Street
London

Foreword

It is with very real pleasure that I write the foreword to the first edition of the *Manual of Paediatric Intensive Care Nursing*. I welcome this addition to the family of paediatric nursing care texts. The arrival of a new child in a family is a cause of celebration and this one is particularly welcomed.

Paediatric intensive care is a relatively new speciality which reflects the availability and appropriateness of new technology, and of scientific and medical developments for the care of critically ill children and young people. However, all these advances would be ineffective without the skills of the paediatric intensive care nurse in meeting and appreciating the needs of the child and family.

It is in recognition of these skills that this book has been written, providing an easily accessible knowledge base for the student and newly qualified nurse practitioner entering this paediatric speciality. It will also provide interesting and useful material for those paediatric nurses working in wards and departments which refer children to, and receive children back from, intensive care situations.

Partnership in care is a reality throughout the text. Teamwork is the hallmark of quality care, and such teamwork is mirrored in the list of contributors to the text. I congratulate them all.

Barbara Weller MSc, RSCN, RGN, RNT
Independent Paediatric Nurse Adviser
Lecturer at Norfolk College of Nursing and Midwifery

The ethos of paediatric intensive care

1

Steve Campbell and Frances Clarke

Paediatric intensive care is a specialty which is made more arduous by the innate variety of the potential users of the service. Children will vary in age and so have differing physical and developmental characteristics, but the age of the child does not define the state of physical and pyschological development. The cause of the child's visit to the paediatric intensive care unit and need for other critical care services will be either acute or chronic in nature, and the resources of the family, both psychosocial and material, will be diverse.

The ethos of paediatric intensive care has responded to the nature of the client it serves and the historical perspective from which it has developed and continues to develop. Technical developments and reactionary responses to crisis have shaped paediatric intensive care, and it is therefore highly appropriate to review the history of the specialty.

A BRIEF SELECTIVE HISTORY

A nurse in training (Laurence, 1912) wrote of her experiences at a General Hospital in London in 1896:

> Soon after I took charge we had a run of tracheostomies; the first was a dear, fat baby of thirteen months, but it had diphtheria very badly, and was not a hopeful case from the first; not many hours after it was operated upon another came in – a sweet little boy of three called 'Alex'. He was much relieved by the operation, and got on so well; but the poor baby ran a temperature of 106° all through the second day, and died late that evening with a temperature of 108°, in spite of all we could do for it. I believe we were much more cut up about losing it than the mother was; she did not seem to mind a bit, and apparently had made all her plans for the funeral beforehand – and it was such a pretty baby too!
>
> The special nurses I had for these tracheostomies had never nursed one before, so you can imagine I could not leave them alone, and was thankful I had a good many to nurse when I was a lady pupil...
>
> (Laurence, 1912: 89–90)

Modern medicine, technology and a deeper understanding of the physiological processes would suggest that Alex would survive in today's health service. Much has changed in paediatric care over last 100 years, but Laurence (1912) in her letter to person(s) unknown touched unwittingly on three areas central to paediatric care today; standards of care, psychological support for families, and staff training and educational needs (Rosenthal and Connors, 1989)

In 1896 (Laurence 1912) nurses and doctors were making advances in the fight against crippling disease and ill-health, and it is interesting to look back in time, even before 1896, and see how the specialty of intensive care has developed. Goldsmith and Karotkin (1988) remind us that the earliest recorded description of mouth-to-mouth resuscitation occurs in the Bible (II Kings 4: 34). It also involves a child:

> Then he went and lay upon the child, putting his mouth upon his mouth, his eyes upon his eyes and his hands upon his hands; and as he stretched himself upon him the flesh of the child became warm.

The literature generally refers to experimentation with intubation occurring around the sixteenth and seventeenth centuries, but Goldsmith and Karotkin (1988) suggest that Hippocrates (400BC) was the first medical investigator to document his experience with intubation of the trachea to support respiration. Nearly two thousand years were to pass before further work by Paracelsus (1493–1541) involving bellows and a tube. Better known is the work of Vesalius (1555) and Hook (1667) (cited by Mushin *et al.*, 1967), who both demonstrated that even though the chest wall was open it was still possible to ventilate an animal's lungs using bellows to sustain life, effectively providing controlled intermittent positive pressure ventilation (IPPV). Problems persisted, however, as it was one thing to intubate an animal in a laboratory but quite another to intubate humans. Pioneering efforts to operate within the abdomen were largely successful, but intrathoracic surgery remained largely futile owing to the problems of lung collapse and only 'a hurried conclusion of the operation ensured the patient's survival' (Mushin et al., 1969).

Goldsmith and Karotkin (1988) report that by 1667 simple forms of continuous and regular ventilation had been developed, along with an improved understanding of the basic physiology of pulmonary ventilation. Early attempts at neonatal resuscitation of asphyxiated infants were described by Chaussier, the Professor of Obstetrics in the French Academy of Science. Goldsmith and Karotkin (1988) cite Chaussier's successors as developing the *aerophone pulmonaire* in 1879, the first device designed purely for use with newborn infants. This consisted of a tube, which was introduced into the infant's upper airway, connected to a rubber bulb which was alternatively compressed and released. Direct intubation of the larynx was still limited and there were few reports of intubation being performed.

Sykes (1962) suggests that interest in intubation only developed on a large scale because of the bizarre efforts of Manuel Garcia, who was born in Madrid in 1805 and was appointed Professor of Singing at the Paris Conservatoire in 1835. Garcia was obsessed with discovering how his vocal cords worked. In 1854 he bought a dental mirror for six francs and practised with the aid of another mirror until he could see his own vocal cords and establish what they did. The outcome was a presentation to the Royal Society in 1855 entitled 'Observation on the human voice'. Garcia's method of indirect laryngoscopy helped to create interest in the larynx, which spread rapidly, commencing in Vienna and Budapest. Although the first direct-vision laryngoscope was described by Kirsten in Berlin in 1895, laryngeal cannulae were by and large introduced by touch alone. Mushin et al. (1969) write that 'not even Kirsten envisaged the routine use of his "Autoscope" for intubation of the larynx'.

Because difficulties in intubation persisted, efforts to provide mechanical ventilation centred around negative pressure devices applied either to the chest or to the whole body (Mushin et al., 1969). Woollam (1976a,b) gives a comprehensive account of the development of intermittent negative pressure ventilation from its first description in 1832 through various refinements and developments to 1976. He cites a story of Alexander Graham Bell, the inventor of the telephone, who also developed a vacuum jacket in 1882 to aid respiration. The death of his infant son a year earlier may have acted as the catalyst (Woollam, 1976a). Negative pressure persisted in various forms and was to dominate the first 30–40 years of the twentieth century. Even Sir Ivan Magill, who refined endotracheal intubation techniques in 1929, believed that intrathoracic operations gave better results when gases were administered under positive pressure with a facepiece rather than endotracheal tubes (Duncalf, 1978). Robson (1936) described intubation of the trachea in infants and young children using rubber tubes. Further sophistication of techniques came with the development of a paediatric laryngoscope, the Shadwell (Gillespie, 1939) and recognition that the material used in endotracheal could be harmful to the trachea (Guess and Stetson, 1968).

By the end of the Second World War, a prototype of a mechanical ventilator, the Blease Pulmoflator, was in use on Merseyside at the Wallasey Cottage Hospital. Initial scepticism about the apparatus was replaced by appreciation. Further refinements and developments ensued (Mushin *et al.*, 1969).

Events moved rapidly in Europe after the catastrophic poliomyelitis epidemic in 1952 in Denmark. Early patients were treated with tank ventilators, mostly without tracheostomy, resulting in 87% dying largely because of inadequate ventilation and retained secretions. Over 300 other patients treated with manual IPPV synchronized with the patient's own breathing via a tracheostomy did much better, with only a 25% mortality rate. Fourteen hundred medical students were co-opted to assist with the hand ventilation, necessitating the suspension of teaching activities until the epidemic was over (Grenvik *et al.*, 1980; Mushin *et al.*, 1969).

The epidemic resulted in contingency programmes being established in other European countries. Mushin *et al.* (1969) write:

> As the winds of alarm at the approaching catastrophe fanned the embers of inventive genius an abundance of new solutions to the manpower problems were forged in flames.   (1969: 209)

Mechanical ventilators flooded the market; within 3–4 years, accepted methods of ventilating patients had been radically challenged and changed. The result was that the USA still had patients being treated in 'tank respirators' while in Europe they had virtually become obsolete.

Donald and Lord (1953) described the use of mechanical ventilation delivered via a face mask for newborns with respiratory distress. Initial efforts had a limited degree of success, and progress was hampered by the lack of suitable ventilation for children. Mushin *et al.* (1962) identifying problems of automatic ventilation in infants and young children, wrote:

> In general automatic ventilators designed for adults do not work satisfactorily for small subjects. Either the flow is too large, the respiratory rate too slow, the tidal volume too large or the cycling pressure too high.   (1962: 514)

Another problem resulted from work by André Cournard in the late 1940s (Goldsmith and Karotkin, 1988). Cournard demonstrated that a prolonged inspiratory time could result in impaired thoracic venous return and decreased cardiac output. It was normal for ventilators to have a short inspiratory phase which was thought to be appropriate for adults but was not helpful to infants with respiratory distress syndrome.

It seems incredible that, as recently as 1970, Behrman stated:

> ... evidence is still not strong enough and the indications for treatment are not sharply enough defined to establish the effectiveness of assisted ventilation for all premature infants with severe hyaline membrane disease.   (1970: 172)

Incredible, in view of the great advances in neonatal and paediatric ventilation made over the last twenty years. Progress came with the work of Gregory *et al.* (1971), who published encouraging results on the use of continuous positive airway pressure (CPAP) in respiratory distress syndrome. Reynolds and Taghizadeh (1974) demonstrated that, by delaying the opening of the expiratory valve, inspirational time could be prolonged, and that this was beneficial to the infant with respiratory distress syndrome.

Downs *et al.* (1973) published a paper on intermittent mandatory ventilation (IMV), which for the first time allowed patients to breathe spontaneously and delivered a mechanical inflation at preset intervals. Further sophistication of IMV enabled synchronization with the child's own breathing. When a mandatory breath is due, the ventilator delays delivering air until the child begins a natural inspiration; if the child does not initiate a breath within a certain time, the ventilator delivers a mechanical inflation (Ellington, 1989).

Initially, many infants and children received respiratory support via modified adult ventilation. During the 1970s, great advances in the design of ventilators specifically for neonatal and paediatric use were made, based on Ayre's T-piece system modified by Rees (Rees, 1950; Inkster, 1978; Sumner, 1986).

One of the earliest paediatric intensive care units was opened at the Alder Hey Children's Hospital in 1964. Advances in cardiac surgery and anaesthesia ensured that a large percentage of children were recovering from cardiac surgery (Duncalf, 1978; Steward, 1989). Steward (1989) writers of a new collaboration between anaesthetists and paediatricians during the 1960s, which allowed new boundaries to be breached in the care of children with pneumonia, asthma, upper airway disease, poisons and so on.

Parallel to respiratory care development, there has been an advancement in the use of inotropic drugs and neuromuscular blocking agents, with increasing understanding of the need and use of analgesia. Monitoring equipment, both invasive and non-invasive, has become increasingly more sophisticated, with links to computer systems. The skills to use these technologies and the background comprehension of life science theory are clear requirements of the modern paediatric intensivist (Kidder, 1989) and are covered substantially in subsequent chapters. The ethos of care that has developed as a result of these technologies is the business of this chapter.

It is the child and the family who are confronted by these little-known and frightening environments. Paediatric care can be regarded as a highly dynamic area, such as in the case of paediatric oncology (Thompson, 1990) but can also be an area where improvements in care strategies have taken considerable time to come to reality (Department of Health, 1959).

The care of children in critical care can be in a variety of settings: the special care baby unit, the neonatal intensive care unit, the paediatric intensive care unit, the adult high-dependency unit, or the adult intensive care unit. This list is far from exhaustive. Specialist courses have existed for nurses for some years for the care of the neonate. However, it is only within the last 5 years that paediatric intensive care nursing courses have come about, notably at the Birmingham Sick Children's Hospital. The drive for this course was brought about by the deficiency of appropriately trained paediatric intensive care nurses. Such courses have dealt with the diversity of need of these children and their families. The resultant practitioners must be innately flexible in their approach to families, as well as dealing with a variety of technologies.

TWO CASE STUDIES

The following two case studies are presented to exemplify the different nature of clients of the paediatric intensive care unit and their impact on the nature of the service and its philosophy. They will be used in the further analysis of the ethos of paediatric intensive care.

George: a child with a congenital heart defect

George was a 2-year-old who was born with a congenital heart defect. The parents also had a 3-year-old daughter, Lisa, at the time of George's birth and lived in the vicinity of George's mother's family, who were very supportive. John, George's father, came from the south of the country, 200 miles away, and his parents came to stay at the family home at the time of George's birth. However, they were elderly and became tired and a worry to John, while they were in the north. Julie's family, in contrast, took over a lot of household tasks, such as washing, and Lisa was cared for by her aunts and uncles, along with her cousins of a similar age.

The management of George's heart defect was problematic. He was duct dependent, and the dosage of drugs required to keep the duct open seemed to vary from day to day in the initial period. This was complicated by George being prone to vomiting until he moved on to a mixed diet. As a result, although George did not require specific care on a paediatric intensive care unit, he was critically ill for periods during his first 6 months of life.

Julie stayed with George while he was on the paediatric cardiology ward. After the discovery of George's heart defect and the initial stress of going through this period of stabilization, Julie was exhausted and went home to rest. From this point, the family settled into a pattern of care. Julie would stay during the week and go home at the weekend to spend time with Lisa. John would visit his wife and son, sometimes with Lisa and other relatives during the evening.

Julie was initially reluctant to provide physical care for George. However, the family's primary nurse worked patiently and carefully with the family and her team to facilitate Julie's involvement. Julie started off by changing George's nappies and keeping him clean. Feeding George was not easy; he became cyanosed very quickly and the recurrent vomiting episodes were potentially dangerous. To a great extent George tended to be tube fed, and Julie started to be involved in the feeding by cuddling George while his nurse tube fed him. Ultimately, Julie was able to carry this out on her own and felt comfortable giving supportive oxygen therapy.

It became increasingly apparent that George was not going to be very old before surgery would be necessary. The cardiologist always included the parents in the discussion about the timing of surgery, but the decision was made with the cardiac surgeon. The family found the surgeon to be an aloof character, in contrast with the more relaxed approach of the paediatric cardiologists.

Julie, in particular, became familiar with many of the other families of children with heart defects. She appreciated the supportive conversations she had with other mothers in the evening when the children had gone to sleep. They all supported the parents of children who had undergone surgery and who were critically ill on the paediatric intensive care unit. Julie had known parents who had lost children and parents whose children had undergone successful surgery. She had a well balanced approach to the imminent surgery, knowing that it was potentially dangerous, but that it was the only hope for George to have some semblance of a normal life.

The immediate postoperative period was without problems; however, it soon became evident that George's temperature was elevated, and it remained high. There were also signs of cerebral irritability. John was very angry that something was going wrong and blamed the doctors for their incompetence. Julie sought the support of her friends on the cardiology ward and John disappeared for 2 days, but when anger gave way to despair John returned allowing Julie to comfort him. George's temperature finally subsided, but the neurological symptoms persisted and he required anticonvulsant drug support. George's heart defect appeared to have been corrected satisfactorily, but the malignant high temperature had caused brain damage.

Maria: a child with a head injury

Maria was a 12-year-old girl. She was an only child who was born to her mother when she was in her late thirties and had largely given up hope of having a family. Maria had to fight for her independence; she had difficulty in getting out to parties and trips with her friends.

Maria had been in hospital before only when she had her tonsils and adenoids removed at 6 years of age. Her mother, Doris, was not allowed to stay and the whole experience was remembered by the family as being unsatisfactory. Doris's husband, Ernest, had chronic heart problems and was on the waiting list for a triple coronary artery bypass graft.

Maria was brought to the paediatric intensive care unit by ambulance. She had been picked up after being knocked down by a car, having run out from between two parked cars. It was suspected that Maria might have fractured her femur, and she had a head injury but was breathing spontaneously. It was fortunate that the paediatric intensive care unit was in the same hospital as the neurosurgical service. Shortly after arriving at the emergency department, Maria became apnoeic and required intubation and ventilation.

Neither of the parents had ever been in an intensive care unit and so despite a doctor and the nurse in charge explaining what they were about to see and the state of their daughter, they were still shocked by the environment and the appearance of their daughter in particular. Doris was also worried about Ernest, who had recovered his pallor after taking some glycerine trinitrate.

Mothers of other children on the unit were a lot younger than Doris. However, it was noticeable that despite Doris's natural disposition, which was not friendly, one of the mothers, whose son was in the bed by Maria, made a point of offering support during the first few hours of Maria's admission.

Maria was found to have had a large intracerebral haemorrhage as a result of a tentorial tear. She underwent neurosurgery for drainage, which reduced the intracranial pressure. However, she never regained consciousness and was found to satisfy the brain death criteria. These events occurred over a period of about a week, leaving the parents to bury and grieve for their only child.

FRAMEWORKS OF CARE

The British Paediatric Association Working Party on Paediatric Intensive Care (1987) defines the function of a paediatric intensive care service as providing 'for the needs of the critically ill child requiring constant individualised nursing care and immediately available skilled medical help'.

This definition establishes some limited criteria of paediatric intensive care services. Each child will differ in chronological and development age, in cause of the initiating problem whether acute or chronic, and in the psychosocial and material resources of the family. The interpretation of the expression, 'constant individualised nursing care' will vary in time, as well as the potential qualities of the individuals providing this care. In a similar manner, immediately available medical help may vary from an experienced consultant paediatric anaesthetist to the senior house officer on his or her first experience of paediatrics.

Rushton (1990) suggests that 'Critical care nurses and other professionals caring for ill or injured infants and children struggle to balance the effects of technology with caring'. This balance need not just be a qualitative one, but may also be one of quantity, when the time demands of technical care are so great for the critical care nurse.

Shelton *et al.* (1987) list the Association of Children's Health Care's elements of family-centred care as the following:

1. recognition that the family is the constant in the child's life while the service systems and personnel within those systems fluctuate;
2. faciliation of parent–professional collaboration at all levels of health care;
3. sharing of unbiased and complete information with parents about their child's care on an ongoing basis in an appropriate and supportive manner;
4. implementation of appropriate policies and programmes that are comprehensive and provide emotional and financial support to meet the needs of families;
5. recognition of family strengths and individuality and respect for different methods of coping;
6. understanding and incorporating the developmental and emotional needs of infants, children and adolescents and their families into health-care delivery systems;
7. encouragement and facilitation of parent to child support;
8. assurance that the design of health-care delivery systems is flexible, accessible and responsive to family needs.

The framework of family-centred care represents one of the few written descriptions of this much-discussed style of care. The background of these elements is North American, and so the framework comes from a fee-paying privatized system of health care. However, since the advent of NHS trusts and the purchaser–provider relationship, the North American experience does not seem to be so far removed from the UK mode of delivery of care.

There seems to be a potential for the use of this framework for paediatric intensive care units, intensive care units with child patients or areas where critically ill children are nursed, to assess the family-centred nature of their care. The framework could be adapted to become a quality assurance tool within the intensive care unit. Nurse teachers, who are asked to help to prepare staff for the unit or update members of the team, could use this framework to analyse the care of the unit or the care delivered by the nurse in a self-reflective manner.

The elements of family-centred care appear to be complementary to the National Association for the Welfare of Children in Hospital Charter (Hogg, 1989). This charter is child-centred, but three of the rights outlined refer to parents and all of them can fit into an element of family-centred care.

Rushton (1990) presents a brief description of each of these elements of family-centred care and suggests that potential strategies be identified to implement family-centred care. This structure represents a useful one to analyse the potential of such an ethos within the UK.

Element 1: recognizing the family as the constant in the child's life

The family has the ultimate responsibility for responding to the child's emotional, social, developmental, and health care needs. To treat the critically ill child respectfully, to acknowledge and value who they are outside of the medical context in addition to the relationships that are central to their lives. This means making the family the unit of care instead of isolating the child's needs from those of the family. (Rushton, 1990: 196).

This element of family-centred care conflicts with the philosophy of medical dominance. A unit that regards the medical and health professionals as having the final responsibility for the health care needs of the child will be in immediate conflict. This attitude is patronizing to the members of the family. It is a truism that the child's loved ones are those that care for him most. They will therefore, almost without exception, choose the best option for the child's health. The role of the health professional becomes one of educator as the family learns about the complexities of the problems.

A good example of such partnership is when a child of a known doctor is admitted to the paediatric intensive care unit. In these circumstances of great stress for both the PICU staff and the family, a natural partnership develops. The family is more often included in the discussions about potential decisions about the treatment and the care of the child. Other children within the family may be cared for by staff through informal arrangements. Special measures are often made for communication and sleeping in the hospital. Subsequent analysis of this phenomenon must consider whether it is justified that these families receive special care compared with the majority of clients.

The care of these families is certainly different, because, apart from the fact that an established relationship already exists, there is at least one family member who has a good level of medical comprehension. However, this difference can be compensated for by appropriate education. The special nature of the respect that the care team has for the family could be regarded, quite simply, as family-centred care. It could therefore become a goal of paediatric intensive care units to strive to achieve a level of care at which there are not perceived differences between this special case and the care of any child and his or her family on admission to the paediatric intensive care unit. Indeed, this goal could be applied to any unit, whether paediatric or adult, acute or chronic.

An example of the practice of this aspect of family-centred care would be in the active inclusion of the family in the ward rounds. It is still not uncommon for parents to be excluded, perhaps not physically, but by lack of communication. The professional members of this group will vary from day to day, but the family remains constant. In the special case of the family of the health professional, the family would be included because of the relationship already in existence, as well as the knowledge base of the family. In George's case, it is more likely but not certain that his family would be included. His family would already have been identified for its unique role because of the 2 years of working with the family. However, this may be difficult for some health professionals, who may only have met the family since the crisis (Moore, 1989). Similarly, the family's knowledge base will be known because of the length of time they have been communicating with hospital staff. Maria and her family are less likely to be included actively in discussions, because they are not known by the health professionals, and their medical knowledge is not sufficiently developed. The family may only be included in an active manner if there is a unified philosophy to their inclusion and respect for their ultimate responsibility for the child's health. This situation is currently exemplified by the inclusion of the family in discussion about their child's potential brain death, such as in Maria's case. In these circumstances there are clear guidelines, but the care can be more naturally developed by including the family from admission in the discussion about potential diagnoses and outcomes, at an appropriate level for constructive communication.

By contrast, it is common for health staff to leave the responsibility with the family for their child's emotional, developmental and social needs. However, this may not always be appropriate, nor may the family be aware that this is the case, unless this is verbalized. The child's physical or mental capacity may be restricted and the parents may not have the skills to deal with the new needs of the child. Here, there are clear demands on health professionals to help parents to adapt their skills to the new demands of the child's care. The parents may be afraid to become involved because of the equipment, or they may feel that they are not allowed to play with their child (Rennick, 1986). If the parents are to be involved in an active manner, they need to be empowered to do so. This empowerment may be in informal discussions with the staff about what they can or cannot do, but may be as a result of formal communications within the unit, such as leaflets and posters.

In communication, the staff who believe in the philosophy of family-centred care will be those that are able to get the message over to the families.

The conversion of the care of a unit into one that considers the needs of the family rather than merely the child is fraught with difficulties. It is not possible to see the child functioning normally within the family when that family is removed from its natural environment, or may not be present entirely. There is also a natural tendency to include the parents alongside the child and ignore the rest of the family. There are some good physiological reasons for restricting the number of visitors to a child in some cases, but this restricts the capacity of the family to be present at the bedside, and may also mean that other restrictions are implicit. For example, parents may choose not to bring two siblings because one parent will have to stay out with one of them and it will be therefore impossible for both the parents to be in with the ill child at any one time. These policies need to be examined within the perspective of family-centred care. Whether health professionals recognize the consequences of their behaviour is not clear; the enforcement of such rules will only be seen as just if they are beneficial to the child's recovery and are understood. Enforcement by rote will only alienate the family from the unit and lead to poor care. The rules put the staff, who are already in a position of power, into an autocratic frame which appears to be at odds with the philosophy of family-centred care, with its democratic roots and focus on the rights of the family.

Element 2: faciliating parent–professional collaboration

The cornerstone of successful collaboration between parents and professionals is mutual respect for the unique perspectives and contributions each has to offer the health care relationship. Traditionally, the relationship has been dominated by professionals who determine the extent of parental involvement. This shift to a collaborative partnership between parents and professionals may be particularly challenging in the critical care setting, where professionals have been exclusively responsible for providing intensive care, making rapid decisions, and controlling the flow of information to families. A partnership cannot occur without deliberate assessment of the attitude and expectations of both and a mutual commitment of each to the new relationship. (Rushton, 1990: 196)

This element of family-centred care is a natural extension of regarding the family as the constant in the child's life. However, it cannot be achieved without the commitment of the staff to this aspect of the philosophy. An examination of other strategies in relation to the current system of care, such as the potential of primary nursing (Manley, 1989), may produce some insight leading to resultant changes in behaviour. However, the philosophy is relevant only if all the staff are involved, potentially from the cleaner to the head nurse or consultant anaesthetist.

It has been traditional for the consultant or senior nurse to make the rules within their own team and attempt to give rules to the other professions. There is a climate encouraging audit of services provided, but even these are divided professionally, into medical and nursing audit (Department of Health, 1991). The results of these exercises will be piecemeal, especially in gaining the cooperation of the entirety of the staff of an intensive care unit in one unified philosophy of care. It would seem more reasonable to carry out such audit functions in a multidisciplinary manner, and in family-centred care teams, with the cooperation of the families or their representatives. The families will demand this in a 'bottom-up' approach. Professional carers who provide direct care for families will be able to see the power of the arguments, as they are close enough to the bottom to see that these relationships will facilitate higher quality care. However, it may be that individuals in positions of power, such as consultants and head nurses, will feel threatened by the collaboration of families from the bottom to the top of the organization; these collaborations mean that they will have to become more democratic and so lose some of their autocratic powers. The senior nurse or consultant who is threatened by such a new relationship with the family can easily undermine its enactment. However, the resultant care provided by the philosophy of family centredness would reflect well upon all those involved in its enactment, from the cleaner to the senior nurse or consultant.

Element 3: sharing unbiased and complete information with parents

Sharing information between parents and professionals is the first step toward establishing a collaborative relationship. During a child's critical illness, opportunities for optimal communication and information sharing may be deficient or inadequate. Parents cannot fully participate in decision making or care if they fail to understand what they are told. The crisis and stress created by the child's critical illness or injury and the nature of the critical care environment may impose additional barriers to good communication. (Rushton, 1990: 196–197)

The stressful nature of the critical care environment (Etzler, 1984) will naturally produce blocks to successful communication. These blocks may be as simple as the noise of high-technology equipment and noise from other staff or families (Carter *et al.*, 1985; Lybarger, 1979). In Maria's case, the trauma to the parents of discovering that their child had been knocked down would have made it unreasonable for the family to have been given full information about their child's condition. However, it would have been expected that the child's immediate state and current expectations would have been related to the family. Similarly, the equipment that Maria had been connected to would have been explained, and there would have been an expectation that this information would need to be explained repeatedly while the parents were in a state of shock. However, it would also be necessary to give the family full and complete information about their child's state. It is all too easy to leave such information at the level of banal statements about not having identified the problem, rather than informing the family of the potential diagnoses as the tests are carried out. This latter approach adds a natural dimension to the development of the family's knowledge of the child's problem.

On the admission of the child to the paediatric intensive care unit, an assessment of the knowledge of the family and of their willingness to listen to such information must be made. There appears to be a continuum in attitude to medical or nursing control, from the family who want the health professionals to have complete control to those that will not let the professionals make the best decisions for the family. Fortunately, most families fall between these two extremes. However, it is a reflection on the nature of the professional caring relationship that the family that lets the care fall entirely to the health professionals cause fewer problems to the health professionals than the family that maintains its control over the child's welfare. Both extremes cause difficulties, one of which is related to communication. The family that surrenders responsibility to the practitioners will be difficult to establish natural partnership with through the sharing of information; the family that maintains control over the child will form similar difficulties, because its demands for information will be considerable and possibly never ending. In both cases, an assessment of the style of parenting will help the professional to decide the style of communication to be adopted. The family that lets go control of the child will need to be encouraged to become involved and understand that it is in the child's best interest for them to be involved; the family that insists on keeping control represent a difficult problem, but the strategy could be argued to be similar in that it is to bring the family's style of parenting nearer to the centre of the continuum of style. It is impracticable to provide never-ending amounts of information at all times, even if all of the care team is involved. It would seem invidious in a discussion about equal and progressive communication with families during the child's illness to suggest that these families need to alter their style of parenting through communication. However, the immediate demands of the family will need to be dealt with until the relationship with the team has produced sufficient trust for the family to give up some aspects of decision making to the care team and to feel that they need less communication.

Other families may not wish to hear information because they are not yet prepared to cope with potentially traumatic information.

Element 4: providing emotional and financial support

> A child's critical illness, injury, and potential disability will have an
> impact on the child, parents, siblings, extended family and on finances,
> career goals, and marriage. Support needs are multi-dimensional, varied,
> and change over time. Thus, policies and programs must be comprehen-
> sive and responsive to the changing needs of the child and family during
> the critical care experience and beyond. (Rushton, 1990: 197)

The ability of each family to cope with crisis will depend on the resources
of the family and their circumstances. The two families in the case studies
differed greatly in their capacity to cope with the admission of their child to
an intensive care unit. Maria's family was older and, in particular, the father
was a great source of worry because of his health. The family had little
experience of having a child in hospital, let alone being in an intensive care
unit. However, George's family had been in hospital on a regular basis since
his birth. This situation might have exhausted the family but they had adapted
already to the systems within the hospital. They had systems already developed
for the care of their two children, such as visiting in the evening with the
sibling and swapping over at the weekend to give each other a rest as well
as to ensure that both children had time with each parent. An assessment of
the capacity of a family to manage their own needs is particularly difficult.
In the case of Maria, her needs superseded those of her father. It became
the mother's responsibility to monitor the state of Maria's father and her judge-
ment could have been affected by the sudden and unexpected events (Eberley
et al., 1985). The staff would not have known Maria's family; however,
George's family would have visited the paediatric intensive care unit and
possibly met the nurse who was to care for him during the immediate
postoperative period. The preoperative visit(s) would have covered the
adaptations that the family would have to make to the new care environment.
Ward nurses might already have drawn the attention of the family to the
different styles and organization of care on the paediatric intensive care unit.

Rushton (1990) suggests that needs may include crisis intervention, food
and lodging, transportation, sibling and parent to parent support, mental health
services, financial assistance, and arrangements for child care. Strategies to
deal with these problems may be handled by the nuclear family or the extended
family. There may be a professional role for social work or psychiatric support,
or voluntary arrangments through friends who are perhaps family members
of children who have spent time on the paediatric intensive care unit. Primary
nursing provides a useful framework on which to base such strategies.
The time spent developing the initial relationship with a family of a child
on a paediatric intensive care unit is an important time for informed and
astute assessment of the needs of the family. Repeated and unnecessary

introduction of new health professionals will be likely to lead to inconsistency in the manner in which these needs are dealt with, and to alienate the family from the care team. The allocation of a primary nurse allows for the sensitive anticipation of parental needs. Without a strong and well founded relationship, the anticipation of parental needs will be non-existent or introduced without subtlety.

The needs of siblings cannot be dealt with if they are not included in the care or in the time when the parents are caring for the sick child. Policies are important in allowing or denying the inclusion of siblings into this process. Visiting times and the number and kind of visitors need to be examined to discover whether they allow the true participation of the family in family-centred care. Similarly, these policies need to be examined to ensure that health professionals have the capacity to assess and be involved in the needs of the entire family. It may be necessary to provide play facilities within the paediatric intensive care unit, or a supervised play area outside it. The siblings and parents then have the capacity to decide whether the siblings should visit the unit with their parents without being constrained by the potential boredom for the siblings or by concern about whether they might cause harm to the high-technology equipment or to themselves. They can also include the siblings in the care of the child, for the benefit of all the children. Such policies are the business of the families and it would seem appropriate, although administratively difficult, to include parents and families in the decision-making process.

Element 5: recognizing family strengths and individuality

> The entire family system will be affected during the child's critical illness (Hedenkamp, 1980). Each family member will interpret and respond to the situation differently. Recognizing the child's and the family's individual strengths is an important prerequisite for respecting their unique coping strategies. Nurses are in a pivotal role to recognize the coping strategies and the methods of adaptation of family members to the child's illness and to intervene appropriately (Philichi, 1989). (Rushton, 1990: 197).

In the same manner as families have different needs and resources, they have different strengths and styles of coping. George's family's reactions to the various crises show some of the potential reactions (Miles and Carter, 1983; Miles et al., 1984). John started off passively accepting the expertise of the health professionals and had blind faith in them. However, the aggression he showed when Julie suggested that there was a possibility of failure and of losing George would suggest that this was merely a protective measure (May, 1972). John's aggression when he realized that something had gone badly wrong with George might have been out of helplessness. The fact that John left might have been seen as inappropriate, but perhaps he knew that staying would cause more problems.

These strong emotions are difficult for the professional to handle, and family-centred care, where there is a clear partnership between professionals and family, should allow some sharing of the responsibility. Facilities need to be available for parents to spend some time on their own without fear of interruption, as well as rooms where the carers can talk away from the bedside (Hansen *et al.*, 1986).

There are cultural and social variations in reaction to crisis, and the health professional needs to respect these. Hospitals in the UK tend to be able to cater for traditional religions of the country, but the professionals and the facilities tend to be more difficult to obtain, for instance, for Middle Eastern faiths. Families under crisis should not have to work to obtain the religious support that they require; these opportunities should be available as a matter of course.

Element 6: understanding developmental and emotional needs of infants, children and adolescents

A comprehensive, family-centred approach to critical care involves devising strategies to address the physiologic, social, emotional, and developmental needs of the child. At times, the critical care environment may preclude optimal attention to the child's developmental issues. Critical care interventions typically focus on restoring the child to optimal physiologic condition, often at the expense of developmental considerations. Moreover, critical care professionals may be unfamiliar with normal developmental patterns and with interventions to facilitate or restore developmental progress. (Rushton, 1990: 198)

The developmental needs of the child are often given little priority and effort at times of physiological crisis. This would seem to be a reasonable decision, especially when the child's life is at risk. However, the persistence of this lack of effort long after the crisis suggests either that there is a lack of perception of the need or that the professionals involved do not have the skills to provide the stimulation necessary. These skills are highly complex and do not follow the norms. For instance, it would not be totally appropriate to call in a 6-year-old's primary school teacher for ideas on activities for a child who has been rendered quadriplegic by an accident. There may be some skills that she can bring, apart from the pleasure of the visit for the child; however, the teacher is used to normal children who can play as normal, not one who is bedbound and unable to move a limb. At 5 years of age, children will amuse themselves to a certain extent and within the limits of safety. Children's nurses specializing in the care of children in paediatric intensive care settings may have greater skills because of their greater understanding of child development and specialist techniques. However, their approach is likely to be piecemeal, because this area of practice is not fully developed and probably requires the provision of specialist hospital play workers.

Playing with children is often handed over to families as a result of such problems. However, it is of equal difficulty for the parents, although they will be able to alter play that they know their child enjoys for the critical care setting. A holistic approach to the assessment of the child's play needs is necessary for continued development, especially if the child is hospitalized for some time. Play will need to be developed to encourage the natural development of the child within the restrictions of the unit and the physical capacity of the child. These assessments are highly specialized, but potentially within the scope of the paediatric intensive care nurse.

Parents and other relatives sometimes feel that they have to play with a child in hospital at all times. It is as though this is their justification for being resident. From about 5 years of age, children do not spend most of the day with their parents and older relatives. It is therefore not necessary for the parents, to feel that they should be playing with the child at all times.

Element 7: encouraging parent-to-child support

> Support by professionals should be augmented with parent to parent support (Winch and Christoph, 1988). Recognizing the role of other parents as 'veterans' of the ICU experience can help to reduce isolation by creating a social network. Support groups can provide mutual support and friendship, information gathering/sharing, problem solving and exploring ways to improve the systems of care (Nathanson, 1986). (Rushton, 1990: 198).

The parents of children who were former users of the paediatric intensive care represent a large potential resource for the families and care team. Support for families may come from families of other children on the unit, but these families are already under stress, and it is unfair to expect this to happen as a matter of course.

The case studies show two families with dissimilar support structures within the hospital. George's family would have had the support of the parents on the paediatric cardiology ward. They would have been able to leave the paediatric intensive care unit and seek out friends and fellow parent sufferers whom they had known for some time. These other families might be expecting their children to undergo cardiac surgery in the near future, or the children might be recovering from surgery. They would therefore have genuine empathy with George's family in the support that they offered as well as benefiting from a reciprocal relationship in which they prepare themselves for future experiences. George's family would also have had the support of the other families on the intensive care unit. For Maria's family, these families would have been the only natural form of support from other families.

This support occurs in an informal manner, and most staff have approached a group of parents, usually mothers, talking late after their child has gone to sleep, and realized that as a member of staff they are not welcome. The reasons for this must come from some dissatisfaction with their child's progress or the care system, but one would suspect that a family-centred style of care would lead to parents having a forum to discuss such problems directly. This parent-to-parent or family-to-family support is vital to the continued healthy coping of these families. The introduction of a stressed family which has been volunteered for the purpose of supporting another family is a recipe for disaster; the giver will feel abused and the receiving family will be made to feel that they are the abuser. However, the parents of children who were formerly treated in the unit are keen to be involved, and if selected appropriately, for their role in supporting the families, rather than their ability to maintain the status quo, will be invaluable in providing humanistic support that can only lead to higher standards of care (Oksala and Merenmies, 1989; Stevens, 1981). Such supporters may facilitate communication about unspoken problems or worries, and these concerns can be fed into policy making to improve the general quality of care.

Element 8: assuring that health care is flexible, accessible and responsive to family needs

> To make family centred care a reality in the critical care setting it will be necessary for parents, professionals, and administrators to collaborate to redesign the services and the care delivery system to ensure optimal responsiveness to the needs of children and their families. (Rushton, 1990: 199).

The parents and families of the children are currently omitted from the design of, and policy making about, care settings in general and paediatric intensive care unit in particular. The UK is fortunate to have an organization which promotes the welfare of sick children: Action for Sick Children (formerly known as the National Association for the Welfare of Children in Hospital). Health professionals have long been members and supported this organization. It is high time that health professionals invited parents into their managerial or *ad hoc* meetings to help in the analysis of care systems for the improved care of children and their families. This open approach will not just produce the hybrid vigour of such a natural combination of families (parents), professionals and administrators, but will also give a very clear message to the future users of these service about the style and attitude of the care team.

These new systems cannot be forced on an established team; the care team should, in the majority, feel that they want to take on this style of care. An example of a consistent style of nursing is that of primary nursing (Manley, 1989). The patient is able to say that one nurse is his or her primary nurse. These allocations are inevitably stressful for the nurses, but the potential for a high-quality relationship is greatly enhanced. Some critical settings will not take on such primary nursing, because it means that each nurse will be 'stuck' with one patient and the nurses will not enjoy the variety that they prefer. In such circumstances, these actions can be seen as self-protective; they prevent the nurse from getting too close to the patient and the family, and are natural in critical care settings where there is a high mortality rate (May, 1972). The introduction of such a care style would therefore seem to need some kind of increased support network of the primary nurse, so that the nurse can risk joining in such a relationship with the family.

Olds and Daniels (1987) suggest a number of facilities which should be assessed, especially if the paediatric intensive care unit intends to introduce family-centred care:

1. lodging and sleeping facilities within the institution or nearby;
2. places for parents to take care of personal needs;
3. waiting rooms that are easily accessible to unit staff;
4. places for private conversations with staff or family members;
5. facilities for families to 'room in';
6. methods for providing privacy within the critical care setting.

These practical requirements are potential barriers to providing high-quality care to the family. Despite the best intentions of the staff, the compromising of these facilities can only limit the quality of care that can ultimately be provided. These requirements were developed by professionals and it is likely that parents would alter this list in emphasis, priority or number. This is yet another situation where the inclusion of the family in policy decision making will produce high-quality care.

CONCLUSION

Innovation in paediatric intensive care is likely to continue to be led by the technology. A recent example is the ability to monitor the state of children using machinery. Computer systems have until recently not been notably user friendly, and the user in this case is the professional. The family-centred style of care requires that these system be not just usable for the professional, but assimilable for the family in general.

The nurse needs to be conversant with the new technologies to make them more friendly for the family.

The inclusion of members of the families of former clients in policy-making groups could drive the ethos of paediatric intensive care. These families have a natural human need to return the care that the professionals offered and to use their experience to benefit other families. A less radical manner might be the use of family members for support purposes, whether in direct contact or in the provision of services. It seems to be a natural development for many families to be more involved in fund raising, but care should always be taken to ensure that the families are not being exploited.

The ethos of family-centred care may appear to be an aspiration which any critical care unit catering for children might wish to achieve, but an evaluation of the effectiveness of such a philosophy in providing quality care is yet to be completed. Indeed, the ability of such a system of care to succeed requires the full enthusiasm of the care team. Success within the paediatric intensive care unit has long been measured in terms of mortality and morbidity figures. Oncology care has been led by the achievement of yet higher 5-year survival rates (Thompson, 1990). However, it is becoming increasingly apparent that these rates are not likely to continue improving as they did in the 1970s. Therefore, the quality of the processes of care and cure will become more important in measuring the success of care regimens. The design of such measures should reflect this change and deal with them in an inductive manner. It is likely that such measurement of success will be carried out by medical colleagues, even though the qualitative paradigm is not as familiar to the medical profession as to the nurse. It is important that the nurse should be involved in these studies, which will provide information on all aspects of nursing care.

REFERENCES

Behrman, R.E. (1970) Commentary: the use of assisted ventilation in the therapy of hyaline membrane disease. *Journal of Paediatrics*, **76**, 172.

British Paediatric Association (1987) *The British Paediatric Association Working Party on Paediatric Intensive Care.*

Carter, M.D., Miles, M.,S. Burford, T.H. and Hassaneinn, R.S. (1985) Parental environmental stress in pediatric intensive care units. *Dimensions of Critical Care Nursing*, **4**(3), 180–8.

Department of Health (1959) *The Welfare of Children in Hospital.* (Chairman H. Platt), HMSO, London.

Department of Health (1991) Guidance on the Welfare of Children and Young People in Hospital, HMSO, London.

Donald, I. and Lord, J. (1953) Augmented respiration with head seal and face mask: studies in atelectasis neonatorum. *Lancet*, **i** (6749), 9–17.

Downs, J.B., Klein, E.F. *et al.* (1973) Intermittent mandatory ventilation: a new approach to weaning patients from mechanical ventilators. *Chest* **64**, 331–5.

Duncalf, D. (1978) History of anesthesia for pediatric cardiac surgery, in *Anesthetic Considerations for Pediatric Cardiac Surgery*, (ed. P. Radney), *International Anesthesiology Clinics*, **18**.

Eberley, T.W. Miles, M.S., Carter, M.C., Henessey, J. and Riddle, I. (1985) Parental stress after the unexpected admission of a child to the intensive care unit. *Critical Care Quarterly*, **8** (1), 57–65.

Ellington, M.I. (1989) Respiratory care of the pediatric patient, in *Pediatric Intensive Care*, 2nd edn, (ed. E. Nussbaum), Futura Publishing, New York, pp, 557–80.

Etzler, A.C. (1984) Parents' reactions to pediatric critical care settings: a review of the literature. *Issues in Comprehensive Pediatric Care Nursing*, **7**, 319–31.

Gillespie, N.A. (1939) Endotracheal anaesthesia in infants. *British Journal of Anaesthesia*, **17**(1), 2–12.

Goldsmith, J. and Karotkin, E. (eds) (1988) Introduction to assisted ventilation, in *Assisted Ventilation of the Neonate*, 2nd edn, WB Saunders, Philadelphia, pp. 1–21.

Gregory, G.A., Kittermann, J.A. and Phibbs, R.H. (1971) Treatment of the idiopathic respiratory distress syndrome with continuous airway pressure. *New England Journal of Medicine*, **284** (24), 1333–40.

Grenvik, A., Gross, B. and Poliner, D. (1980) Historical survey of mechanical ventilation, in *Intermittent Mandatory Ventilation*, (eds. R. Kirby and G. Graybar), International Anesthesiology Clinics, **18**.

Guess, W.L and Stetson, J. (1968) Tissue reaction to organotin-stabilised polyvinyl chloride (PVC) catheters. *Journal of the American Medical Association*, **207**(7), 118–22.

Hansen, M., Young, D.A. and Carden, F.E. (1986) Psychological evaluation and support in the pediatric intensive care unit. *Pediatric Annals*, **15**(1) 60–9.

Hedenkamp, E. (1980) Humanising the intensive care unit for children. *Critical Care Quarterly*, **3**(63), 63–73.

Hogg, C. (1989) *NAWCH Quality Review: Setting Standards for Children in Health Care*. National Association for the Welfare of Children in Hospital, Cambridge.

Inkster, J. (1978) Paediatric anaesthesia and intensive care, in *Recent Advances in Anaesthesia and Analgesia*, (eds, C. Hewer and R. Atkinson), International Anesthesiology clinics, pp. 58–91.

Kidder, C. (1989) Re-establishing health: factors influencing the child's recovery in pediatric intensive care. *Journal of Pediatric Nursing*, **4**(2), 96–103.

Laurence, E.C. (1979) The intensive care enviroment. *Issues in Comprehensive Pediatric Nursing*, **3**(6), 50–7.

Manley, K. (1989) *Primary Nursing in Intensive Care*, Scutari, London.

May, J.G. (1972), A psychiatric study of pediatric intensive therapy unit. *Clinical Pediatrics*, **11**,(2), 76–82.

Miles, M.S. Spicher, C. and Hassaneinn, R.S. (1984) Maternal and paternal stress reactions when a child is hospitalised in a paediatric intensive care unit. *Issues in Comprehensive Pediatric Nursing*, **7**, 333–42.

Miles, M.S. and Carter, M.C. (1983) Assessing parental stress in intensive care units. *Maternal Child Nursing*, **8**, 354–9.

Moore, A.C. (1989) Crisis intervention: a care plan for families of hospitalised children. *Pediatric Nursing*, **8**, 354–6.

Mushin, W., Mapleson, W. and Lunn, J. (1962) Problems of automatic ventilation in infants and children. *British Journal of Anaesthesia*, **34**(8), 514–22.

Mushin, W., Rendall-Baker, L., Thompson, P.W. and Mapleson, W. (1969) Historical background to automatic ventilation, in *Automatic Ventilation of the Lungs*, 2nd edn, Blackwell Scientific, London, pp. 185–213.

Nathanson, M. (1986) *Organising and Maintaining Support Groups for Parents of Children with Chronic Illness and Handicapping Conditions*, Association for the Care of Children's Health, Washington.

Oksala, R. and Merenmies, J. (1989) Children's human needs in intensive care. *Intensive Care Nursing*, **5**, 155–8.

Olds, A. and Daniels, P. (1987) *Child Health Care Facilities: Design Guidelines – Literature Outline*, Association for the Care of Children's Health, Washington.

Philichi, L. (1989) Family adaptation during a pediatric intensive care hospitalisation. *Journal of Pediatric Nursing*, **4**(4), 268–76.

Rees, G.J. (1950) Anaesthesia in the newborn. *British Medical Journal*, **ii** (4694), 1419–22.

Rennick, J. (1986) Reestablishing the parental role in a paediatric intensive care unit. *Journal of Pediatric Nursing*, **1**(1), 40–4.

Reynolds, E. and Taghizadeh, A. (1974) Improved prognosis of infants ventilated for hyaline membrane disease. *Archives of Disease in Childhood*, **49**,(7), 505–15.

Robson, C.H. (1936) Anesthesia in children. *American Journal of Surgery*, **34**,(3), 468–73.

Rosenthal, C.H. and Connors, C. (1989) Pediatric/neonatal graduate internship: a collaborative effort. *Pediatric Nursing*, **15**, (27, 194–6.

Rushton, C.H. (1990) Strategies for family-centred care in the critical care setting. *Pediatric Nursing*, **16**(2) 195–9.

Shelton, T., Jeppson, E. and Johnsen, B. (1987) *Family Centred Care for Children with Special Health Care Needs*, Association for the Care of Children's Health, Washington.

Stevens, K.R. (1981) Humanistic nursing care of critically ill children. *Nursing Clinics of North America*, **16**, (4), 611–22.

Steward, D. (1989) History of pediatric anesthesia, in *Pediatric Anesthesia*, Vol. 1, 2nd edn, (ed. G. Gregory), Churchill Livingstone, New York, pp. 1–13.

Sumner, T. (1986) Ventilatory support in children. *Care of the Critically Ill*, **2**, (4), 134–6.

Sykes, W.S. (1961) *Essays on the First Hundred Years of Anaesthesia*, Vol, 2, Churchill Livingstone, Edinburgh.

Thompson, J. (1990) *The Child with Cancer*, Scutari, London.

Woollam, C.M. (1976a) The development of apparatus for intermittent negative pressure respiration, 1832 to 1918. *Anaesthesia*, **31**,(4), 537–47.

Woollam, C.M. (1976b) The development of apparatus for intermittent negative pressure respiration, 1919 to 1976. *Anaesthesia*, **31**,(5), 666–85.

<table>
<tr><td>2</td><td>

Care of the child with compromised immunology and infection

</td></tr>
</table>

Susan Maxwell

Nurses caring for critically ill children, many of whom have infectious diseases and/or develop secondary infections during the course of therapy for another illness, must be aware of the ways in which particular organisms may affect the host, potentially threatening their therapy. It is also essential to be aware of and seek to avoid conditions that make infections more likely, and above all to be aware of the reasons why children are at greater risk.

CHILDHOOD IMMUNOCOMPETENCE

The development of immunocompetence requires the interaction of many genetically determined variables which code for the expression of both specific and non-specific host defences. Traditionally it has been accepted that babies, especially neonates, are generally more suceptible to infection (Table 2.1).

Table 2.1 Immature immunological mechanisms changing the patterns of infectious disease in childhood

Age group	Characteristic susceptibility	Underlying immature immunological mechanism
Newborn	Escherichia coli Staphylococcus aureus Streptococcus haemolyticus Streptococcus pneumoniae	Acute inflammatory response T and B cell cooperation and immunological memory function Reticuleondothelial clearance
1–6 months	Viruses Acute inflammatory bacteria* Candida	Acute inflammatory response T and B cell cooperation and immunological memory function Mucosal antibody production
7–18 months	Viruses Acute inflammatory bacteria*	Immunological memory, e.g. to polysaccharide antigens Switch from IgM to IgG antibodies Mucosal antibody production
Over 18 months	Viruses Acute inflammatory bacteria* Immunological hyperactivity Immune complex disease Autoimmunities	Immunological memory to polysaccharide antigens Disturbed immunological feed-back and 'tuning' Over-active helper activity T or accessory cells Reduced suppressor T cell function

*Staphylococcus aureus, Streptococcus haemolyticus, Streptococcus pneumoniae, Haemophilus influenzae type B and Neisseria meningitidis.
(Source: Pabst, H.F. and Kreth, H.W. (1980) Ontogeny of the immune response as a basis of childhood disease. *Journal of Paediatrics* **97**, 519.)

However, advances in immunology now make it clear that babies are relatively deficient in some areas of immune expression although competent in others.

Non-specific immune path

The non-specific immune path is concerned with:

1. protective mechanical mechanisms such as coughing, sneezing, wafting of cilia in the tracheobronchi, intact skin and mucous membranes;
2. the presence of substances in secretions which help destroy bacteria, e.g. hydrochloric acid in the stomach and enzymes in tears;
3. cells capable of destroying foreign material as soon as it enters the body, e.g. circulating neutrophils and tissue macrophages;
4. circulating substancces such as interferon, which are important in the prevention of viral infections;
5. complement, which is a complex of not less than nine components (C1–C9) that combine with the antigen–antibody complex in a definite sequence; all nine seem to be required for immune lysis and the first seven for chemotaxis (the undirectional movement towards an increasing gradient of attractant), but only the first four are involved in immune adherence of phagocytosis or fix to conglutinins.

Specific immune path

This path is concerned with the recognition of certain foreign materials known as antigens and how the immune system can be stimulated to produce a very specific immune response leading to their destruction. The path can be divided into the humoral system and the cell mediated system.

Humoral system

The humoral system is concerned with the production of circulating proteins known as immunoglobulins or antibodies. The cells of the humoral system are B lymphocytes. Under certain circumstances, these become plasma cells, which produce and release immunoglobins into the circulation. B lymphocytes and plasma cells are important in the prevention of many bacterial infections.

Immunoglobulin G (IgG) is the only immunoglobulin passed transplacentally. It requires previous exposure to specific antigens and, although levels are high at full term, the child only begins to produce IgG at approximately 4–5 months.

Immunoglobulin M (IgM) is predominantly intravascular presumably because of its physical size. It is the initial antibody produced in response to infection. This acute response is of particular importance in septicaemia and in the newborn.

Immunoglobulin A (IgA) is the predominant immunoglobulin of secretions in the gastrointestinal, respiratory and urinary tracts, tears and milk in humans. IgA also prevents absorption of antibodies across the respiratory tract mucosa.

Immunoglobulin E (IgE) is the immunoglobulin that responds to allergic reaction, e.g. in asthma, eczema and urticaria.

Pre-B cells are seen in the liver by 5–8 weeks of gestation, and by the middle of the second trimester have reached almost adult levels. Despite this, the capacity to synthesize specific immunoglobulins is limited.

Serum IgG levels are as great as or exceed those of the mother because of transplacental passage of IgG in the final trimester, so that IgG levels in the preterm baby are low and directly proportional to gestational age. IgG levels fall in the first 4 months of extrauterine life and adult levels are reached by 4–6 years of age. During the first 6 months of life maternal IgG provides some degree of passive immunity, but the presence of these antibodies may inhibit the ability of the newborn to mount an antibody response.

, By 10 weeks, the fetus is able to mount an IgM response. The non-infected newborn baby has an IgM concentration of approximately 10% of the adult value and reaches a mature level at 1–2 years.

IgA activity is very limited in the infant and does not reach adult levels until puberty. Secretory IgA appears later than serum IgA, which accounts for the easy sensitization to ingested allergens and infections of mucosal surfaces in the first year of life.

Cell-mediated system

This system is concerned with the activity of cells know as T lymphocytes, which are capable of specifically destroying antigenic material, e.g. foreign material such as microorganisms, which are either fixed in the tissues or inside cells. Therefore T lymphocytes are important in the prevention of many viral infections.

Lymphocytes are first found in the liver at around 40 days of gestation. The newborn has a cellular immune incompetence, as demonstrated by anergy, failure to produce certain lymphokines (e.g. interferon and monocyte migration inhibitory factor) and an abnormal interaction between T and B cells. In addition, because both humoral and cellular immune competence depends on previous exposure to offending antigens and immunological memory, the neonate has some impairment of both arms of immunity on this basis alone.

To summarize, both limbs of specific immunity are impaired in the newborn, making the baby susceptible to a number of microorganisms. Non-specific mechanisms are also impaired (phagocytosis is inefficient and chemotaxis impaired), making localization of infections difficult. Preterm and full-term babies are deficient in complement, and they have a limited ability to produce specific immunoglobulins, especially towards encapsulated organisms such as *Haemophilus influenzae* type B, which requires the presence of IgG_2. This ability is limited until after 2 years of age.

CATEGORIES OF IMMUNOCOMPROMISED PATIENTS

In addition to specific defects of immune function seen in primary immuno-deficiency disorders, a large percentage of patients admitted to paediatric intensive care units are immunocompromised as a result of acquired defects in immune function resulting from injury, surgery, anaesthetics, drugs or primary infection.

Anaesthesia

Specific anaesthetics are known to have a depressant action on immune function.

1. Nitrous oxide can cause bone marrow depression. It also suppresses both T and B cell function.
2. Halothane suppresses the bone marrow and decreases phagocytosis and chemotaxis. T-cell function is also impaired.
3. Thiopentone and other short-lasting barbiturates can produce granulocytopenia.
4. Morphine sulphate can depress leucocyte chemotaxis.
5. Pancuronium and tubocurare can impair chemotaxis.

Surgery

In patients undergoing surgery, the non-specific defence mechanism of intact skin is altered. Blood levels of B and T lymphocytes decrease in response to surgical stress, but the immunological concentrations do not change appreciably.

The nature of the surgery will alter the extent of the immunological compromise to follow; splenectomy, for example, places the patient at a permanent disadvantage. However, certain patients who are stressed by disease, immaturity, malnutrition or immune compromise will have increased rates of postoperative local or systematic infection, regardless of the type of surgery performed.

Trauma

It is sometimes difficult to separate the effects of accidental trauma on immune function from those of the surgery and anaesthesia that may be required, exposure to organisms at the site of trauma, and the underlying state of the patient's health. However, severe trauma appears to depress various components of the immune response, some general and others specific to the tissue most involved.

Phagocytosis is impaired in the recently traumatized individual, as is B cell function. More pronounced effects are seen with injury to or rupture of the spleen, kidney or liver.

Complement components may be non-specifically consumed as part of the body's general response to stress. Levels of specific immunoglobulins are lowered, especially where there is damage to the reticuloendothelial system.

Specific problems are encountered when disruption of the normal barriers to invasion by colonizing bacterial species occurs due to, for example, penetrating or deep blunt abdominal trauma that results in perforation of any portion of the gastrointestinal tract, central nervous system trauma that disrupts the meninges, or open fractures or burns.

Burns and scalds

Burns and scalds suppress all aspects of specific and non-specific immune function. Chemotaxis, opsonization (which occurs when the antigen is coated by its specific antibody and complement), phagocytosis and bacterial killing are all inhibited. Complement activation is reduced and immunological levels are decreased (mainly because of leakage into damaged tissue). Circulating factors such as endotoxins, leukotrienes and prostaglandins impair immunity. There is some evidence that hyperglycaemia impairs immunity by affecting neutrophil function. In addition, the burned and devitalized tissue forms an excellent culture medium.

Acute infection

The immunological response in acute infection produces an initial rise of IgM with a more gradual rise in IgG. As IgG rises IgM levels decrease, although immunological memory remains. The extent of generalized immunodepression is dependent on age, type of bacteria or virus and the underlying health of the patient.

The degree to which haematological changes occur depends on the virulence of the pathogen and the ability of the host to respond. Acute bacterial infection is usually characterized by leucocytosis, neutrophilia and eosinopenia. Pyogenic bacteria and cocci generally cause a more marked leucocytosis than other bacteria, counts being especially high in pneumococcal pneumonia. Some severe infections, such as staphylococcal pneumonia and bacterial meningitis and sepsis, tend to be associated with marked haematological changes. The bone marrow reserve pool of neutrophils is about 13 times greater than that of the peripheral blood. This pool is rapidly dispersed until there is an over-compensation for the outflow of neutrophils to the tissue and leucocytosis develops. In severe infection, the bone narrow pool may become depleted and neutropenia may develop. Neutropenia is a poor prognostic sign (McKenzie, 1987).

Chemotherapy

Unfortunately, in an attempt to treat many illnesses and infections, the chemotherapy used may further compromise the patient's immune response. The immunodepressant effects of steroids and cytotoxic drugs are well known, but some other drugs inducing neutropenia and blood dyscrasias are less well recognized. Drugs with an immunodepressant effect include captropril, isoniazid, tetracyclines, vancomycin, cefotaxime, cephradine, sulphadimidine and sulphadiazine.

ADMINISTERING BLOOD AND BLOOD PRODUCTS TO THE IMMUNOSUPPRESSED

Blood and blood product transfusions are commonplace in paediatric intensive care units, being used to replace blood loss secondary to haemorrhage, to correct deficits resulting from sepsis, and in neutropenic children whose bone marrow function is depressed as a result of cytotoxic therapy.

As with all forms of therapy, the risks of blood transfusion must be weighed up against the benefits to the individual patient. Nurses should be aware of the adverse effects that blood transfusion may present, the factors considered and the precautions taken when medical staff decide to transfuse the immunosuppressed child. The factors considered include the following:

1. Has the child been previously exposed to blood products?
2. Why does this child require transfusion?
3. What type of blood product is required?

Whether the child is mildly immunocompromised or neutropenic, it must be acknowledged that blood transfusion is an immunosuppressant. Previous exposure to blood and blood product transfusion may have produced high levels of antibodies; therefore, these children are more likely to develop fever, urticaria and more pronounced anaphylactic reactions.

Medical staff may prescribe antihistamines and steroid cover prior to the administration of blood products to safeguard the child from adverse reactions. Side-effects of platelet transfusion can be minimized by administering specially prepared *compatible* platelets.

Infection

Risk of infection, especially viral infections such as cytomegalovirus, hepatitis A and B and human immunodeficiency virus (HIV), is very real in the immunosuppressed child. For this reason, blood products given to immuno-suppressed children after bone marrow transplantation should be irradiated. Irradiation of blood products destroys viral substances present in donor blood, and aids compatibility by removing the lymphocytes' ability to respond to the recipient's antigens.

Although rare, bacteria may contaminate red cells, whole blood or platelets. *Pseudomonas fluorescens* and *Staphylococcus* may contaminate blood products Therefore, sterile technique and blood filters should always be used. Platelet filters are now available.

The type of blood product given also influences the prospective risk of infection because of the number of donors involved. Cyroprecipitate may have been prepared from as many as 20 donors, and factor VIII concentrate from approximately 1000 donors, although each unit of red cells, whole blood and fresh frozed plasma will be from one donor, and platelets may be supplied either as a single-donor unit or as a pack containing a pooled product (usually of 4–6 units).

The medical staff will recognize non-acceptable values of full blood count and coagulation screening, but nurses can also explore and promptly report possible explanations for deficits. For example, in a child who has undergone cardiac bypass surgery, large amounts of chest drain loss and fresh blood oozing from wound and puncture sites may indicate insufficient reversal of heparinization with protamine sulphate. A child exposed to excessive blood replacement during surgery will have a lowered platelet concentration, and so additional platelets may be required.

INFECTION CONTROL

The therapeutic battle against life-threatening diseases is constantly expanding and yet despite this, or perhaps because of it, infection is still the main cause of death in the compromised host (Gurevich and Tafuro, 1986).

Although it is recognized that some infections are caused by the patient's own endogenous flora, especially in the immunosuppressed, there are others which arise from exogenous sources, which may be either inanimate (e.g. food, equipment) or animate (e.g. visitors, health care personnel).

Many infections can be prevented, and responsibility lies with everyone having either direct or indirect contact with patients. Everyone with a respon-sibility for infection control must therefore be educated, supported and motivated in their response to protecting vulnerable children during their time in the intensive care unit.

An overwhelming contribution is made by the infection control team, who can provide a wealth of information and advice and play an important role in heightening awareness in all the staff involved. Access to this team of experts should be considered vital to the smooth running of the unit. All levels of clinical, ancillary and service staff should be involved in the examination of existing policies and development of new strategies so that a higher degree of quality can be assured.

In-service education of all staff is essential, so that often limited knowledge can be developed and improved. If education sessions involve a wide range of staff involved in infection control, a broader appreciation of the difficulties and solutions can be achieved.

All staff should be aware of the latest infection control policies and be sure that they are followed correctly. Staff should be encouraged to view the issues surrounding infection control with a high degree of professional interest and ensure that this motivation and commitment is sustained.

Part of the nurse's role lies in ensuring that all staff coming into contact with the child are well informed and educated in respect to infection control matters. The nurse is also responsible for ensuring that clear instructions and prominent notices inform staff what protective measures must be taken to protect the child and/or the worker. An important aspect is to make sure that all female staff, in particular, are aware of infections that may endanger pregnancy and the unborn child, as this may affect them personally in addition to any pregnant visitors to the unit.

Visitors must be advised of the infection control practices that exist in the unit. Any guidelines that they must adhere to should be made clear at the beginning of the admission and gently but firmly reinforced throughout the stay. If they understand the reasons for particular actions, families are happy to help to protect their child from infection.

Common bacteria found in hospitals

Although the bacteria discussed are by no means the only bacteria responsible for hospital infections, they are the most frequent in the compromised patient.

Critical environments such as intensive care units provide an excellent setting for studying the spread and prevention of infection. One consequence of the ever-increasing sophistication of treatments (many of which are invasive) and equipment is an increase in the problems of treating and preventing infection. Children requiring intensive care now are more likely to:

1. receive broad spectrum antibiotics, which alter normal body flora;
2. have undergone major surgery, altering normal anatomy and physiology;
3. have received cytotoxic and/or steroid therapy, altering normal host defence mechanisms.

Table 2.2 Common hospital bacteria

Pathogen	Port of entry	Disease	Exit	Usual source of infection	Comments
Staphylococcus aureus Staphylococcus pyogenes Coagulase positive Staphylococcus	Local, by contact or inhalation	Wound infection	Pus from lesions	Human carriers' hands, equipment, bedding and clothing	Capable of remaining airborne for long periods of time
	Surgery	Abscesses	Pus following incision		
	Blood stream	Oestomyelititis	Pus following incision		
	Respiratory tract	Pneumonia	Sputum		
	Ingestion of infected food	Vomiting (food poisoning)	Faeces and vomit	Enterotoxin strain in staff handling food, e.g. septic finger	
	Skin or deep infection	Septicaemia	Initial lesion		
Proteus mirabilis	Urethra	Urinary tract infection	Urine	Cut, nasal and external ear carriers	Usual sources: nose, gastrointestinal tract and external ear
	Contact transmission	Wound and respiratory infections	Discharges		
Pseudomonas aeruginosa Pseudomonas pyocyanea	Contact transmission	Infection in tissues damaged by disease, accident or surgery, e.g. burns, tracheostomy wounds and urinary tract infection	Secretions and discharges	Organism often present in the gut; reservoirs in wet situations e.g. humidifiers, sink traps, flower water, contaminated medications	
Klebsiella spp.	Some strains normally present in respiratory tract	Respiratory tract infection e.g. pneumonia	Nasal and bronchial secretions	Endogenous, easily transmissible via wet hands and instruments	Normally commensals, but become pathogenic if they stray from normal site
	Contact transmission	Wound infections	Discharges		
	Via urethra	Urinary tract infection	Urine		
Escherichia coli	Via urethra	Urinary tract infection	Urine	Cuts and faecal contamination	Normally harmless commensals which become pathogenic if they stray from normal site
	Contact transmission	Infection of wounds, burns	Discharge from lesions		
Enteropathogenic strains	Ingestion	Diarrhoea	Faeces	Human cariers or cases	
Candida spp.	Damaged tissue	Candidiasis, oral thrush, skin, septic fingers, vagina, systemic	Exudates	Opportunist organism often found in mouth, vagina and intestines	Often appear as suprainfection after prolonged antibiotic therapy

Therefore, children receiving intensive care are more susceptible to infection, and it must be acknowledged that caring for increasing numbers of such compromised hosts in specialized areas can produce high and unacceptable levels of infection.

To understand microbiological problems in intensive care it is first necessary to become familiar with the ways in which microbes spread and the reasons why the compromised host is more susceptible. Then action can be taken to prevent many potential infections from occurring.

Of the countless bacterial species, five or six appear to be responsible for the majority of hospital infections. Although the spectrum of infection varies from hospital to hospital and from time to time, these changes seem to be minor fluctuations in the pattern of major pathogens. (Gaya, 1979). More than two-thirds of all hospital infections are caused by *Staphylococcus aureus, Escherichia coli, Klebsiella, Pseudomonas aeruginosa, Proteus,* and *Candida.* The origin of any infection may be endogenous or exogenous; that is, the offending pathogens may originate from the patient's own bacterial flora or may come from an outside source. In hospital, however, patients may become colonized by hospital strains of *Staphylococcus aureus, Escherichia coli, Klebsiella* and *Pseudomonas aeruginosa*, which may subsequently cause infection. These apparently endogenous infections are in reality exogenous, the patient's alimentary tract, nose or skin being the final pathway to infection (Gaya, 1979).

The intensive care environment

It has been suggested that intensive care units should be divided into both two-bedded cubicles and single isolation cubicles. There should be separate clean and dirty utility rooms. Wash basins should be within easy reach of each bed. Toilet and changing facilities should be situated at the entrance of the unit, thus encouraging hand washing on arrival.

Ventilation should be maintained at positive pressure, with the unit receiving about ten air changes per hour, with temperature and humidity control. Containment isolation areas should be exhaust ventilated (negative pressure) and protective isolation plenum ventilated (positive pressure) with respect to the rest of the unit. Some modern designs of intensive care units use plenum-ventilated dual-purpose cubicles, each of which is separated from the rest of unit by an exhaust-ventilated vestibule and interlocked doors.

Clean areas such as the central sterile supply department (CSSD) and preparation rooms should be plenum ventilated and the sluice and toilets exhaust ventilated (Gaya, 1979).

Provided the environment is kept reasonably clean, dry and free from spillage of human excretions and secretions, it can be considered low risk. The organisms present will usually be similar to those found in the air (Ayliffe *et al.*, 1982). Bacteria do not readily adhere to walls and ceilings, and counts tend to be low. Counts of floors will be higher and related to the number of people present (Collins and Jose, 1987).

Good domestic services are of paramount importance in intensive care units, with particular attention to sinks, wash bowls, kitchen areas and horizontal surfaces. The nurse also has a role to play in domestic services, with regard to damp dusting of equipment in use. Dusty equipment provides an ideal contact for transmission of bacteria. Correct cleansing of blood and fluid spillages, and the cleaning of Baby Therms and incubator units, are also important.

Cleaning inanimate objects

In an ideal intensive care unit, disposal of all equipment that comes into direct contact with patients would occur. Although many items of equipment are now available for disposal after use, many are not and expense is a major issue. Therefore, sterilization and disinfection remain necessary practices. Choices of sterilization methods may differ throughout the country, as will disinfection policies. Recommended policies should be adhered to.

Items requiring sterilization tend to be those which directly invade the patient's non-specific defence barriers, breaking the skin (including contact materials) and entering vessels, cavities, etc. Sterilization is the complete destruction of all types of microorganisms and is usually achieved by the use of heat, ionizing radiation or ethylene oxide gas.

Chemical agents cannot reliably sterilize in short exposure time and therefore physical methods should be used in hospitals where possible. Heat, whether dry or moist, is the most efficient and cheapest method of sterilization. There is an inverse relationship between the temperature used and time required to sterilize; high temperatures necessitate shorter times. Bacteria in the vegetative state (non-sporing) are killed by heat at 100°C after a few seconds. Spores are destroyed only by longer and more intensive application of the various methods used to destroy bacteria.

Disinfectants

There is no such thing as a perfect all-purpose disinfectant. Disinfection is intended to produce extensive though not total, removal of harmful organisms. Cleaning with detergent is often sufficient to remove a large proportion of organisms and is often preferable to using a disinfectant. Vegetative bacteria, but not spores, are killed by most disinfectants. Hypochlorite is recommended for inactivation of viruses.

In many intensive care units, nurses are responsible for the disinfection of everyday equipment. It is important to remember the following points.

1. Disinfection is no substitute for cleaning. Articles should be cleaned thoroughly prior to usage of chemical disinfectants.
2. Hospital policies must be adhered to when selecting disinfectants.
3. Disinfectants should be used at the correct concentration.
4. No two disinfectants should be mixed as they may react with each other becoming inactivated, e.g. Savlon and soap.
5. Bacteria can grow in disinfectants, therefore, solutions should not be used for longer than recommended.
6. Once cleansed, items should be dried completely and not left to dry.
7. Sterile solutions should be used immediately after opening the container and unused solution discarded.

Disposal of waste and linen

All nursing staff should be aware of and practice the correct disposal of waste and linen. Each hospital will differ in ways of indentifying each category, although the principle of safe disposal is the universal objective. Guidelines for disposal of waste and linen are laid down by the Department of Social Security (DSS) in England and Wales and the Scottish Home and Health Department (SHHD) in Scotland. Linen by be categorized as:

1. *used*, i.e. domestically dirty;
2. *foul or infested*, i.e. contaminated with blood and/or other body fluids or used by infested patients;
3. *infected*, i.e. used by a patient with infectious disease;
4. *high-risk*, i.e. contaminated with blood, secretions and other body fluids from patients in high-risk categories.

The first three categories should be purposefully bagged and laundered. The fourth category requires incineration.

Each hospital has its own indentifiable system for waste disposal based on DSS or SHHD guidelines. Suggested categories include the following.

1. *Household waste* consists of paper and packaging, leftover foods and floor sweepings.
2. *Other clinical waste* includes surgical dressings, nappies, stoma and urine bags, materials from infectious patients other than linen and disposable clothing. Human tissue should be double bagged. Radioactive waste should be identified by a radiation hazard symbol.
3. *'Sharps'*, such as used needles and syringes, should be placed in the containers provided. Needles should not be resheathed after use. Sharps containers should be disposed of when three-quarters full and should be securely sealed before removal.
4. *Glass*, non-returnable pharmacy bottles and *aeorsols* should be place in

containers. Broken glass and crockery on which liquid is still present must be placed in a polythene bag first.

Isolation techniques

All forms of isolation should be instituted in an enclosed area separate from the general unit.

Source isolation, previously known as barrier nursing, applies to most infections requiring isolation.

Protective isolation, previously known as reverse barrier nursing, applies to patients requiring protection from infection.

Strict isolation, applies to patients who are placed in the high-risk category. In some hospitals, this may be restricted to patients with HIV and hepatitis B infections. At present, there is an awareness of children who are HIV antibody positive. However, there is still a relatively limited experience of providing intensive care to the child who is HIV positive or has acquired immune deficiency sydrome. It must be emphasized that local guidelines and good practices must be followed to ensure the protection of all staff and visitors regardless of known HIV or hepatitis status.

Handling of blood and body fluids

Suggested guidelines are as follows.

1. Scrupulous attention to detail and personal hygiene is required. Non-sterile gloves are necessary.
2. Cuts and abrasions should be covered with a waterproof plaster or dressing.
3. Receptacles for blood and blood products should, whenever possible, be made of plastic. Containers should be securely fastened.
4. Syringes and needles should be disposed of by the person using the equipment in suitable puncture-proof containers. Needles should not be resheathed.
5. An appropriate sluice system should be used to dispose of body fluids whenever possible. With certain types of equipment or drains this is not possible; this equipment should be double bagged and the contents clearly marked to inform the person collecting the waste of its nature. Care must be taken to protect clothing, eyes and mouth when emptying blood and body fluids if splashback is a danger.
6. Blood remaining in transfusion bags should be sealed (if already removed from the giving set) and double bagged. Blood should not be emptied down either the sluice or sinks.
7. The sluice area should be kept clean and free from blood and other fluid spillages.

In the event of blood spillages, the following procedure is recommended.

1. Always wear a plastic disposable apron, non-sterile disposable gloves (and eyeshields and/or mask if indicated).
2. Pour the disinfectant directed by hospital policy onto the contaminated area, placing paper towels over the spill.
3. Gently pour more disinfectant on top and wipe the area thoroughly.
4. Discard towels, gloves, apron, etc., into the recommended disposal bag.

Note that hypochlorites (e.g. neat Milton) are extremely corrosive and will damage metals, some plastics, rubbers and fabrics. All traces of disinfectant must be removed with water before any items are reused. Care should be taken, when using such substances for cleaning, to avoid contact with the skin and mucous membranes. Excessive inhalation of fumes should also be avoided.

Collecting and recording specimens

Infection screening is of vital importance and must be performed efficiently. Often set days are allocated to ensure that specific specimens are routinely sent, according to the established policy of each unit.

Great care must be taken to ensure that full and accurate information accompanies the specimens. This would include the patient's name, address and date of birth, unit and hospital number, consultant, date and time the specimen was obtained, examination required, clinical details and any other specific information required. Full information will assist the microbiologist in correctly interpreting the results of the tests.

An important issue to consider prior to the collection of any specimens relates to the correct collection and transportation of the specimen itself. Any special transport medium or requirements for the collection of the specimen should be ascertained.

Once the specimens have been collected and appropriately transported, the nurse must note that the specimen has been taken in the nursing notes or on an infection screening flowchart. Basic information kept on such a chart quickly identifies the types of specimen taken, the result, the action taken and other comments.

Bacteriological findings must be evaluated and discussed with all the staff involved and possible trends in infections must be explored and eliminated.

High-risk or suspected high-risk specimens should be clearly marked in the recognized manner. Failure to inform laboratory staff is not only inconsiderate but negligent and could lead to legal action.

Transporting specimens

Many specimens may be transported in sterile unprepared containers; however, some specimens for virology or bacteriology require special preparation of the patient and/or transportation in a specific medium. The nurse must ensure that the specimen is collected and transported correctly.

Once requested specimens have been collected and sent to the appropriate department, some form of documentation should be kept and should be easily accessible for nursing and medical reference. Infection screening Flowcharts such as that shown in Figure 2.1 are very useful.

Date	Type of specimen	Examination required	Result	Comment
1.1.91	Endotracheal aspirate	Culture and sensitivity	3.1.91 Streptococcus pneumoniae	On erythromycin since 29.12.90

Figure 2.1 Infection screening flowchart.

The microbiology department may issue the unit with a weekly print-out of specimens and results. This helps to identify common bacteria and any evidence of cross-infection or colonization taking place. If this facility is not available, time should be allocated to collate results on a weekly basis. It must be remembered that well-documented information, properly transported specimens and correctly recorded results assist diagnosis, treatment and hopefully the child's recovery. Bacteriology findings must be evaluated and discussed with all the staff involved so that any trends of infection may be explored. Research projects can be carried out on infection control and the findings may indicate a need to evaluate or alter present practices.

Handwashing

Hand washing is the single most important procedure in preventing cross-infection in hospital. This is a well known fact (Lowberry, 1975), although it is so basic that some people act as though they have outgrown it (Taylor, 1978). In a clinical emergency, no-one is expected to consult the Infection Control Manual, as prompt responses undoubtedly save lives. However, if infection control does not become instinctive, the child may succumb to infection as a result. Compromise between the need for speed and the need to minimize infection may at times be necessary, but this compromise should be agreed and practised by all grades of staff (Collins and Jose, 1987).

Good hand washing and drying technique is more important than the type of solution used. An excessive demand for hand washing may result in poor technique and will increase the risk of skin damage. Therefore it is important that procedures for thorough hand washing are established.

Physically clean hands can be disinfected effectively using 70% alcohol, which should be available at each bed and space and can save crucial time. It is not suggested that alcohol rubbing should be an alternative to washing, but that it can be effective between procedures requiring hand washing.

It has been suggested that hand creams should only be used at tea breaks and in off-duty hours, as they may provide an excellent medium for multiplication and transmission of residual bacteria on hands.

Rings and other jewellery must not be worn.

Protective clothing

Much controversy surrounds the issue of what should be worn when working in intensive care areas.

The *overgown*, although still widely used, has not been established as an effective way to prevent the spread of infection. Gowns are traditionally used by staff working with patients who require wound, skin, enteric or strict isolation. If nothing else, they are thought to remind staff of the need to take care. However, recent literature fails to support this (Donowitz, 1986).

The single-use plastic apron is also advocated as a means of protecting the wearer's uniform, rather than protecting the patient. If an apron is used, consideration should be given to the extent of coverage it provides.

Gloves should always be worn when handling or having contact with blood and body fluids. Gloves help to protect the nurse from the child and the child from the nurse. Incorporating glove wearing into everyday practice is not difficult. Changing nappies, changing suction flasks and disposing of linen can all be carried out wearing gloves. Potential opportunities for self- and cross-infection can be partially eliminated if gloves are worn.

The effectiveness of *overshoes* as a measure of infection control is unproved (Daschner *et al.*, 1978). Wearing of *masks* may be indicated in the protective situation where there is a large breach of skin surface or where the patient is suffering from a disease that is highly contagious by droplet infection. Some units suggest that, when the child requires protective isolation, those spending lengthy periods caring for the child do not need to wear a mask but those making short or frequent visits should do so.

Unnecessary movement in and out of isolation cubicles should be firmly discouraged.

Good, careful, planned nursing care is more likely to prevent the spread of infection than gowns, masks, cap and overshoes. Plastic aprons and disposable gloves are usually the only protective clothing required.

INVASIVE THERAPY

Ventilation

In most intensive care units the need for ventilation is a criterion for admittance. Ironically, intubation and ventilation, along with all the invasive lines and equipment critically ill children may require, may increase their risk of succumbing to infection.

Intubation

Although the intial procedure is often performed in an emergency, experienced staff should be able to carry out intubation in a manner which is not only efficient but also as clean as possible. Endotracheal and tracheostomy tubes should be sterile, as should lubricating jellies (preferably packaged as single-use sachets). Laryngoscopes and Magill forceps should be thoroughly disinfected after use. Hands should be clean; it takes only a few seconds, to disinfect physically clean hand with alcohol, but longer to treat secondary chest infection. Whether the child requires ventilation as a result of an established chest infection or is being electively ventilated as part of the therapy, it is important to obtain endotracheal secretions as soon as possible as part of the initial infection screen. Baselines must be established.

Infection control

The aims of infection control in the ventilated child are to:

1. prevent the transfer of organisms from ventilator to child and vice versa;

2. ensure aseptic technique when assembling and disconnecting circuits and when carrying out invasive procedures;
3. limit the multiplication of bacteria within the circuit to prevent it reaching infective level;
4. ensure adequate decontamination of the ventilator after use.

Suctioning of secretions

Suctioning of endotracheal and tracheostomy tubes is a regular nursing task performed on the ventilated child. An aseptic technique using sterile gloves and single-use catheters should be used. Consideration must also be given to the cleaning of rebreathing circuits used for hand-ventilation during this procedure. The positioning of the disconnected ventilator circuit should be considered; it should not be draped over the child's bed or the ventilator.

The contents of suction bottles should be disposed of in the sluice. The changing of tubing, disinfecting of suction bottles and cleaning of other equipment should be carried out as a final task at the end of a shift, when all direct patient handling has been completed. Disposable suction units are preferable.

The ventilator

Much controversy regarding the frequency of changing ventilator tubing continues. Callwaller *et al.* (1990) stated that present evidence suggests oral and stomach flora as the main sources of secondary chest infection. Bacterial filters should be used, and disposable filters changed at the intervals recommended by the manufacturers, or more often if waterlogged. If the ventilator has an inbuilt filter, adequate disinfection is necessary.

Ideally, filters should be placed at both the inspiratory and the expiratory ends of the ventilator (provided this does not interfere with ventilatory pressures), thus protecting both patient and ventilator from contamination.

If the water in the *humidifier basin* is maintained at 60°C, bacteria will be killed; above 50°C, bacteria cannot multiply (Glover, 1966). It is imperative to measure the heated inspired gas as close to the patient as possible, as the length of tubing from basin to patient will alter the temperature of the gas inspired. Sterile water within the humidifier basins should not be topped up, but should be changed completely, thus avoiding cooling the potentially contaminated reservoir. The humidifier should be switched off while the patient is disconnected from the ventilator, avoiding overheating of the tank.

Condensed water drainage from ventilator tubing should be 'tapped' into *in situ* water traps and the circuit broken as infrequently as possible in an aseptic fashion.

Most paediatric ventilators now have disposable circuits. However, sterilization can be achieved by ethylene oxide or formaldehyde gas or by autoclaving. Anaesthetic tubing, bags and suction apparatus may be efficiently disinfected by a purpose-built washing machine, or may be decontaminated in low-temperature disinfector.

Whatever frequency of changing ventilator tubing and cleaning methods is adopted, careful surveillance and monitoring of infection rates are necessary.

Ventilation pneumonia

The ventilated patient has a non-functioning cough reflex, which allows secretions to pass freely into the lower respiratory tract. Other possible causes of ventilation-associated pneumonia include stress ulcer prophylaxis and retrograde pharyngeal colonization by pathogens originating from the stomach, which represents an essential factor in pathogenesis of nosocomial pneumonia in intensive care patients receiving ventilation.

Because there is a strong link between gastric pH and bacterial growth, it is of particular importance to know whether stress ulcer prophylaxis with histamine-type H2 blockers, which neutralize the gastric acids, enhances the risk of ventilation pneumonia (Daschner and Kappstein, 1988).

Driks *et al.* (1987) and Tryba (1987) have shown that maintaining the natural acid barrier of the stomach by use of sucralfate for stress ulcer prophylaxis effectively reduces the incidence of ventilator-associated pneumonia. However, sucralfate may reduce the bioavailability of digoxin and may also alter the absorption of other oral drugs. Its side-effects include constipation and diarrohoea, and its safety and effectiveness for use in children has not yet been established.

Selective antimicrobial decontamination

In some intensive care units, selective antimicrobial decontamination of the oral cavity and gastrointestinal tract is used to help prevent endogenous respiratory infection. Ledingham *et al.* (1988) have shown in preliminary studies that gram-negative bacilli can be almost eliminated from these sites with the indigenous anaerobic flora remaining.

Intravenous therapy

Intravenous therapy is associated with appreciable risk of life-threatening septicaemia. Although it is unlikely that infusion-associated infections can be completely eliminated, they can be minimized if physicians, nurses and other hospital personnel adhere to establish infection control measures when administering intravenous fluids (Goldman *et al.*, 1973).

The mode of access required in a critically ill child should be seriously considered. Nystrom (1983) demonstrated an increase in hospital-acquired bacteraemias in patients with intravenous devices. Where peripheral access was used, 3.7 per 1000 patients developed bacteraemia, whereas 44.8 per 1000 patients with central venous lines developed bacteraemia (Nyston, 1983).

Central venous access is indicated for:

1. facilitation of long-term usage;
2. administration of total parenteral nutrition;
3. administration of drugs unsuitable for peripheral infusion;
4. monitoring central venous pressure.

Peripheral access would suffice for:

1. transfusion of blood and blood products;
2. administration of most intravenous drugs;
3. maintenance or correction of urea and electrolyte balance;
4. facilitation of intravenous access in case of emergency.

Contamination may be caused intrinsically, i.e. before use, in infusion sets, infusion fluids, contaminated cannulae or antiseptic ointments used in dressing the cannula site, or extrinsically in contaminated intravenous additives or by poorly practised technique by those changing giving sets and administering intravenous therapy, who may too frequently interrupt closed circuitry by means of three-way taps, etc.

Reducing the risks

It is now accepted that the patient's normal skin flora is capable of causing sepsis and that adequate skin cleansing is necessary before the insertion of cannulae and lines. Hands should be washed, the patient's skin prepared thoroughly, and good aseptic technique practised.

In the emergency situation, when a cannula is sited without such precautions, the initial cannula should be removed once aseptic access is gained elsewhere. When intravenous cannulae and lines are inserted, the date should be recorded and access sought elsewhere after an agreed interval of time.

The infusion site should be covered with a sterile dressing, which should be renewed when necessary. Using a transparent dressing allows easy observation; many materials now have the added bonus of being permeable to moisture but impermeable to bacteria.

Where possible, the daily task of renewing intravenous lines should be organized so that all infusions are simultaneously commenced on the renewed, sterile, closed circuit and not staggered throughout the day, thus repeatedly interrupting the circuit. Aseptic technique should always be practised, and unnecessary stopcocks and three-way taps avoided as they have been identified in numerous studies as a cause of contamination.

The use of filters in intravenous lines is advocated, although they are not an alternative to good aseptic technique.

Intravenous drugs should be reconstituted and administered in a sterile manner. If possible, drugs should be administered without using a three-way tap, and injected before a bacterial filter. Reconstituted drugs should be discarded after use or stored directly in accordance with manufacturers' instructions. Reusage of opened ampoules may be cost effective, but presents a risk to the patient. Ampoules must always be discarded once opened.

The patient receiving intravenous therapy should be observed for pyrexia and for any signs of cannula or line site inflammation, and medical staff must be informed immediately should pyrexia develop. Where the central venous or arterial catheter is suspected to be the source of infection causing the pyrexia, differential blood cultures should be performed. Once access is obtained elsewhere, the tips of these lines should be sent for culture and sensitivity test along with swabs from the puncture sites.

Other invasive lines and tubes

As well as the invasion of intravenous and intra-arterial lines, children requiring intensive care are often subjected to invasion by many other lines, catheters and tubes. However, the fundamental principles of care to prevent infection are the same:

1. sterile technique and adequate skin preparation on insertion;
2. continuous observation and care of entry site;
3. infrequent interruption of closed circuitry;
4. monitoring for signs of possible infection.

Although, when necessary, the child in intensive care is invasively monitored, it is important to recognize promptly when lines and tubes are no longer necessary. Invasive equipment should be removed as soon as possible. The nurse caring for the patient can be invaluable in assessing and suggesting to medical staff when urinary catheterization or central venous access is no longer required and where bag collection of urine and peripheral venous access could suffice.

ENTERAL FEEDING

Care and attention must be given to the storage and administration of milk feeds given to the child in intensive care. The high environmental temperature in intensive care can provide an excellent opportunity for enteral feeds to sour, causing unnecessary gastric upset. Feeds prepared in the hospital milk kitchen should be removed from the fridge only in time to allow them to reach an acceptable feeding temperature. Each feed prepared should be bottled separately, thereby avoiding multiple opening and closing of a larger flask. All bottled feeds should be examined for obvious signs of contamination before use.

Where continuous nasogastric feeding is used, there should be an agreed unit policy regarding the interval at which feed flasks and administration sets are renewed.

Any child who develops diarrhoea and/or vomiting should be investigated thoroughly before simply attributing this to antibiotic therapy.

REFERENCES AND FURTHER READING

Ayliffe, G.A.J., Barry, D.R., Lowberry, E.J.L., Roperhall, M.J. and Walker, W.M. (1966) *Lancet*, **i**, 1113.

Ayliffe, G.A.J., Collins, B.J. and Taylor, L.J. (1982) *Hospital Infection. Principle and Prevention*. John Wright, Bristol.

Buxton, A.E. (1979) *The Intensive Care Unit, Hospital Infections*.

Callwaller, H.I., Bradley, C.R., Auliffe, G.A.J. (1990) Bacterial contamination and frequency of changing ventilator circuitry. *Journal of Hospital Infection*, **15**, 65–75.

Collins, B.J. and Jose, E.D. (1987) Infection in intensive therapy units. *Care of the Critically Ill*, **3**, 3–5.

Cloney, D.L. and Donowitz, L.G. (1986) Overgown use for infection control in nurseries and neonatal intensive care units. *American Journal of Disease of Children*, **140**, 680–2.

Dascher, F. and Kappstein, I. (1988) Infections in intensive care. *Current Options*, 1, 735–8.

Daschner, F., Borneff, G., Jackson, M. and Parker, T. (1978) Detection, prevention and control of hospital acquired infection. *Infection*, **6**, 194–6.

Data Sheet Compendium (1989–90), Datapharm Publications Ltd, London.

Donowitz, L.G. (1986) Failure of the overgrown to prevent nosocomial infection in paediatric intensive care unit. *Paediatrics*, **77**, (1), 35–8.

Driks, M.R., Craven, D.E., Celli, B.R. and Manning, M. (1987) Nosocomial pneumonia in intubated patients given sucralfate as compared with antacids or histamine type 2 blockers. The role of colonization. *New England Journal of Medicine*, **317**, 1376–82.

Forfar, J.O and McCabe, A.F. (1958) Gowning and masking in nurseries for the newborn infant; effect on staphylococcal carriage and infection. *British Medical Journal*, **i**, 76–9.

Gezon, H.M., Rogers, K.D and Thompson, D.J. (1960) Some controversial aspects in the epidemiology of hospital nursery staphylococcal infections. *American Medical Journal*, **50**, 478–84.

Glover, W.J. (1966) *Pseudomonas Aerupinosa* cross infection. *Lancet*, **i**, 203.

Goldman, D.A., Maki, D.G., Rhame, F.S. and Kairser, A.B. (1973) Guidelines of infection control in intravenous therapy. *Annals of Internal Medicine*, **79**, 848–50.

Gurevich, I. and Tafuro, P. (1986) The compromised host: deficit-specific infection and the spectrum of prevention. *Cancer Nursing*, **9**(5), 263–75.

Knoben, J.E. and Anderson, P.O (1983) *Handbook of Clinical Drug Data*. 5th edn, Hamilton Press, Illinois.

Koda-Kimbel, M.A., Katcher, B.S. and Young, L.Y. (1983) *Applied Therapeutics*, 3rd edn, Applied Therapeutics Inc., Spokane.

Kominos, S.D., Copeland, C.E. and Gosiak, B. (1972) *Applied Microbiology*, **23**, 309.

Ledingham, I., Alcock, S., Eastway, A. and McDonald, J. (1988) Triple selective decontamination of the digestive tract, selective cefotaxime, and microbiological surveillancce for prevention of acquired infection in I.T.U. *Lancet*, **i**, 785–90.

Lowberry, E.J. (1975) *Control of Infection. A Practical Handbook*. Chapman and Hall, London.

McClelland, D.B.L. (1989) *Handbook of Transfusion Medicine*, 2nd edn. HMSO, London.

McKenzie, S.B. (1987) Haematological changes in infectious disease. *Journal of Medical Technology*, **4**, July/August, 159–60.

Millar, S., Sampson, L.K., Soukup, M. and Weinberg, S.L. (1980) *Methods in Critical Care A.A.N.C.*, W.B. Saunders, Philadelphia.

Nystrom, B. (1983) Bacteraemia in surgical patients with intravenous devices: a European multicentre incidence study. *Journal of Hospital Infection*, **4**, 338–49.

Parker, M.J. and Stucke, V.A. (1982) *Microbiology for Nurses*. Bailliere Tandale, London.

Phillips, I. (1966) *Lancet*, **i**, 347.

Phillips, I., Eykyn, S. and Laker, M. (1972) *Lancet*, **ii**, 258.

Price, D.J.E. and Sleigh, J.D. (1970) *Lancet*, **ii**, 1213.

Rogers, M. (1987) *Textbook of Paediatric Intensive Care*, Vol. 2. Williams and Wilkins, Baltimore.

Shooter, R.A., Cooke, E.M., Gaya H. *et al.* (1969) *Lancet*, **i**, 1227.

Sleigh, J.D. and Timbury, MC. (1986) *Notes on Medical Becteriology*, 2nd edn. Churchill Livingstone, Edinburgh.

Speight, T.M. (1987) *Avery's Drug Treatment*, 3rd edn. A.D.I.S.

Spiers, R., Shooter, R.A. Gaya, H. and Patel, N. (1969) *Lancet*, **ii**, 233.

Stedman, J.L. (1982) *Medical Dictionary*, 24th edn. Williams and Wilkins, Baltimore.

Taylor, L.J. (1978) An evaluation of handwashing techniques. *Nursing Times*, part 1, January, 54–5.

Tryba, M. (1987) Risk of acute stress ulcer bleeding and nosocomial pneumonia in ventilated intensive care patients: sucralfate *versus* antacids. *American Medical Journal*, **8**, 117–24.

Williams, C.P.S. and Oliver, T.K. (1969) Nursery routines and staphylococcal colonization of the newborn. *Paediatrics*, **44**, 640–6.

Care of the neonate

Mary Wallis

In recent years there have been many advances in the care of neonates and their families. Increasingly sophisticated technology now allows the neonate to be supported through many crises. Most neonates are nursed in neonatal units attached to maternity units, although a few may be transferred to a neonatal unit or a paediatric intensive care unit. Some of the babies that are transferred are those commonly referred to as 'surgical babies'.

Major congenital abnormalities are now able to be corrected in the neonatal period and a proportion of babies with these abnormalities will need intensive care facilities. Some babies will also require admission because of 'medical' problems such as severe cardiac problems, birth asphyxia, microthorax and cerebral problems. Whatever the reason, it is essential that members of the family are fully aware of all that is happening. Initially they will be very shocked at the sight of their baby, the equipment and the unit. Parents will wish to ask the staff many questions about the cause of their baby's problems, prognosis, long-term problems and possible risks for future pregnancies. All the staff should be prepared to discuss these questions and try to find answers even if the questions cannot be completely answered. Honesty and compassion are essential at all times.

Each family will require a comprehensive and appropriate explanation of the baby's condition and an honest plan of action. Explanation of the equipment is also important.

ACTIVITIES OF LIVING

The activities of living are a useful way of looking at the general needs of the neonate.

Maintenance of a safe environment

In most cases, the safest environment for a baby is *in utero*. However, for babies admitted to intensive care, the aim must be to make their surroundings as safe as possible. This includes good emergency systems and highly trained staff.

One of the biggest potential problems is the risk of cross-infection. Routine screening on admission (umbilical, nasal and throat swabs) should be performed. Any baby with potential infection should be isolated until deemed 'clear'.

Communicating

Communication must be maintained with the baby, the family and the unit staff. Babies communicate their needs through non-verbal cues, which the staff must be able to recognize and respond to. However, if the baby is very unwell, these cues can be masked. Parents should be encouraged to touch, handle, cuddle and talk to their baby as appropriate. Families react in different ways to their baby's illness. Some may withdraw, become angry or aggressive, or seem to act inappropriately. Gaining the family's trust and encouraging communication is vitally important. Staff, including all members of the multi-disciplinary team, must also communicate effectively with each other. Handovers should include details of the baby's history, medical condition and family and social circumstances where appropriate.

Breathing

Most babies breathe normally at a rate of 40–60 breaths per minute with a regular and quiet pattern. Babies with noisy or irregular breathing, or who are using accessory muscles, need investigation. Babies are obligatory nose breathers, so if their nostrils become blocked they develop cyanosis and apnoea. The nurse should also be aware of the baby's Apgar score, as this is an important indication of the baby's initial competence in cardiovascular and neuromuscular activity (Table 3.1). Apnoeic attacks should be recorded and their characteristics, such as accompanying bradycardia and need for stimulation, noted. The cause of such attacks should be determined and appropriate treatment such as aminophylline or caffeine commenced. Minimal handling and nursing the baby prone may help to reduce the risk of apnoea attacks.

Table 3.1 Apgar score

Sign	Score		
	0	*1*	*2*
Heart rate	Absent	<100/min	>100/min
Respiratory effort	Absent	Weak, irregular	Strong, regular
Muscle tone	Limp	Some flexion	Active movement
Reflex response to stimulation of feet	None	Weak movement	Cry
Colour	Blue or pale	Body pink, blue extremities	Completely pink

This is usually done at 1 and 5 min. Further later assessment may be required in unwell babies.

Most babies in intensive care units need some form of ventilatory support. In mild conditions, the use of an oxygen-enriched environment may be adequate and humidified oxygen can be delivered via a headbox. The environment is analysed hourly and regulated in response to apnoeas, oxygen saturation or transcutaneous P_{0_2}. As the baby improves, the amount of oxygen can be decreased until they are nursed in air.

Respiratory support can also be given by using nasal prongs and/or continuous positive airways pressure (CPAP) of 2–4 cm. The former system can be used for babies who require long-term oxygen therapy. Many babies, however, require full ventilatory support. Neonates appreciate pressure-limited continuous-flow ventilators. These machines give many variables and are easily adjusted. Endotracheal tubes can be positioned either orally or nasally, although the oral tubes are perhaps less secure and can cause damage to the palate. A variety of home-made 'bonnets', tube holders and harnesses are useful in keeping the tube in position. Dental plates can be used and may help prevent damage to the palate. Nasal tubes are more secure but may be more difficult to insert and can cause damage to the nostrils and nasal septum. The ventilated neonate is at risk from ventilation for a number of reasons, including dislodgement of the tube due to inadequate securing, tube blockage, pneumothorax, bronchopulmonary dysplasia and damage to nasal passages.

Most ventilated babies have an arterial line *in situ*, and umbilical vessels are often used. However, these are not suitable in the long term and can predispose to necrotizing enterocolitis. Paralysis and sedation may also be required to facilitate satisfactory ventilation.

As their condition improves, babies may be weaned from the ventilator using intermittent mandatory ventilation (IMV) and CPAP.

Eating and drinking

From the 36th week of gestation the sucking reflex is present and most babies express their need for food volubly from the time of birth. The most suitable milk for babies is breast milk because it is nutritionally correctly proportioned for the baby, contains maternal antibodies, and is warm and clean. Above all, it gives the mother great satisfaction to feed the baby and it helps to establish a bond between them. Mothers of babies who are unable to feed can express their milk, which can be stored for later use.

Modified milk can be a satisfactory alternative. Babies with a history of allergy in the family can be fed on a soya-based feed such as Wysoy (John Wyeth). Lactose-free feeds such as Pregestimil are of value in babies with malabsorption problems.

Ventilated babies will need nasogastric or nasojejunal tubes passed to allow the feeds to be delivered safely. Nasogastric tubes also help to keep the stomach deflated.

Many babies will require total parenteral nutrition to support them until they can manage enteral feeds. Total parenteral nutrition is not without problems; the biggest risk is that of sepsis.

Eliminating

Fluid balance is an essential aspect of intensive care in babies, and due consideration must be made of insensible water losses. These losses are increased for babies under phototherapy and/or radiant heater, but can be reduced by using humidification or plastic sheeting. Normal losses vary from 65 ml/kg per day in babies weighing less than 1kg to 12 ml/kg per day in babies over 2 kg. Allowances may need to be increased by 50% for preterm infants under radiant heaters. These allowances can be decreased by 25% for infants nursed under a heat shield or thermal blanket.

Urinary losses can be measured using adhesive urine bags or weighing nappies, or by using the finger of a glove to catch baby boys' urine. Catheters may be required if very accurate measurement and monitoring is vital.

Stools will often need to measured, recorded and tested. Again, imagination can help collection of the specimen; placing the baby on bubble film (bubble side up) may prove helpful.

Personal cleansing and dressing

Even in intensive care babies must be kept clean, although it may be difficult when the baby is connected to tubes. Parents can be encouraged to do mouth and face care and nappy changing, and often enjoy supplying their own baby's clothes. Colour coordination is still seen to be important!

Controlling body temperature

Temperature-controlling mechanisms are immature in the newborn and they have a limited ability to produce heat by shivering. Catabolism of brown fat (located mainly in the middle to upper thorax) is the main mechanism for heat production and, as this mechanism increases in response to cold, oxygen requirements increase. Acidosis occurs as glucose is metabolized and the production of surfactant is decreased, leading to further respiratory distress.

Newborns have a large surface area in relation to size, and their reduced subcuticular fat for insulation makes careful heat regulation essential. Energy consumption can be reduced by nursing the baby in a thermoneutral environment. This is defined as the range of environmental temperature over which heat production, oxygen consumption and nutritional requirements are minimal provided the body temperature is normal. This varies according to gestational age and whether the baby is nursed in an incubator or overhead (radiant) heated cot. (See Table 3.2.) Heat loss can be reduced by using a heat shield or bubble plastic.

Mobilizing

Unless a baby is sedated and paralysed it is surprising how much spontaneous movement can be made. Regular turning is essential and this should

Table 3.2 Mean incubator air temperatures needed to provide a suitable thermal environment for healthy naked infants

Birth weight (kg)	Temperature (°C)			
	35	34	33	32
1–1.5	for 10 days	after 10 days	after 3 weeks	after 5 weeks
1.5–2	for 10 days	for 10 days	after 3 weeks	after 4 weeks
2–2.5	for 10 days	for 2 days	after 2 days	after 3 weeks
over 2.5	for 10 days	for 2 days	for 2 days	after 2 days

In a single-walled incubator the environmental temperature needs to be increased by 1°C difference between room and incubator temperature. Very-low-birthweight infants (below 1 kg) need higher air temperatures and a humidified incubator in the first week (Wheldon and Hull, 1983: Sauer *et al.*, 1984). These values are average ones, but there is considerable individual variation. (Source: Hey, 1975)

be coordinated with other nursing care. When handling the baby, staff should assess the baby's tone and reaction to stimuli. Preterm babies enjoy lying prone and may find respiration easier in this position. Passive movements of the limbs may prove helpful if the baby is paralysed.

Working and playing

The main work of any baby is to maintain breathing, feeding and rest patterns. Babies are sometimes said to be 'working hard', which means that they are using effort to breathe; this needs careful assessment and assistance may be required. Babies need to be stimulated, and staff and family can provide this stimulation by talking to them, touching them and using mobiles and toys.

Expressing sexuality

If the baby has not been named, it is important for staff always to refer to the correct sex when talking to the family about the baby. 'Appropriately' coloured bonnets and bootees can be a helpful reminder. Cultural beliefs and customs should be respected. Occasionally, babies are born of indeterminate sex and this can be very difficult for the family; confidentiality must be maintained throughout, especially if surgery effects a change in sex which the parents do not wish to be divulged to other family members.

Sleeping

Babies need rest and sleep even if it seems impossible in an intensive care unit. Care should be coordinated, ward lights dimmed, minimal handling adhered to, to ensure that the baby has the opportunity to rest for reasonable periods.

Dying

The loss of a newborn baby is one of the most difficult and traumatic times for any family. Feelings of shock, guilt, disbelief, anger and fear will surface at times. Some families can express their feelings openly; others will bottle them up and express them in anger and irritability on the ward and at home. All families require support either from the professional support services or from family members. The nursing staff should be aware of the unique and individual needs of families during this time and must make every effort to meet these needs. The administrative details must also be dealt with competently and compassionately.

SPECIAL PROBLEMS OF THE PRETERM BABY

By definition, low-birthweight babies weigh 2.5 kg or less, regardless of their gestational age. About half of these babies are born before 37 weeks and are therefore preterm. The overall incidence of low birthweight is 6% of all births in the UK. This varies regionally and according to ethnic background.

About two-thirds of all perinatal deaths (i.e. deaths occurring in the first 7 days of life) occur in the low-birthweight group, but most deaths occur in those weighing less than 1.3 kg. Babies surviving below that weight are those most likely to suffer handicap.

There are two main types of small baby: those 'born too soon' and those 'born too small' i.e. babies whose growth has been limited *in utero*. These babies may be called 'small for dates' or 'light for dates'.

The weight needs to be plotted on a growth and development chart, which gives normal ranges of growth and weight for gestational age. A baby is said to be light for dates if the weight falls below the 10th centile value. Some babies (e.g. Asian babies) are small for genetic reasons, but healthy. Other reasons for low birthweight include primiparity mothers, maternal age less than 18 years, poor socioeconomic status, pre-eclampsia, chronic maternal ill health, smoking, alcoholism and intrauterine infection.

About 50% of cases of low birthweight occur because of spontaneous preterm onset of labour; others occur following induction. Regular scans during pregnancy help to assess intrauterine growth, multiplicity and congenital anomaly. This growth, in conjunction with the date of the last menstrual period, helps to assess the gestational age. After birth, the Dubovitz score is one method of confirming this.

Most low-birthweight babies are nursed in neonatal units in maternity hospitals. However, a proportion may be admitted to paediatric intensive care units because they also have other problems.

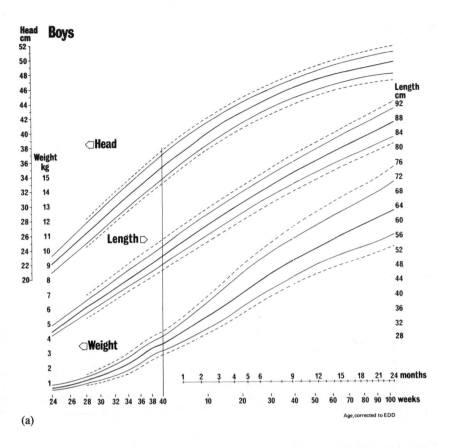

(a)

Figure 3.1 Growth and development charts, (a) boys, (b) girls. Centiles: ------ (upper) 97th, _____ (upper) 90th, _____ 50th, _____ (lower) 10th, ------ (lower) 3rd.

The low-birthweight baby faces many problems, the most common of which will now be explored in more detail.

Risk of infection

Severe bacteriological infection affects 0.3–0.5% of live births. However, this rises to 2–4% in the preterm baby in special care, and up to 30% in babies in intensive care.

Newborn babies have reduced defences against infection because some immunoglobulins do not cross the placental barrier, and because they have an immature immune system. Babies who are not breast fed are at added risk

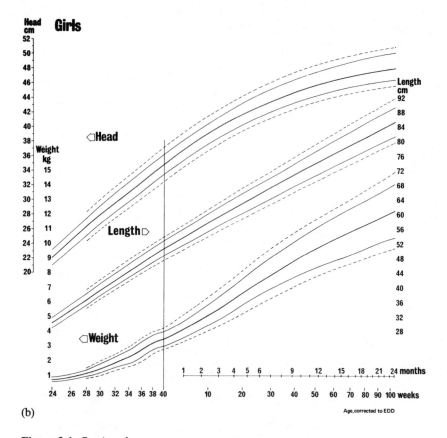

(b)

Figure 3.1 *Continued.*

as they do not benefit from the immunoglobulin secreted in colostrum and breast milk.

Those most at risk from infection are:

1. babies born to mothers who had prolonged rupture of membranes (over 24 h);
2. babies whose mothers have infection;
3. babies born to mothers with antepartum haemorrhage (especially abruptio placenta);
4. babies with respiratory distress.

Routes of infection:

Congenital infection may occur from ascending infection e.g. early membrane rupture, the transplacental route, e.g. cytomegalovirus, toxoplasmosis, and aspiration of infected material before or at delivery.

Infection can be acquired thought the umbilical cord, skin lesions and on aspiration. Nosocomial infection from inadequate hand washing and cleaning of apparatus can also be a problem.

Signs of infection include:

1. lethargy and general ill-health;
2. increasing apnoeas with respiratory difficulty;
3. unstable temperature;
4. tachycardia and tachypnoea;
5. local signs, e.g. redness and tenderness, particularly of the umbilical stump;
6. hepatosplenomegaly;
7. poor feeding and/or vomiting;
8. increasing jaundice;
9. abdominal distension;
10. blood in stools and diarrhoea;
11. kidney enlargement;
12. seizures;
13. schlerema;
14. haematological problems, including bleeding from mucous membranes and petechiae.

Any baby showing signs of infection should receive an infection screen. This will include blood sampling for culture and sensitivity, full haematological and electrolyte estimations, and blood gas analysis. Bacteriological swabs are taken from the nose, throat, umbilicus, ear, rectum and any other place showing obvious sign of a local problem. Samples of urine and gastric aspirate are sent for microscopy and culture. A lumbar puncture is performed and the cerebrospinal fluid investigated for microscopy culture and sugar content. Chest and abdominal radiographs are taken. Further blood tests may include acute phase reactant (i.e. C-reactive protein), erythrocyte sedimentation rate and coagulation studies.

Once all investigations are initiated, broad-spectrum antibiotics are required until cultures reveal more information.

Appropriate supportive intervention will be needed to supplement antibiotic therapy. Specific antibiotics are required to treat the various organisms and doses are determined by the baby's weight.

Nephrotoxicity and ototoxicity can occur, especially when using aminoglycosides such as gentamicin. Regular trough and peak blood levels are taken to ensure the effectiveness of these antibiotics and to prevent toxicity. Babies with poor renal function need very careful monitoring.

To prevent the spread of infection, meticulous care is required when handling the babies. Handwashing technique, isolation of infected, or potentially infected, babies and absolute cleanliness or all equipment are *mandatory* in any intensive care or neonatal unit.

Poor temperature control

Preterm babies have difficulty in maintaining a stable temperature. This is due to an immature heat-regulating centre, inability to shiver, a large surface area in relationship to weight, poor fat stores for insulation, and inadequate nutrition in conjunction with an immature liver and resultant delay in metabolism.

Preterm babies need to be nursed in their thermoneutral environment, and adequate calories must be given to help maintain blood sugar and allow the baby to grow.

The aim is to keep the baby's temperature around 36.5°C. Very preterm babies (i.e. below 28 weeks) may also need humidity in the incubator.

Hypothermia can cause increased oxygen consumption, vasoconstriction, acidosis, increased fatty acid production, hypoglycaemia and coagulation disorders. *Hyperthermia* can cause apnoea, tachycardia, tachypnoea, and restlessness. An *unstable* temperature may be the manifestation of neonatal sepsis, brain injury or brain anomaly.

Idiopathic respiratory distress syndrome (IRDS)

This condition is caused by lack of surfactant, which is responsible for reducing surface tension in the lung alveoli, preventing alveolar collapse on expiration.

The active ingredients of surfactant are lecithin (60%), phosphatidylglycerol and phosphatidylinositol. These substances are produced at 24–26 weeks by pathways very sensitive to changes in temperature and pH. By 35 weeks, surfactant is produced by a second route which is less sensitive to these changes.

Deficiency in surfactant leads to alveolar collapse, reduced lung volume and decreased lung compliance. Ventilation and perfusion problems occur and in severe cases pulmonary hypertension with right-to-left shunting occurs.

Radiologically, areas of collapse appear as diffuse reticulogranular mottling with air in the major bronchi causing air bronchograms. Hypoxia from ventilation/perfusion abnormalities leads to metabolic acidosis, and alveolar hypoventilation causes respiratory acidosis. Acidosis and hypoxia reduce cardiac output and arterial blood pressure. Perfusion is reduced in the kidneys and gastrointestinal tract, so oedema and electrolyte disturbances occur. It is therefore essential that hypoxia and acidosis are corrected with ventilatory support.

In uncomplicated cases, surfactant is produced after 48 h and, as the baby stabilizes, the oedema reduces and the urine output improves.

There is a predisposition to respiratory distress syndrome when there is a history of IRDS in a previous sibling, maternal diabetes, rhesus incompatability, or antepartum haemorrhage. It also occurs more frequently in male infants, the second twin, those born by lower segment Caesarian section and those with birth asphyxia.

Early signs and symptoms include:

1. increasing tachypnoea;
2. grunting respirations;
3. use of accessory muscles (alae nasae/abdominal).

Radiography confirms diagnosis. Later signs include:

1. increasing apnoeas with cyanosis;
2. increasing bradycardias requiring stimulation;
3. apnoeas requiring ventilatory assistance.

The baby is nursed in an incubator with a head-up tilt, assessed constantly and monitored using an oxygen saturation monitor in conjunction with blood gas analysis. Rest is essential and care is kept to a minumum and coordinated. If grunting respirations and tachypnoea increases, headbox oxygen is given. Full ventilatory support via endotracheal tube may be needed in severe cases.

Surfactant replacement therapy has proved helpful, often dramatically reducing symptoms and the length of time ventilatory support is required, and is now becoming more freely available.

Most babies progress well, improve over 3–4 days and can gradually be weaned off their ventilatory support. The main long-term problem is oxygen dependency with bronchopulmonary dysplasia.

Nutritional needs

Neonates need nutrition to grow and maintain body temperature. Preterm babies are unable to suckle, so alternative methods are required until they can feed by themselves. The frequency and volumes of feeds used will depend on the gestational age and overall condition of the baby. As a general rule, very small babies require frequent (or continuous) feeds of high calorific content. If a continuous feed of expressed breast milk is used, the syringe must be placed with the nozzle upwards to ensure that the cream is delivered to the baby.

Low-birthweight formula of modified milk is now widely used. These milks contain higher protein and caloric values volume for volume. The high sodium content may not be suitable for all babies, and regular checks of their serum and urine sodium levels should be made. The mean urine sodium level in a preterm baby is 6 mmol/l (Tables 3.3–3.5).

Vitamin supplements may also be required, although using a modified milk this is not mandatory. Babies of very low birthweight or those on expressed

Table 3.3 Composition (per 100 ml) of milks for normal nutrition in infants under 6 months

	Energy		Protein (g)	Carbo-hydrate (g)	Fat (g)	Sodium (mmol)	Potassium (mmol)	Osmolality (mOsmol/ kg)
	kcal	kJ						
Human milk (mature)	69	289	1.3	7.2	4.1	0.6	1.5	264
SMA Gold	66	275	1.5	7.2	3.6	0.7	1.4	300
Premium	66	275	1.5	7.3	3.6	0.8	1.7	290

The mother's own milk should be given as first choice, by breast feeding or by the mother expressing her milk. If breast milk is not available, a whey-based infant formula must be used.
Other whey-based formulas are Aptamil and Ostermilk. Casein-based formulas are White Cap SMA, Cow & Gate Plus, Milumil and Ostermilk 2. Any infant admitted on these feeds may be given Ready-to-Feed Gold Cap SMA or Premium.

Table 3.4 Composition (per 100 ml) of supplemented human milk for preterm and low-birthweight infants

Quantity of supplement added to 100 ml mature human milk*	Energy		Protein (g)	Carbo-hydrate (g)	Fat (g)	Sodium (mmol)	Potassium (mmol)	Osmolality (mOsmol/ kg)
	kcal	kJ						
3 g Pregestimil	82	345	1.7	9.0	4.6	0.9	0.9	
5 g Pregestimil	91	383	1.9	10.3	5.0	1.1	2.1	391
3 g SMA Gold	84	353	1.7	8.9	4.9	0.7	1.8	
5 g SMA Gold	94	396	1.9	10.0	5.5	0.9	2.1	
3 g Caloreen	81	339	1.3	10.2	4.1	0.6	1.5	348

*Composition of unsupplemented mature human milk is given in Table 3.3.

breast milk are recommended to have Abidec (Warner-Lambert) 0.6 ml daily. Vitamin D 800–1600 units may also be given to very preterm infants.

Much discussion occurs with regard to iron supplements. It is generally agreed that supplementation is required for babies born before 36 weeks. Supplements are usually started at 4–6 weeks (iron stores are high at birth), although with constant blood sampling they may be commenced earlier in some cases.

A recommended dose of iron is 2.5–5mg/kg per day. Medications suitable are ferrous sulphate or Sytron (sodium iron edetate, Parke, Davis; a sugar-free mixture).

Folic acid may help to prevent macrocytic anaemia. The dose recommended is 50 ug/kg per day.

Total parenteral nutrition (TPN) and the preterm baby

Many very preterm babies will be unable to tolerate enteral feeds. Total parenteral nutrition is now available in most hospitals and is made up

Table 3.5 Composition (per 100 ml) of low-birthweight formulas and supplemented infant milk formulas for preterm and low-birthweight infants and those failing to thrive on fluid restrictions

	Energy		Protein (g)	Carbo-hydrate (g)	Fat (g)	Sodium (mmol)	Potassium (mmol)	Osmolality (mOsmol/ kg)
	kcal	kJ						
Low-birthweight SMA	80	335	2.0	8.6	4.4	1.4	1.9	268
Low-birthweight SMA + Caloreen to 12% carbohydrate	93	389	2.0	12.0	4.4	1.5	1.9	
13% SMA + Caloreen to 12% carbohydrate + Calogen to 5% fat	96	403	1.6	2.0	5.0	0.7	1.4	
15% SMA	76	320	1.8	8.4	4.2	0.9	1.7	332
15% SMA + Caloreen to 12% carbohydrate + Calogen to 5% fat	97	408	1.8	12.0	5.0	0.9	1.7	

Other low-birthweight and preterm formulas are Nenatal, Prematalac, Prematil and Osterprem. Infants admitted on any of these formulas will receive one of the above feeds, after discussion with the dietitian.

centrally. This helps to prevent line infection and is cost effective.

Regular checks of blood sugar (6–8 hourly) and urine sugar levels (daily) are needed during the introduction of TPN, because some small babies cannot tolerate the high input of concentrated dextrose. A BM stick level of 9 mmol/l or above on more than two occasions is considered high. It may be an early sign of sepsis or stress. Concurrent solutions of insulin are required in some cases.

Inefficient liver function

Glucose metabolism

Hypoglycaemia is defined as a blood sugar level below 1.5 mmol/l in the first 24 h, and below 2 mmol/l thereafter. Blood sugar levels are mainly estimated at the bedside using capillary blood and one of the 'strip' methods, e.g. Dextrostix (Ames) or BM Sticks (Boehringer). It is essential that a large drop of blood is used. Where possible, fingers or toes should be used although the fleshy part of the heel is most frequently used in the neonate.

Hypoglycaemia can occur if there are depleted glycogen stores (e.g. in a small-for-dates baby or a preterm baby) of if there is delayed feeding, asphyxia or hypothermia. Another cause is fetal insulinaemia, which may occur in an infant of a diabetic mother, if there is rhesus incompatibility, or in Beckwith's

syndrome. Adrenal insufficiency, sepsis, congenital heart disease and galactosaemia can also cause the problem.

Symptoms of hypoglycaemia include lethargy, hypothermia, apnoeas, jittery
movements, seizures, cyanosis and heart failure.

Extra sugar given in the form of glucose water should be adequate in
asymptomatic babies until feeds are fully established. If symptoms occur,
intravenous dextrose 25%, 2 ml/kg should be given at once and followed
by intravenous 10% dextrose 5 ml/kg per hour until sugar levels are normal.
Glucagon (300 mg/kg), adrenalin and hydrocortisone may be required in
extreme cases.

Hyperglycaemia is defined as a blood sugar level of more than 8 mmol/l.
It can occur in preterm babies receiving high dextrose concentration intravenous
fluids, and may be an early sign of sepsis or related to stress.

In many cases, reduction of the concentration and/or volume of infusate
is sufficient treatment. Occasionally an infusion of insulin is required (0.1
unit/kg per hour). This is given as a continuous infusion using a sliding scale
according to blood sugar estimations.

Jaundice

Jaundice (hyperbilirubinaemia) occurs in about 30% of all babies in the first
week of life. If levels of bilirubin (the yellow pigment that shows as jaundice)
become high, severe long-term problems can result.

Bilirubin is formed by the normal breakdown of haemoglobin as the red
cell dies. Bilirubin is fat soluble, but is rendered water soluble by the action
of the liver enzyme glucuronyl transferase in a process known as conjugation. This conjugated form is then excreted via the bile into the gut. It is often
2–3 days before sufficient glucuronyl transferase is available to cope with
the process, and during this time the serum bilirubin levels rise and the
unconjugated yellow pigment becomes evident. This is known as physiological
jaundice and in most cases little treatment is necessary apart from ensuring
an adequate fluid intake and monitoring bilirubin levels. A glucose solution
can be given between breast, bottle or tube feeds.

Breast-fed babies are more likely to develop jaundice, because they have
a lower fluid intake and an abnormal progesterone metabolite in breast milk
competes with bilirubin for conjugation, so that bilirubin levels rise. The
unconjugated form causes kernicterus.

Predisposing factors to jaundice include:

1. preterm delivery;
2. haemolytic disease due to blood incompatibility with the mother, e.g.
    rhesus, ABO problems;
3. inadequate fluid intake;

4. infection, e.g. sepsis, urinary infection, viral infection;
5. haemolysis, e.g. cephalhaematoma, polycythaemia, excessive bruising;
6. cystic fibrosis;
7. rarer diseases, e.g. thalassaemia, spherocytosis, galactosaemia, biliary atresia.

Charts (Figure 3.2) can assist in alerting staff to the need for phototherapy and/or exchange transfusion.

It is important to ensure that bilirubin levels do not reach levels that cause damage. Levels as which damage can occur depend on two main factors: the gestational age of the baby and the general condition. Any sick baby is very much at risk.

Treatment
If bilirubin levels are rising, check the haemoglobin level and blood groups, conduct a Coombs test, and regularly monitor and record serum bilirubin levels. 10% extra fluid/kg per 24 h is given either orally or intravenously. This is usually given as 5% dextrose. If bilirubin levels continue to rise, phototherapy is commenced and an infection screen is performed to exclude and monitor any sepsis. Exchange transfusion may be required if serum bilirubin levels continue to rise.

In phototherapy, light from the blue end of the spectrum converts bilirubin into the water-soluble form, which can then be excreted via the kidneys and bowel. In conjunction with this, extra fluids are given at 10%/kg per day. Regular estimations of bilirubin levels are taken during the treatment.

Phototherapy is not without its problems. These include fluid depletion from extra insensible losses, thermal instability and masking of sepsis, irritability, restlessness and insecurity. Problems from the eye bandages include asphyxia (when the bandage covers the nostrils) and irritation to the cornea. Skin bronzing and loose stools may also occur. Family anxiety can be alleviated by careful explanations, and when possible the light should be turned off for part of their visit.

Nursing the baby in an incubator will help to reduce insensible water losses. Allowance for this is suggested as: 25 ml/kg per day for babies under 1 kg, 20 ml/kg per day for babies of 1–1.25 kg and 10 ml/kg per day for babies over 1.25 kg.

Babies with increasing bilirubin levels not responding to phototherapy and extra fluids may need *exchange transfusion*. For this procedure, babies are most easily nursed in an overhead heated cot. Monitoring equipment must be in use, and resuscitative measures at hand.

Venous access is usually by the umbilical vessels, although other vessels are sometimes used. Blood is exchanged at 180 ml/kg (i.e. twice the circulating blood volume) in 5, 10 or 20 ml aliquots. Samples of blood for bilirubin

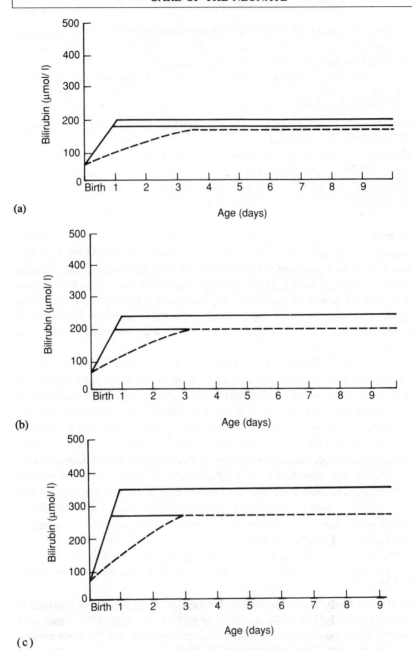

Figure 3.2 Bilirubin charts for preterm infants born at (a) less than 29 weeks, (b) 29–33 weeks, (c) 34–37 weeks. Any value above the top line indicates a need to consider exchange transfusion in a well infant. Any value above the lower solid line indicates a need for exchange transfusion in a sick infant. Any value above the broken line indicates a need for phototherapy.

estimations are taken regularly. The bilirubin level should fall by 60% during the procedure.

Complications of exchange transfusion include:

1. collapse, metabolic acidosis;
2. cardiac arrhythmias;
3. electrolyte imbalance;
4. hypoglycaemia;
5. sepsis;
6. hypothermia;
7. abdominal distension;
8. bowel ischaemia causing necrotizing enterocolitis;
9. air embolism.

More than one exchange transfusion may be required, and a strict aseptic technique is essential.

Any baby who remains jaundiced needs further investigation. Other possible problems are sepsis, neonatal hepatitis and obstructive problems, e.g. biliary atresia. Congenital hypothyroidism, virus infections (e.g. toxoplasmosis) and metabolic disorders (e.g. galactosaemia) are also seen.

Impaired renal function

In preterm babies, the kidney is usually able to excrete urea and water adequately, but may not be able to cope with excess amounts, and so metabolic acidosis and oedema may result. It is also less able to retain sodium than the kidney in more mature babies; therefore, a higher sodium intake may be needed.

Babies most at risk include those with IRDS, history of birth asphyxia and excess antidiuretic hormone.

Preterm babies often have low albumin levels, which will also increase oedema. Excessive fluid intake should be avoided. Fluids may need to be restricted and a diuretic may be required. The minimum adequate urine output for all babies is 1 ml/kg per hour.

Sclerema

This affects mainly very sick babies. Those having asphyxia, septicaemia, hypovolaemia or hypothermia are most at risk. The woody appearance and feel is due to the hardening of the subcutaneous tissue. It usually starts around the buttocks and then spreads throughout the body. Supportive treatment is required and, when the cause is due to infection, an exchange transfusion is helpful. With improvements in the care of neonates, this condition is now less frequently seen.

Impaired bowel function

Some preterm babies have problems in passing meconium after birth, which may be due to an immature bowel. Associated reasons are asphyxia, hypothermia, sepsis or diabetes in the mother.

Although there is no anatomical anomaly, the baby fails to pass meconium; the abdomen becomes distended and there may be bilious vomiting. This condition may also be called a 'functional obstruction' or 'meconium disease of the preterm'.

Treatment consists of stopping feeds and passing a nasogastric tube for deflation and aspiration of the stomach. A septic screen is usually done and intravenous fluids commenced. In some cases a rectal examination may be sufficient to stimulate a bowel action. In more severe cases, a gastrografin enema may be necessary to clear the plugs. This hygroscopic radio-opaque fluid can cause excessive fluid loss, so volume expanders should be given during or immediately after this procedure.

In many babies, this treatment will prove effective and, after some hours of bowel rest and intravenous fluids, enteral feeds can be slowly introduced. Occasionally surgical intervention is required. (Meconium ileus and Hirschsprung's disease rarely occur in preterm babies, but they may need to be considered.)

Haematological problems

The main problems seen in the preterm are:

1. anaemia (early or later);
2. polycythaemia;
3. haemorrhagic disease of the newborn;
4. disseminated intravascular coagulation (DIC);
5. inherited disorders, e.g. thalassaemia, haeomophilia, thrombocytopenia (which occur in all gestational ages).

Some of these are manifested by bleeding. When this occurs, the following investigations are required:

1. *History*: family history, maternal drugs, obstetric history;
2. *Examination*:
    (a) in an ill baby, suspect infection, DIC or severe liver disease;
    (b) in a well baby, suspect platelet defect or haemorrhagic disease of the newborn; if there are petechiae, suspect thrombocytopenia; if ecchymoses, suspect DIC, haemorrhagic disease in the newborn, liver disease;
3. *Gastrointestinal bleeding*: differentiate between maternal blood and the baby's blood;

4. *Other investigations*: platelet count, prothrombin time, partial thrombo-plastin time, bleeding time, fibrin degradation products in urine and blood, fibrinogen.

Vitamin K deficiency (haemorrhagic disease of the newborn)

This is due to a deficiency of prothrombin and other vitamin K-dependent blood clotting factors. Vitamin K, which is needed for hepatic synthesis of factors II (prothrombin), VII, IX and X, is synthesized in the gut by intestinal bacteria. As cows' milk contains four times as much vitamin K as breast milk, this problem is more common in breast-fed babies.

Predisposing factors are chronic diarrhoea, prolonged antibiotic therapy, and TPN in preterm babies. Maternal drug therapy with phenobarbitone, salicylates and anticoagulants can also predispose to vitamin K deficiency.

The sign is bleeding, which may occur from mucous membrane, in the gut (haematemesis or malaena), via the cord, or into the skin (petechiae).

Treatment is to give 1 M vitamin K 1–2 mg. This may need to be repeated if the symptoms do not subside. Local application of pressure with topical coagulants to the umbilical stump may also be necesssary. Fresh frozen plasma or blood transfusion will be needed in severe cases and to correct resultant anaemia.

All babies requiring surgery must receive intramuscular vitamin K 1 mg before the operation begins unless otherwise indicated.

Retinopathy of the newborn (retrolental fibroplasia)

This condition occurs in preterm babies exposed to high concentrations of oxygen. Therefore, avoidance of P_{aO_2} of over 12 kPa at all times is essential, and environmental oxygen should be measured at all times and monitored closely. High P_{aO_2} values cause initial retinal vessel constriction. This may be follow-ed by proliferation of new capillaries if ischaemia of the retina has occurrred. The growth of these vessels causes fibrosis and scarring, which can lead to detachment and blindness (cicatricial stage). All babies who have received added oxygen should have their eyes examined at 32 weeks and prior to discharge.

Predisposing factors include low gestational age, multiple pregnancies in the mother, acidosis and blood transfusion.

Possible treatment at present includes large doses of vitamin E and adrenocorticotrophic hormone, cryotherapy to the peripheral retina in the early proliferative stage, and laser treatment.

Separation problems for the family

With all the modern technology of caring for the preterm baby, it is important not to lose sight of the family and their relationships with each other and with the baby. In 1907, Pierre Budin (cited in Brimblecome *et al.*, 1978) wrote in *The Nursling* in Paris:

> Unfortunately a certain number of mothers abandon their babies whose needs they have not had to meet, and in whom they have lost all interest. The life of the little one has been saved, it is true, but at the cost of the mother.

Nowadays, staff of baby units are very aware of this problem and every effort is made to encourage the family to get to know their new member. Free visiting should be encouraged for all the family (including siblings).

Much encouragement is needed for the family, and nursing staff should be alert to their needs. The family can be encouraged to assist in the assessment, planning, implementation and evaluation of their baby's care. Families should be encouraged to handle and touch the baby at each visit, even when the baby is very poorly. Times that the care is given can be coordinated to assist the family.

ADMISSION OF THE NEONATE TO ITU

Preparation

It is essential that adequate preparation is made for the baby. An update of the baby's condition at the referral hospital (or other ward) is essential, as this should ensure that equipment is available and the admission procedure is efficiently completed.

Details of the pregnancy, delivery and history of the disorder are required. Where possible, a family member should be encouraged to accompany the baby.

In many units, babies requiring intensive care are nursed in overhead heated cots. Preterm babies and those not requiring ventilation may be nursed in closed incubators, thereby giving good observation facilities, helping to assist with heat regulation and reducing insensible fluid losses.

The following should be available for each baby:

1. facility for giving oxygen and air (piped or by cylinder);
2. suction equipment and catheters;
3. a hand ventilating circuit attached to an oxygen supply;
4. toilet requisites;
5. equipment for measuring blood sugar levels;
6. stethoscope and paper tape measure;
7. blood pressure cuff;

8. nursing care charts according to unit policy;
9. monitoring equipment and leads (cardiac, temperature, transducer for blood pressure monitoring, pulse oximeter for transcutaneous P_{0_2} measurement);
10. bacteriological swabs according to unit policy;
11. leaflets, maps, etc. for parents.

A blood pressure machine (e.g. Dynamap), resuscitation equipment and weighing scales should also be available.

When it is known that the baby is ventilated, equipment should be prepared to facilitate a smooth transfer.

Admission

An immediate assessment should be made as the baby arrives and resuscitative measures undertaken if necessary. Where appropriate, the baby can be weighed before placing into the cot or incubator as this will minimize disturbance and handling.

Baseline observations are taken and blood for BM sticks tests. The baby is attached to unit monitoring equipment and support. In some cases this may involve reintubation.

The following are required at the time of admission and should be checked before referral staff leave:

1. history of previous pregnancies and this pregnancy;
2. history of this baby, including details of labour, type of delivery and condition at birth, Agpar scores and any resuscitative measures, and the presentation of the problem;
3. details of management of the baby up to and during transfer;
4. details of family circumstances (for completion of hospital documentation), including address and telephone numbers and any religious requests;
5. record of whether vitamin K has been given;
6. signed anaesthetic consent form (if relevant and if the family is not present);
7. sample of maternal blood (to aid cross match);
8. relevant radiographs, charts and letters.

Once the baby's immediate needs have been met, staff can examine the baby in more detail and a plan of action can be made. Venepuncture, radiographic investigations, and the insertion of access lines can then be performed.

During this time it is important that the family are not forgotten. First impressions are very important and families need to feel welcome and part of the admission procedure. As soon as possible, staff should talk to them about the baby, his or her problems, and plans for investigations and treatment. Diagrams are helpful, especially if a baby has complicated congenital anomalies.

Practical arrangements may need to be made to accommodate the family. If the mother is admitted, midwifery cover is required for 10 days. Facilities for expressing milk should be available to ensure that the mother's milk supply is maintained. If the mother is not resident, pumps can be hired from the National Childbirth Trust, or hand pumps should be obtainable.

Honesty at all times is essential when talking to the parents, especially when a complicated problem is evident which may involve staged procedures with long periods of hospitalization.

THE SURGICAL BABY

A high proportion of babies admitted to a paediatric intensive care unit have congenital anomalies that require surgery. Unfortunately, some babies will have several problems and will require repeated admission, staged surgery and a multidisciplinary approach.

General principles of preoperative care

The overall aim is to prepare the baby for surgery and ensure that he or she is in optimum condition. This involves the following.

1. Immediate resuscitative measures: ventilatory support, volume expanders, pharmacological support.
2. Monitoring of vital signs and oxygen saturations.
3. Monitoring and maintainance of body temperature: central, peripheral.
4. Regulation of fluid balance: measurement of serum glucose levels, measurement of urine output.
5. Medications: vitamin K (if not already given), antimicrobials, premedication as boarded.
6. Weight (if condition permits).
7. Specific needs, e.g. intubulation and ventilation: passage of large nasogastric tube (intestinal obstruction), passage of Replogle tube (oesophageal atresia).
8. Information for the family: anaesthetic and operative consent form to be signed, handouts as relevant to the condition.

General principles of postoperative care

The overall aim is to ensure a smooth and comfortable recovery from surgery and to enable the baby to be integrated fully into the family. This involves the following.

1. Prepare the cot area to ensure that all equipment is to hand.
2. Check the overall condition and observe the baby closely.
   (a) Ensure that ventilatory support is optimum.
   (b) Reconnect monitoring equipment to check vital signs and oxygen saturation.
3. Regulate fluid balance. Surgical babies require fluid restriction to prevent fluid overload following the stress of surgery. Guidelines which can be used are: one-third requirements on day 1, two-thirds requirements days 2 and 3, and full requirements on day 4.
   (a) Consider insensible losses.
   (b) Monitor urine output (1 ml/kg per h is acceptable).
   (c) Monitor blood sugar level.
4. Monitor and regulate temperature control.
   (a) Nurse in thermoneutral range.
   (b) Record central and peripheral temperature, and report a temperature gap of 2°C or more. Volume expanders may be required.
5. Ensure that all tubes and drains are well secured.
6. Give pain relief.
7. Ensure that family needs are met.

Specific care for some common anomalies requiring surgery

The following conditions will be looked at in greater detail: oesophageal atresia with or without tracheo-oesophageal fistula, meconium ileus, Hirschsprung's disease, and necrotizing enterocolitis.

Oesophageal atresia with or without tracheo-oesophageal fistula
It has become customary to group the babies by weight and associated anomalies. There are five main varieties of this condition (Figure 3.3), which has an incidence of one in 2500–3000 live births. The most common (87%) is that of the blind oesophageal pouch with a distal tracheo-oesophageal fistula (TOF). Pure oesophageal atresia occurs in approximately 8% of cases, and an H-type TOF is in approximately 4% of cases. The remaining 2% have the other two varieties of which the upper pouch TOF is most common.

Wide variation (0.5–5 cm) is found in the length of the gap between the upper and lower pouches of the oesophagus. The upper is usually thick walled and the lower may be small and hypoplastic, making surgical repair difficult even when the pouches are close to each other. The biggest gaps occur in babies with pure oesophageal atresia (or those with only an upper pouch TOF), when the lower pouches extend only a short distance upward above the diaphragm. This causes a 'long gap' problem and it is often these babies who require staged surgery to effect continuity of the oesophagus.

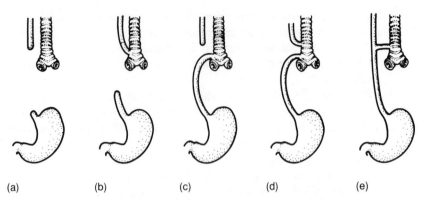

Figure 3.3 Types of oesophageal atresia: (a) isolated; (b) with proximal tracheo-oesophageal fistula; (c) with distal tracheo-oesophageal fistula; (d) with proximal and distal tracheo-oseophageal fistula; (e) tracheo-oesophageal fistula (H type) without associated atresia.

This condition is sometimes diagnosed antenatally by ultrasonography. A high proportion of mothers have hydramnios and some may deliver preterm. The baby presents with a history of excessive secretions from the mouth, often in association with cyanosis and/or apnoea. The diagnosis is made by the inability to pass a large nasogastric tube (i.e. Fr 8 or 10). Radiography confirms the diagnosis, showing the nasogastric tube coiled in the upper oesophagus, and also reveals whether there is gas in the stomach. Absence of gas suggests that no tracheo-oesophageal fistula is present. The condition of the lungs (including whether aspiration has occurred) and the size and shape of the heart should also be observed. A 'double bubble' suggests duodenal atresia (an associated anomaly).

Preoperative care The main objective is to ensure a clear airway and prevent further aspiration. A double-lumen suction tube is inserted (Replogle tube, Figure 3.4) into the upper pouch of the oesophagus and attached to a low-pressure suction pump. Alternatively, the baby can be nursed head-up to prevent reflux through the fistula. Every 15 min, 0.5 ml is instilled to ensure that the tube is kept patent. Regular suction is given to the oropharynx and physiotherapy is commenced. Once the Replogle tube is working, the baby can be nursed on a head-up tilt. This should help to prevent gastric content refluxing via the TOF into the lungs.

For transfer, if a Replogle tube is not available, a large nasogastric tube can be passed into the upper oesophagus and aspirated frequently (at least every 5 min). The baby is best nursed flat and prone during transfer.

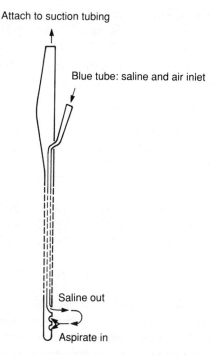

Attach to suction tubing

Blue tube: saline and air inlet

Saline out

Aspirate in

Figure 3.4 Replogle tube. (Not to scale, as indicated by the broken line.)

Surgery for types 1–4 The aim is to join the oesophagus and close the fistula (when present) to enable the baby to feed, grow and develop normally. In most babies this operation will be attempted within 24 h of admission. Anastamosis of the oesophagus and closure of the fistula will be effected through a thoracotomy.

Postoperative care Recovery is often excellent, and feeds via a nasogastric tube may be used initially until oral feeds are possible. Breast or bottle feeds should be given as soon as possible to ensure that the oesophagus does not stricture. Where the anastomosis is easy, oral feeds may be commenced in 2–3 days to the mutual benefit and comfort of the mother and baby.

Babies who have a tight oesophageal anastomosis may benefit from having paralysis, sedation and ventilatory support for several days, as this helps to prevent leakage from the newly repaired oesophagus. The baby is allowed to wake up after several days and oral feeds can be commenced once the condition is satisfactory. If there is anxiety about the patency of the oesophagus, contrast studies can be performed before oral feeds are commenced; some units may prefer to do this routinely prior to oral feeding.

'Long gap' problems These babies pose a bigger problem. If a TOF is present, it is closed soon after birth, but when the gap is long an anastomosis may not be possible. There are two main courses of action.

1. A feeding gastrostomy may be fashioned and a Replogle tube placed in the upper oesophageal pouch. The baby is then fed via the gastrostomy to allow weight gain and development. The upper pouch is kept clear with continuous Replogle tube suction. At a later date, a delayed anastomosis of the oesophagus is performed, or occasionally the stomach is pulled up (gastric interposition). Ventilatory support is usually required when this surgery is undertaken.

   The advantage of this method is that the oesophagus is preserved, but the disadvantage is that the baby has to remain in hospital for many months. During this time oral feeding is not possible, and the baby may have difficulty in feeding by mouth later. Vigilant care of the Replogle tube is essential to prevent overspill of secretions with aspiration.

2. A feeding gastrostomy is fashioned and the oesophagus is brought out through the neck to form an oesophagostomy. Feeds are given both by the gastrostomy and by mouth. The oral feeds, with the saliva, drain out via the oesophagostomy. The baby is then able to gain weight, enjoy oral feeds, and learn to associate sucking with a full stomach. When the baby is 6–9 months old, a gastric interposition or colonic replacement of the oesophagus is performed. Ventilatory support is usually required when this surgery is undertaken.

   The advantage of this approach is that the baby is able to enjoy oral feeds early and to be nursed at home and integrated into the family, but the disadvantage is that the baby's oesophagus is abandoned.

Long-term results have still to be fully evaluated. Each family's situation should be taken into consideration when the decision about the course of treatment is made.

Complications of surgery Feeding difficulties and tracheal malacia are two major areas of complication.

Assessment of the reason for feeding difficulties is essential to ensure that the baby receives the correct treatment.

1. *Gastro-oesophageal reflux.* The baby is nursed on a head-up tilt or in a chair. The feeds are thickened. Metoclopramide (to encourage gastric emptying) may also prove helpful. Nissen fundoplication is required in severe cases.

2. *Oesophageal stricture.* Regular oesophageal dilatations may be needed. It is essential that the families encourage these toddlers to chew food well, and discourage them from putting other items, such as buttons and toys, in their mouths.

3. *Anastomotic leak.* Oral feeds must be stopped, contrast studies performed, and tube feeds recommenced until the leak has healed. Occasionally, if the leak is very large, enteral feeds are stopped and total parenteral feeding commenced. In extreme cases the oesophagus disrupts and an oesophagostomy and gastrostomy have to be fashioned. Further surgery is then attempted at a later date.
4. *Recurrent TOF.* Choking on feeding with abdominal distension are the signs of this problem. Surgical intervention is required.

Tracheal malacia usually occurs at the site of the repaired TOF as the tracheal cartilage is soft and allows the trachea to collapse. The baby has noisy expiratory breathing and may have sudden collapse 'death attacks', which are usually associated with feeding.

Surgical intervention involves aortopexy, i.e. stitching the trachea to the aorta, thereby giving it support and stopping the tracheal cartilage collapsing.

H-type tracheo-oesophageal fistula (type 5) Choking on feeds, recurrent chest infections and gaseous abdominal distension are manifestations of this problem. Not all babies are diagnosed in the neonatal period.

Surgery involves ligation and division of the fistula and the baby is fed by tube for several days. Some of these babies also have tracheal malacia and require aortopexy.

Anomalies associated with all types of oesophageal atresia All midline anomalies are associated with TOF and oesophageal atresia, and most deaths occur in babies with multiple problems. The mnemonics VATER (or VACTERL) and CHARGE may assist one in remembering the problems:

Vascular, vertebral	Vertebral
Anorectal anomalies	Anorectal anomalies
TOF	Carciac
Etresia of oesophagus	TOF
Radial/renal	Etresia of oesophagus
	Renal
	Limb

Colomba (an opening of the pupil which extends into the iris on one side)
Heart anomalies
Atresia choanae
Retardation
Genitourinary problems, e.g. micropenis
Ear deformity and hearing loss

The prognosis for babies with charge association is not good and many babies die within the first year of life.

Categorization and prognosis of oesophageal atresia Waterson *et al*. (1962) categorized babies with this condition to assess their prognosis and this is still the internationally accepted classification.

A   Babies over 2.5 kg and well;
B_1 Babies 1.8–2.5 kg and well;
B_2 Babies over 2.5 kg with moderate pneumonia or congenital anomaly;
C_1 Babies under 1.8 kg;
C_2 Babies of any weight with severe pneumonia and/or other severe congenital anomaly.

They found that most of the deaths occurred in babies with multiple anomalies or those born preterm, i.e. group B_2 or C. This remains true today.

Babies who undergo primary surgery have a very good outlook and have few problems. Some may need occasional dilatations. Babies with long gap problems and those who had difficult initial surgery may need repeated admission with staged surgery. Much support is required for the family under these circumstances and it is essential that they are aware of the complications that may arise. The support group TOFS is helpful and branches exist throughout the country.

Intestinal obstruction

Any baby who vomits bile needs careful observation and investigation. Other signs of intestinal obstruction are delay or failure to pass meconium and abdominal distension.

Reasons for intestinal obstruction include:

1.   functional problems (also sometimes called meconium disease of the preterm);
2.   intestinal pyloric atresia, a rare problem with an association of epidermolysis bullosa; duodenal, jejunal, ileal or colonic (also rare) atresia;
3.   malrotation with volvulus;
4.   meconium ileus;
5.   milk plug obstruction;
6.   Hirschsprung's disease.

Two intestinal problems will be looked at in greater detail: meconium ileus and Hirschsprung's disease.

Meconium ileus

This intraluminal obstruction (incidence one in 600 live births) is due to thick inspissated meconium blocking the mid ileum. In most cases the distal ileum and colon is narrow and underdeveloped (microcolon). In some babies there is an intrauterine perforation of the bowel; the meconium calcifies in the peritoneum and can be diagnosed on antenatal scan. In other cases there is an associated volvulus and the necrotic intestine and meconium form a meconium cyst.

Almost all babies with meconium ileus have cystic fibrosis. This is carried by an autosomal recessive gene and mainly affects Caucasian races.

Cases present with:

1. calcification and obstructed bowel on antenatal scan;
2. failure to pass meconium
3. abdominal distension, fluid levels on radiography;
4. vomiting which becomes bile stained;
5. history of cystic fibrosis in the family.

Preoperative and medical care Blood should be sent for trypsin levels if possible. An immunoreactive trypsin (IRT) level of 80 ng/ml requires further investigation (Hodson *et al.*, 1983).

Unless bowel perforation has occurred, a Gastrografin enema is done to try to clear the sticky meconium. Gastrografin is a radio-opaque, hyperosmolar, hygroscopic fluid which helps to draw fluid into the sticky meconium, thereby making it more liquid so that it can be passed rectally. In view of the mode of action of the contrast material, the baby must be kept well hydrated. Volume expanders are given during this procedure.

If the enema is successful, feeds can be commenced when the baby's bowel is deflated and gastric aspirates are minimal.

Pancreative enzymes are required in most cases, but if the baby is breast fed they are not always necessary.

Surgery If the enema does not clear the meconium, a laparotomy is performed and in some cases the sticky meconium can be milked and washed out of the bowel. In others, a resection is needed at the site of the obstruction or perforation. Occasionally a stoma is fashioned, but this is now rare.

Postoperative care When the bowel starts to function and gastric aspirates decrease, the baby can be fed. Pancreatic enzymes help the milk to be absorbed and assist the baby to gain weight.

A sweat test is performed to confirm the diagnosis; a sweat sodium level of over 70 mmol/l is considered diagnostic. The test may need to be repeated if there is inadequate sweat with an ambiguous result.

Chest physiotherapy is commenced early. The parents must be given a full explanation of cystic fibrosis and offered as much help as possible. The diagnosis will bring much sadness to the family and they will need support from hospital staff, the primary health care team and the Cystic Fibrosis Trust.

Prognosis Once the diagnosis is confirmed, the baby should receive all supportive care. With regular pancreative enzymes, chest physiotherapy and the use of antimicrobials if there are signs of infection, the outlook is fairly good. Many children live into their late teens and some to adult life. Males are sterile but girls are not, so before they become pregnant (if possible) they should be counselled. The risk for the children of a mother with cystic fibrosis is one in 40–50 unless the partner also carries the gene, when the risk increases to one in four for every pregnancy. The cystic fibrosis gene has now been identified and research continues to determine whether this gene could be replaced or restored to normal by drug therapy.

Associated anomalies

1. Cystic fibrosis (approximately 10% of children with cystic fibrosis present with meconium ileus).
2. Small bowel atresia.

Hirschsprung's disease

In Hirschsprung's disease (incidence one in 5000 live births), an area of bowel is deficient in nerve ganglia and therefore lacks peristalsis. This agangliotic area usually affects the large bowel and the length affected can be short or long. Occasionally the small bowel is involved. Total agangliosis is rare, but carries a very poor outlook.

Cases present with:

1. delay or failure to pass meconium;
2. increasing abdominal distension;
3. vomiting, becoming bile stained;
4. in short-segment disease there may be intermittent distension relieved by the passage of explosive stools; if this condition continues for some time, the baby shows signs of failure to thrive;
5. passage of explosive stools after rectal examination;
6. if diagnosis is delayed necrotizing enterocolitis may occur;
7. history of Hirschsprung's disease in the family.

To diagnose the condition a careful history is taken. An abdominal radiograph shows distended bowel loops and a barium enema shows a dilated area of large bowel with a narrow agangliotic segment. A rectal suction biopsy confirms the diagnosis, showing the absence of bowel ganglia. Rectal manometry is useful if available; a balloon probe is placed in the rectum and expanded, and the pressure response to the expansion is measured. The area proximal to the atretic area will have a high pressure, as force is required to propel the stool through the atretic area.

Preoperative care Discontinue oral feeds, pass a nasogastric tube and aspirate regularly, and commence intravenous fluids. Instigate investigations but do not give rectal washouts before the contrast enema as this will confuse findings. After the enema, wash out the bowel to encourage deflation. No washouts must be given after rectal suction biopsies, as perforation of the bowel can occur.

Surgery Once the diagnosis is confirmed a colostomy is fashioned. Frozen section biopsies are done to ensure that the colostomy is in the gangliotic segment.

Postoperative care The stoma is observed for colour, bleeding and action. Gastric aspiration is continued with intravenous fluids until the bowel is functioning, then oral feeds can be commenced and increased.

A stoma bag is applied early as this will help to keep the surrounding skin in good condition. Distal loop washouts are needed to clear the distal loop of residual bowel content, which would become solid owing to water absorption.

The parents need assistance in caring for the stoma, with local support from the stomatherapist and primary care team.

Prognosis In most cases prognosis is good, although occasionally babies develop Hirschsprung's enterocolitis and become very unwell. Pull-through operation and closure of colostomy is done at 4–6 months and before toilet training takes place. In long-segment disease with a large resection of bowel, constipation, soiling and incontinence may cause problems.

Associated problems include necrotizing enterocolitis and Down syndrome.

Abdominal wall defects

The main defects seen are exomphalos and gastroschisis. The incidence for both is one in 6000–7000 live births.

Gastroschisis

The defect occurs in the 5th to 7th week of pregnancy when the gut is developing in the umbilical cord. The gut fails to return to the abdomen and continues to develop in the cord.

If the defect lies adjacent to the umbilical cord and there is no sac covering the abdominal contents, it is called a gastroschisis (Figure 3.5). In this condition, the stomach and the bowel are often dilated with thickened oedematous walls. There may be atretic areas in the bowel, which may be

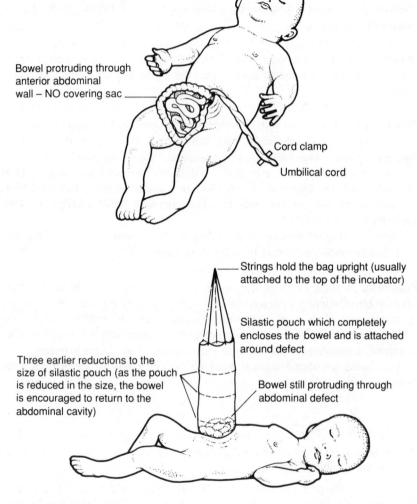

Figure 3.5 Gastroschisis.

gangrenous and, in some instances, short. The liver is usually involved and is also outside the abdomen.

Many babies with this condition are diagnosed antenatally, but if they are not the defect is very obvious at delivery.

Preoperative care The main problems involve maintenance of body temperature, deflation of the gastrointestinal tract and maintenance of fluid balance. The exposed bowel should be placed in clingfilm or in a clear plastic bag so that it can be observed and heat conserved.

A large nasogastric tube is passed, aspirated every 1–2 h and left open at all times. The volume aspirated is replaced ml for ml with normal saline plus potassium chloride 10 mmol/500 ml. The volumes aspirated may be large.

Serum losses from the exposed bowel are replaced with 4.5% human albumin solution ml for ml.

The baby is most easily nursed in an overhead heated cot to give easy access.

Surgery This is attempted as soon as possible. There are two procedures.

1. The bowel is returned into the abdomen as a primary procedure with muscle and skin closure. The abdomen will then be very tight and most babies need ventilatory support at this time.
2. The bowel is placed in a Prolene sac which acts as an artificial peritoneum. In most cases the baby can breathe spontaneously. Tucks are taken in the sac until closure can be done (7–10 days in most cases).

Postoperative care

1. Primary procedure Ventilatory support, careful fluid balance and temperature control is essential.

With increased abdominal pressure the kidneys may be constricted and their function diminished. Careful observation of urine output is required. The lower limbs may become oedematous.

2. Application of Prolene mesh sac Ventilation is rarely required, unless the baby is also preterm.

The main problems are:

1. Large losses of serous fluid around the base of the sac. Gauze swabs in place around the sac must be weighed 6-hourly to estimate losses, which need replacement with 4.5% human albumen solution ml for ml.
2. Gastric losses which need replacement with 0.9% saline + KCl 10 mmol/500 mls. Large volumes often occur.
3. Infection around the artificial sac. Topical and systematic antibiotics may be required.
4. Nutrition – TPN is required until the abdomen is closed. The advantage

of this method is that the baby can breathe spontaneously. However, disadvantages include electrolyte imbalance with hypovolaemia due to excessive serum losses and large gastric aspirates. Infection around the sac and longer hospitalization are other problems.

Babies with a very large defect may need more than one Prolene sac applied until muscle and skin closure can be completed.

In both cases enteral feeds are commenced when gastric aspirates decrease.

Prognosis In most cases this is good unless there has been a major resection of gangrenous bowel. Some babies have problems with gut motility and malabsorption. Adhesion obstruction occurs in some cases.

If hospitalization is extensive the family need much support and encouragement.

There are no associated anomalies with gastroschisis.

Necrotizing enterocolitis
Incidence – it affects 4–5% of all preterm infants. This condition, first accurately described in 1963, is one of the commonest causes for surgery in neonatal units.

The most widely held theory is that when perinatal stress casues hypoxia, blood is shunted to the vital centres of the heart and brain, so that mesenteric circulation is diminished and ischaemia occurs. It is thought that bacterial invasion of the bowel wall occurs. Gas forming organisms cause intramural gas, i.e. pneumatosis intestalis. Organisms grown on culture include: *E. Coli*, *Aerobactur*, streptococci, staphylococci, *Klebsiella*, *Pseudomonas* and *Clostridium*.

Predisposing factors

1. Maternal – diabetes
              – multiple pregnancy
              – intrauterine bleeding (in last 2 weeks)
              – intrauterine infection
2. Prematurity
3. Stress causing bowel ischaemia, e.g.
              – intrauterine or birth asphyxia
              – respiratory distress syndrome
              – sepsis
4. Hypothermia

5. Decreased blood flow to the bowel, e.g.
   - umbilical catheterization
   - patent ductus
   - polycythaemia
   - exchange transfusion
6. The early introduction of artificial milk feeds.

Presentation

A. Early signs

1. A generally unwell baby, lethargic, disinterested in feeds with unstable temperature and increasing apnoeas.
2. Vomiting and/or large bile stained gastric aspirates.
3. Increasing abdominal distension, sometimes with cellulitis.
4. Loose stools becoming blood stained.
5. Haematological changes, i.e. Hb ↓ decreasing;
   WBC ↑ increasing;
   Platelets ↓ decreasing.
6. X-ray changes – distended bowel loops
   – intramural gas.

B. Later signs

1. Pneumoperitoneum, sometimes with gas in portal vein
2. Increasing apnoeas and instability
3. Increasing blood in the stools
4. Increasing WBC count with platelets decreasing
5. Abdominal distension with increasing cellulitis and localized mass due to a walled off perforation.

Immediate care Stop feeds and pass a large nasogastric tube. Aspirate this 1–2 hourly and allow it to drain freely. Commence maintenance IV fluids and give volume expanders, especially if a temperature gap occurs. Take blood cultures and give broad spectrum antibiotics, e.g. penicillin, gentamycin and metronidazole. Vital signs are monitored and the general condition is assessed constantly, especially the respiratory pattern and urinary output. If abdominal distension is noted, 6–8 hourly radiographs may be taken to monitor the course of the disease and observe for increasing intramural gas and/or perforation. The baby may need an enriched oxygen environment or ventilatory support if further deterioration occurs.

Continuing care Maintain circulatory and respiratory support, observing the baby carefully and monitoring vital signs. Continue the antibiotics and commence total parenteral nutrition (TPN) when the electrolytes are stable. If the baby remains well, continue TPN for 10 days, then commence enteral feeds using expressed milk if possible. Increase these slowly and reduce the TPN accordingly. If the baby deteriorates, reassess, repeat radiography and blood cultures, and consider surgery.

The indications for surgery are a general deterioration, with increasing apnoeas or ventilatory requirements and an unstable temperature. The blood picture shows an increasing white blood cell count and reducing platelet count. There is increasing abdominal distension and, in some cases, cellulitis of the abdominal wall, with an abdominal mass. The radiograph shows increasing bowel distension, more intramural gas and/or a bowel perforation with free gas under the diaphragm.

Surgery A laparotomy is performed to show the extent of the disease. For a *localized* problem, a resection and end-to-end anastomosis is done. A *perforation* is closed with excision of the locally affected area. A stoma may be fashioned. In *extensive* disease, a large area of bowel may appear gangrenous. Initially, the black areas are excised and stomas fashioned which are carefully observed. At 12–24 h a 'second-look' operation is done in the hope that some bowel has recovered in the interim. During that time the baby is fully ventilated and kept well saturated with oxygen. In some cases, sufficient recovery occurs, enabling further surgery to be effective.

Unfortunately, in other cases, the bowel does not recover and no further operative treatment can be offered. Many parents wish to be present when treatment is withdrawn. They will need much support and care.

Longer term needs and problems When babies have a stoma fashioned, their parents will need support to assist them with the care. The stoma is usually closed after 1–2 months. If recurrent disease occurs, the feeds are stopped for 10 days to give further bowel rest. Feeds are then recommenced and introduced slowly.

Malabsorption owing to a short gut may occur. Breast milk is usually satisfactory, but in severe cases lactose-free feeds, e.g. Pregestimil, is needed. Immodium to slow gastrointestinal motility is helpful for some babies.

Unfortunately some babies develop colonic strictures; surgical resection is then required.

Prognosis This is very variable. Some babies respond well to conservative treatment and recover fully without surgery. Others undergo major surgery and recover very well. Sadly, some have overwhelming disease and die despite all treatment.

There are no associated anomalies.

REFERENCES AND FURTHER READING

Brimblecome, F.S.W., Richards, P.P.M. and Robertson, N. (1978) *Separation and Special Care Units*. Spastics International Publishers, London.

Department of Health (1988) *Feeding Today's Children*. HMSO, London.

Department of Health and Social Security (1988) Report on Health and Social Subjects 32. *Present Day Practice in Infant Feeding*. 3rd Report. HMSO, London.

Halliday, H., McClure, G. and Reid, M. (1989) *Handbook of Neonatal Intensive Care*, 3rd edn. Balliere Tindall, London.

Hatch, D.J. and Sumner, E. (1986) *Neonatal Anaesthesia and Peri-operative Care*, 2nd edn. Edward Arnold, London.

Hey, E.N. (1975) Thermal neutrality. *British Medical Journal*, **31**, 69–74.

Hodson, M.E., Norman, A.P. and Batten, J.C. (1983) *Cystic Fibrosis*. Ballière Tindall, London.

Jenner, C., Harjo, J. and Brueggemeyer, A. (1988) *Neonatal Surgery: A Nursing Perspective*. Grune and Stratton Harcourt, Brace Jovanovich, New York.

Kelnar, C.J.H. and Harvey, D. (1987) *The Sick Newborn Baby*, 2nd edn. Balliere Tindall, London.

Lister, J. and Irving, I.M. (1990) *Neonatal Surgery*, 3rd edn. Butterworths, London.

Rickham, P.P., Lister, J. and Irving, I. (1978) *Neonatal Surgery*, 2nd edn. Butterworths, London.

Robertson, N.R.C. (ed.) (1986) *Textbook of Neonatology*. Churchill Livingstone, Edinburgh.

Sauer P.J.I., Dane, J.H. and Visser, H.K.A. (1984) New standards for neutral thermal environment of healthy very low birth weight infants in one week of life. *Archives of Disease in Childhood*, **59**, 18.

Spitz, L., Steiner, G.M. and Zachary, R.B. (1981) *A Colour Atlas of Paediatric Surgical Diagnosis*. Woolf Medical, London.

Vulliamy, D.G. and Johnston, P.G.B. (1987) *The Newborn Child*, 6th edn. Churchill Livingstone, Edinburgh.

Waldhausen, J.A., Herenderen, J. and King, H. (1963) Necrotising colitis of the newborn. *Surgery*, **54**, 365–72.

Waterson, D.J., Bonham-Carter, R.E. and Aberdeen, E. (1962) Oesophageal atresia and trachea-oesophageal fistula. *Lancet*, 819–22.

Wheldon, A.E. and Hull, D. (1983) Incubation of very immature infants. *Archives of Disease in Childhood*, **58**, 504.

4

Care of the child with respiratory problems

Margaret Clancy and Eiri Jones

Disturbances in respiratory function are common causes of ill health in infancy and childhood, and as a result children with respiratory problems are seen relatively frequently on intensive care units. Respiratory disease can be either a primary cause of admission or a secondary problem. The child with a respiratory problem provides the nurse with a unique range of challenges.

The nurse as a member of the multidisciplinary team must support the child and the family through the psychological, emotional and spiritual trauma that such an admission creates. Additionally, and more obviously in some respects, the nurse must use considerable skill and knowledge to deliver effective holistic respiratory management. The nurse requires knowledge of the underlying pathophysiology, of the technologies associated with the intensive care of the child with respiratory problems, of the most appropriate research-based nursing practice, and of the child's own needs based on an understanding of development. The nurse also requires good communication skills to involve the family and the child and to coordinate the care delivered by other member of the multidisciplinary team.

ANATOMY AND PHYSIOLOGY

There are some major differences in the structure of the respiratory tract among the infant, the child and the adult. The nurse must be aware of these differences if effective care is to be delivered.

1. Infants up to about 4 weeks of age are obligatory nose breathers; therefore, they are particularly at risk if their nose becomes blocked for any reason.
2. The infant and young child have a relatively narrow upper airway and this can increase airflow resistance. They are therefore at increased risk from anything that may decrease the size of the airway, such as oedema and accumulation of secretions.
3. In the newborn, the diaphragm is not able to contract as much as or effectively as in the older infant and child because it is attached higher at the front and is therefore longer.
4. The infant's glottis is more cephalad than in the older child and the laryngeal reflexes are more active.
5. The infant's epiglottis is longer and extends further posteriorly.
6. The infant and the young child are at increased risk of oedema due to the presence of areolar tissue just below the vocal cords and therefore at increased risk of respiratory problems.
7. The child's C-shaped tracheal cartilages are very elastic and thus the trachea is very flexible.
8. The child's respiratory tract is relatively short, which increases the risk of infection.
9. The infant and young child do not have a full complement of alveoli. This means that they have a relatively small alveolar surface area for gaseous exchange.
10. The infant and child have a relatively round thoracic cavity due to the horizontal position of the ribs. This places increased dependence on the diaphragm and abdomen as the primary means of ventilation.
11. The infant has a relatively high tracheal bifurcation at the level of the third thoracic vertebra, compared with the fourth thoracic vertebra in the adult.

Gas transport and gaseous exchange

The alveolus is the functional unit for gaseous exchange. Diffusion via pressure gradients causes oxygen to diffuse from the alveolar air to the blood and carbon dioxide to diffuse from the blood into the alveolus.

Oxygen is carried in simple solution in the plasma (2.5%) and combined with haemoglobin (97.5%). The combination of the oxygen carried in the plasma and by the haemoglobin is the arterial oxygen content. Heamoglobin is capable of carrying four oxygen molecules and when it does so it is considered to be fully (95–100%) saturated. The haemoglobin accepts the first oxygen molecule with moderate difficulty, the second and third molecule more easily and the fourth molecule only with difficulty. When the oxygen tension is above 13 kPa, the haemoglobin is said to be fully saturated. When the blood is fully saturated and the child has a haemoglobin level of 14.5 g/dl (Table 4.1) each 100 ml of blood carries about 20 ml of oxygen. At the lungs, the PaO_2 is 13.3 kPa; therefore, the haemoglobin in arterial blood is about 95% saturated. At the tissues, the PaO_2 is 5 kPa and therefore the haemoglobin in venous blood is 70% saturated (a 25% loss of saturation). That 25% loss represents 5 ml of oxygen.

Table 4.1 Normal haemoglobin values

Age	Values (g/dl)
1–3 days	14.5–22.5
2 months	9.0–14.0
6–12 years	11.5–15.5
12–18 years	
Male	13.0–16.0
Female	12.0–16.0

Oxyhaemoglobin dissociation curve

Understanding the oxyhaemoglobin dissociation curve (Figure 4.1) is important because it is invaluable in helping the nurse to understand the reasons for changes in therapy and it makes the readout of the pulse oximeter more meaningful. The top part of the curve is flat and runs from about 8 to 13 kPa. It has this flat shape because even relatively large increases in pressure bring about only very small increases in oxygen saturation (SaO_2). It can therefore be seen that normally there is no point trying to achieve very high arterial oxygen tension because it makes very little difference to the amount of oxygen available to the tissues.

The middle steep section of the curve runs from 5.3 to 8 kPa so that greater amounts of oxygen react for smaller changes in pressure. On this section of the curve, increasing a child's inspired oxygen brings about a relatively large increase in oxygen saturation.

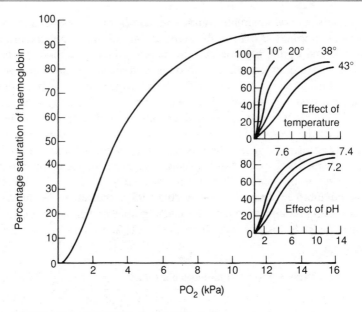

Figure 4.1 The oxyhaemoglobin dissociation curve.

Many factors can alter the shape of the curve. These include the level of metabolic activity, the amount of fetal haemoglobin, the level of carbon dioxide and the temperature.

If the level of metabolic activity increases, the curve is shifted to the right. This means that the 5 kPa constant bisects the curve lower down and cuts across the SaO_2 lower down. This means that increased amounts of oxygen are given up or offloaded to the tissues.

If there is an increase in $PaCO_2$ (from 5.0 kPa), the curve is shifted to the right and less oxygen is carried at a given PaO_2; therefore, more is given up to the tissues.

A right shift means that the haemoglobin has less affinity for oxygen. A shift to the left means that the haemoglobin has a greater affinity for oxygen and therefore holds on to it harder.

Carbon dioxide

Carbon dioxide is carried in three ways: as a simple solution, combined with protein, and combined with bicarbonate. The amount in simple solution increases if the $PaCO_2$ is increased. Carbon dioxide combines with either haemoglobin or plasma proteins and forms a carbamino compound. The amount combined depends on the PaO_2 of the blood. Fully saturated haemoglobin carries 3 ml carbon dioxide as carbamino compound per 100 ml of blood.

Fully desaturated haemoglobin carries 8 ml carbon dioxide as carbamino compound per 100 ml of blood. Most of the carbon dioxide is carried combined with bicarbonate (HCO_3) at 42 ml per 100 ml of blood. It is transported as sodium bicarbonate in the plasma and potassium bicarbonate in the red blood cells.

$$CO_2 + H_2O \rightleftharpoons H_2CO_3 \rightleftharpoons H^+ + HCO_3^-$$

This reaction is towards the H^- and HCO_3^- side of the equation at the tissues but it is reversed at the lungs, where carbon dioxide is liberated and diffuses out into the alveoli. Not all the original carbon dioxide that is converted into H^+ and HCO_3^- is breathed out at the lungs. Much stays within the bloodstream as HCO_3^- and acts as an anion reserve.

pH of the blood

pH measurements of the blood measure the concentration of hydrogen ions. Normally, the pH of the blood is maintained by a variety of homeostatic mechanisms, which include the lungs, the blood buffers and the kidneys. These prevent the blood from becoming too acid from both carbon dioxide and by-products of food digestion. Blood buffers are a short-term defence to prevent radical alterations in the blood pH. There are three main blood buffers: the bicarbonate system, the phosphate system and the protein system.

Acid can be excreted via the lungs and the kidneys. If the respiratory centre detects a decrease in the pH of the blood, the child's respiratory rate is stimulated and increased. This allows more carbon dioxide to be washed out of the lungs. This is a rapid and immediate response to an altered pH. The kidneys play a role in regulating pH but it is a slower process, which may take up to 36 h. The kidneys regulate blood pH by the tubular secretion of H^+. This leads to the renal secretion of H^+ and the regeneration of HCO_3^-, which replenish the buffer system of the blood.

Acid–base balance

There are four states of acid–base balance: respiratory acidosis, respiratory alkalosis, metabolic acidosis and metabolic alkalosis (Table 4.2). There are several causative factors for these imbalances, which include varying concentrations of body fluids. Alteration in renal function causes variation in elimination of certain elements. In the infant or neonate this can be compounded by the low renal threshold for bicarbonate excretion. Functional influences can be immaturity of the lung tissue (as seen in the preterm baby) or small pulmonary alveolar surface area. In the preterm baby the respiratory centre in the cerebral medulla can also be immature. Where there are also other congenital defects, such as cardiac lesion, there may be high pulmonary vascular resistance or restricted pulmonary blood flow.

Table 4.2 Changes in arterial blood gases with acid–base imbalances

	pH	pCO_2	HCO_3
Respiratory acidosis	↓	↑	N
Compensated respiratory acidosis	*N	↑	*↑
Respiratory alkalosis	↑	↓	N
Compensated respiratory alkalosis	*N	↓	*↓
Metabolic acidosis	↓	N	↓
Compensated metabolic acidosis	*N	*↓	↓
Metabolic alkalosis	↑	N	↑
Compensated metabolic alkalosis	*N	↑	↑

↓, decreased; ↑, increased; N, normal; *, compensation complete.

Respiratory acidosis

Respiratory acidosis can be defined as an excess of carbonic acid in the extracellular fluid. This is primarily due to decreased carbon dioxide excretion. Causative factors include hypoventilation, obstructive lung disease, respiratory centre depression, muscular or nerve dysfunction, and thoracic cage abnormalities. In the ventilated child, respiratory acidosis can be seen where there is either inadequate mechanical ventilation or, despite adequate ventilation, poor tissue perfusion due to poor cardiac output.

Metabolic acidosis

Metabolic acidosis can be defined as a loss of bicarbonate with a gain of acid. Poor tissue perfusion, hypoxaemia and infection will all lead to lactic acidosis. Peripheral chemoreceptors sense alterations in tissue pH when there is lactic acid production and increase respiratory rate to increase carbon dioxide excretion. Where there is renal dysfunction, this may contribute to metabolic acidosis by insufficient excretion of acids (Behrman and Vaughan, 1987). Excess excretion of bicarbonate (as seen in the child with diarrhoea) is also a causative factor. This should be borne in mind in the care of children on high-dose antibiotic therapy or continuous nasogastric feeds who sometimes develop diarrhoea.

Respiratory alkalosis

Respiratory alkalosis can be defined as loss of carbon dioxide in the presence of normal lung function at alveolar level. Hyperventilation can cause this state.

It is also seen when there is anxiety and hysteria and in the early stages of salicylate overdose.

Metabolic alkalosis

Metabolic alkalosis can be defined as an excess of HCO_3^- in the extracellular fluid with a loss of acid. This can be seen in the child who has been vomiting excessively, classically pyloric stenosis, and also where there has been prolonged diuretic therapy.

Where the primary disorder is of respiratory origin, the compensatory mechanisms will be renal; and conversely, where the primary disorder is renal, there will eventually be respiratory compensation.

RESPIRATORY ASSESSMENT

Accurate and ongoing respiratory assessment is a critical part of the nurse's role. It is often a vital clue as to the child's condition and can indicate the need for more substantive assessment. The signs observed will to a degree depend on the age of the child and on underlying condition. The nurse assessing the infant or child should possess a knowledge of the expected breathing rate (Table 4.3) and pattern and the stage of maturity and development of the respiratory tract and its associated structures. Assessment can be made in two major ways; observation and physical examination.

Table 4.3 Normal respiratory rates in infants and children

Age	Rate/min
Newborn	30–50
11 months	26–40
2 years	20–30
4 years	20–30
6 years	20–26
8 years	18–24
10 years	18–24
Adolescent	12–20

Source: Weller 1991

Alterations in the child's respiration can indicate underlying changes in the child's blood gases and acid–base balance, and as such require immediate attention.

The preterm infant can be objectively assessed for the level of respiratory distress using a pictorial chart that gives a structured framework (Figure 4.2).

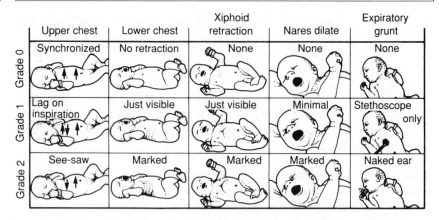

	Upper chest	Lower chest	Xiphoid retraction	Nares dilate	Expiratory grunt
Grade 0	Synchronized	No retraction	None	None	None
Grade 1	Lag on inspiration	Just visible	Just visible	Minimal	Stethoscope only
Grade 2	See-saw	Marked	Marked	Marked	Naked ear

Figure 4.2 Observation of retractions. An index of respiratory distress is determined by grading each of five arbitrary criteria. Grade 0 indicates no difficulty, grade 1 moderate difficulty and grade 2 maximum respiratory difficulty. The retraction score is the sum of these values; a total of 0 indicates no dyspnoea, whereas a total of 10 indicates maximum respiratory distress.

Additionally, observation will involve consideration of the respiratory rate, rhythm, depth, retractions and effort. The nurse should assess whether the respirations are noisy (wheezy, stridor, hoarse, grunting) or quiet, and whether accompanied by a cough, sputum, and other signs of dyspnoea and extra workload. The following terms are used.

1. *Cyanosis* is the blue colour of the mucous membranes, skin, nail beds and/or schlera of the child with arterial oxygen desaturation. The degree of cyanosis depends on a variety of factors including the haemoglobin level and the saturation of the haemoglobin. On its own, cyanosis is not a reliable indicator of the degree of hypoxeamia that a child is experiencing. The degree, site, duration and associated factors should be noted.
2. *Nasal flaring* indicates an increase in respiratory effort. It is a means of enlarging the nostrils and thus decreasing nasal resistance and improving the patency of the nasal airway.
3. *Grunting* is characteristic of respiratory distress syndrome and indicates that the infant is attempting to increase end expiratory pressure and enhance gaseous exchange.
4. *Retractions* refer to the 'sinking in of soft tissue relative to the cartilaginous or bony thorax' (Whaley and Wong, 1991). Retraction can be seen as the intercostal, subcostal, suprasternal, substernal and clavicular sites.

Respiratory assessment can also involve diagnostic procedures such as chest radiography and blood gas assessment via pulse oximetry and capillary and arterial blood gas sampling. Transcutaneous estimates of PO_2 and PCO_2 can also be made, although they have lost favour in recent years because they can cause trauma to the skin; the non-invasive and less traumatic pulse oximeter is now more readily available.

The most useful reliable system of measuring the effectiveness of gaseous exchange is via arterial blood sampling, which allows pH, PO_2 and PCO_2 to be measured. However, this is often technically more difficult to achieve and there are problems associated with indwelling arterial catheters. As a result, other methods may be used routinely with arterial sampling being an option.

Arterial blood gas sampling

This can be achieved by performing intermittent arterial stabs or by siting an indwelling arterial cannula if it is expected that frequent samples will be required for analysis. The most usual sites for arterial sampling are the umbilical artery in the newborn and the radial, brachial and femoral arteries in the infant and child. The radial and brachial arteries are the preferred sites because they are associated with fewer problems. Once the sample has been taken, the nurse must ensure that pressure is applied to the site for at least 5 min for radial and brachial sites or 5–15 min for the femoral site. The nurse should be aware of normal arterial blood gas values so that an accurate interpretation of the results is possible (Table 4.4).

Table 4.4 Normal arterial blood gas values

	Neonate	Child
pH	7.32–7.42	7.35–7.45
PCO_2 (kPa)	4–5.3	4.7–6.0
HCO_3^- mEq/l	20–26	22–28
PO_2 (kPa)	8.0–10.6	10.6–13.3

Extreme care should be taken with arterial sampling because there is the possibility of haemorrhage, haematoma formation, arterial spasm and occlusion of the artery, resulting in compromised perfusion distal to the site.

For the child requiring sequential blood gas sampling, an indwelling arterial cannula attached to a flushing device is needed. The arterial cannula can be used for both frequent sampling and monitoring arterial blood pressure. Several principles apply to the care of arterial lines, regardless of the site. Firstly, nothing should be infused through the line apart from isotonic saline, which is usually heparinized. The distal limb should be checked frequently for colour, perfusion and movement. The arterial cannula requires a continuous infusion (one-way) valve, which is normally a required part of the system.

Additionally, the number of connections and connectors should be kept to a minimum and they should be of the lockable variety to reduce the risk of accidental disconnection.

Capillary blood gas sampling

This can be used to assess pH and P_{CO_2} and to some extent P_{O_2} when it is not appropriate or possible to take an arterial blood sample. The P_{O_2} readings are generally lower than would be recorded if an arterial sample was taken.

Very often nurses are involved in taking capillary gas samples, especially in infants where the preferred site is the heel. Other sites which can be used are the earlobe, finger and toes. Careful preparation for the procedure can enhance the ease with which the sample is taken and reduces the trauma to the baby. The site should be prewarmed to encourage easy blood flow and the puncture should be made with an autolet. The autolet controls the depth of the puncture and is reported to reduce pain experienced by the infant. Alternatively a lancet can be used, but care should be taken

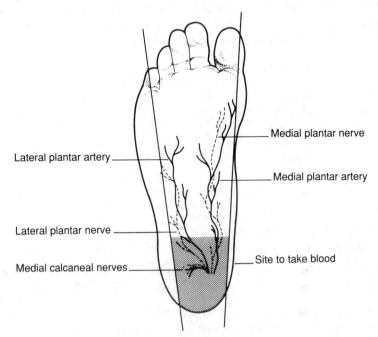

Figure 4.3 Major blood vessels and nerves of the foot and appropriate site for heel stab blood sampling. The shaded area should not be used as a sampling site.

to avoid puncturing the skin too deeply. The heel should not be squeezed in an attempt to stimulate blood flow because this increases the possibility of venous blood mixing with the capillary sample. If using the infant's heel, the safest and most effective site is the highly vascular medial portion of the heel (Figure 4.3).

Pulse oximetry

This is a non-invasive, extremely useful means of continually monitoring the oxygen saturation of arterial blood (SaO_2). The oximeter measures the amount of light absorbed by oxyhaemoglobin and from this it calculates the SaO_2. A range of probes is available which can be used for the infant, child or adolescent. The probe contains a light-emitting and a light-receiving sensor, which, when correctly aligned and gently positioned, effectively measure SaO_2. The nurse can relate the SaO_2 recording to the patient's PaO_2 by using the oxyhaemoglobin dissociation curve. It should be noted that the oximeter is not a reliable tool for detecting hyperoxia and it is not reliable if the child is moving too much.

SUCTIONING

Sputum is produced by the mucosal and submucosal glands in the lungs and it is moved upwards towards the epiglottis by ciliary movements. It is usually expelled by coughing and can consist of cellular debris, inflammatory cells, blood, water, immunoglobulins and glycoproteins.

The aim of suctioning the child is to remove potentially dangerous secretions from the oropharynx, trachea and bronchi to maintain adequate ventilation. As the suctioning procedure is not without adverse effects and complications, techniques must be used to minimize such problems and only used when necessary. A good suction technique aims to be as atraumatic as possible. Coughing can be encouraged to facilitate removal of secretions. Suction can be applied regardless of whether the child is intubated or not.

Adverse effects

The adverse effects of suction must be at the forefront of the nurse's mind so that the procedure is not undertaken unnecessarily. They are:

1. tracheobronchial trauma, including perforation;
2. atelectasis;
3. hypoxia;
4. raised intracranial pressure;

5. cardiac arrhythmias;
6. infection;
7. pneumothorax.

The frequency of suctioning must be determined by the amount of secretions produced and their nature (viscosity and colour). A child producing copious or viscous secretions will require more frequent suctioning. The child's general condition and disease process must also be assessed when determining the amount of suction required. For example, a child with raised intracranial pressure, an unstable condition, or a neonate, may not tolerate frequent suctioning.

Suction catheters

The type of suction catheters used should be pliable enough to minimize trauma and atelectasis, but resilient enough not to collapse when negative pressure is exerted. The catheter should be smooth and open-ended, preferably with two or more side holes. Many small catheters also have fingertip-controlled adaptations which facilitate better control when applying suction; this is preferable to bending the catheter.

The suction catheter size should not be more than half the size of the internal diameter of the endotracheal tube. A rough guide is to double the size of the endotracheal tube to find the size of suction catheter (e.g. a 6 FG suction catheter fits a 3mm ET tube). If too large a suction catheter, relative to the endotracheal tube, is used room air cannot pass around the sides of the endotracheal tube to compensate for gas removed by suction. Increased amounts of tracheal gases are removed and hypoxia and alveolar collapse are more likely to occur. Tidal volumes may fall to 25–75% of presuction tidal volumes (Brandstater and Muallem, 1969).

It has been identified that severe mucosal damage can occur as a result of suctioning. It is thought that the greater the amount of negative pressure applied, the larger the risk of ulceration. Therefore the suction unit must have a manometer attached to measure the pressure exerted. The amount of negative suction pressure used should not exceed 60–90 cm H_2O in the infant, 90–110 cm H_2O in the child or 110–150 cm H_2O in the older child (Hazinski, 1984).

It is thought that mucosal haemorrhage and erosion are caused by insertion of the suction catheter. Good suction technique is vital to minimize the potential for adverse effects. Traditionally the suction catheter was introduced until resistance was met, at the carina. However, histological changes of perforation of the bronchi can occur in the mucosal tissue when this technique is applied. To avoid adverse effects, suction catheters should either be measured or inserted to specific point in the trachea either 1 cm below the end of the endotracheal tube or to the carina (the point where resistance is met) and then withdrawn 0.5 cm before applying suction. When applying suction to a tracheostomy tube, the easiest method of ensuring safe, efficient suctioning is to use the spare tracheostomy tube as a guide to the length of the suction catheter that needs to be inserted.

If damage occurs to the ciliated mucosal tissue, repair results in the formation of granulation and fibrous tissue. In a study by Nagaraj *et al.* (1980) on infants requiring mechanical ventilation and frequent suction over a period in excess of 20 days, obstructive crusting occurred.

Studies have documented that hypoxia is a complication of suction. It is possible that insertion of the catheter and application of negative pressure in the airways results in decreased lung volume and atelectasis. Another study showed that suctioning leads to a fall in the heart rate and an increase in blood pressure. It is also suggested that this may cause intrapulmonary hypoperfusion, leading to physiological shunting and desaturation (Simbruner *et al.*, 1981).

Studies cited by Young (1984) agree that some hyperinflation and hyperoxygenation before and after suctioning minimize the likelihood of hypoxia (Boutros, 1970; Naigow and Powaser, 1977). Hyperinflation means increasing the child's tidal volume, and hyperoxygenation means increasing the fraction of inspired oxygen (FiO_2), usually to 100%. However, some patients have also displayed adverse effects resulting from this procedure; hypotension and bradycardia from increased compression of the great veins due to increased thoracic pressure. It seems, therefore, that hyperinflation and hyperoxygenation is a useful process to avoid hypoxia but must be used with reference to the child's condition and careful observation for any signs of deterioration during the procedure.

Endotracheal suction is known to cause an increase in intracranial pressure in susceptible patients (Tyler, 1982; Fanconi and Duc, 1987; Perlman and Volpe, 1983). Cerebral oedema is increased by hypoxia and cerebral blood volume is increased by cerebral vasodilation. This is caused by an increase in arterial carbon dioxide tension, a decrease in intracranial pressure and a decrease in cerebral perfusion. It would seem sensible to monitor susceptible patients carefully whenever possible and to preoxygenate to try to prevent the rise in carbon dioxide and fall of oxygen levels.

Bradycardias may result during suction because of vagal stimulation. If bradycardia occurs, stop suctioning, hyperoxygenate if necessary or call for medical assistance to administer atropine. This emphasizes the need for close observation during the suctioning procedure and for recordings of the heart rate and oxygen saturation.

As the body's own defence mechanisms – to prevent foreign matter entering the airways – are being overridden, the intubated patient is susceptible to infection from both poor suction technique and poor hand hygiene. It has also been noted that the risk of infection is increased with mucosal damage and destruction of ciliated epithelium as previously discussed. It is therefore important that as sterile a technique as possible is employed, using a sterile glove, catheter and isotonic (0.9%) saline. Any change in the colour or nature of the secretions obtained should be reported and a specimen obtained for culture and sensitivity tests. Sterile saline may need to be introduced into the endotracheal tube before suctioning. This depends on the type of secretions being obtained. Most patients receiving adequate humidity may not require the instillation of saline. However, if the secretions obtained are tenacious or difficult to extract, sterile isotonic saline (0.2–2 ml depending on the child's size) is required.

Principles of good suction technique

The following principles should ensure that the procedure is safe and effective and creates the least amount of trauma possible.

1. Assess the patient's condition, taking note of the observations. Also ascertain whether preoxygenation, postoxygenation and hyperinflation are permissible.
2. Explain to the child and relatives what you are going to do and why it is necessary. Comfort and reassure the child. The nurse should remember that children may become very distressed at the thought of being 'sucked out'. It is a routine procedure for the nurse but often constitutes a real psychological and physical threat to the child.
3. Prepare the equipment required: sterile glove, sterile isotonic saline (if required), sterile suction catheters of appropriate size, water for flushing through the suction tubing.
4. Ensure that all rebreathing equipment is available and working before the commencement of the procedure.
5. Wash hands.
6. Instill sterile isotonic saline if required.
7. Hyperinflate and hyperoxygenate as the child's condition and unit policy dictates.
8. Put on a sterile glove, disconnect the ventilator tubing with a clean hand. Insert the catheter with the gloved hand until resistance is felt (withdraw 0.5 cm) or place the catheter 1 cm below the end of the endotracheal tube or just below the end of the tracheostomy tube.
9. Gently apply intermittent suction as the catheter is withdrawn, rotating the catheter between the fingers. Never apply suction when introducing the catheter. Suction should not be applied for more than 3–5 s (American Heart Association, 1988).
10. If the procedure needs to be repeated, the child should be allowed to

recover by being allowed about five breaths before applying suction again. This can be given by manual ventilation or by reconnecting the child to the ventilator.

11. Once the suctioning is completed, reconnect the child to the ventilator with a clean hand.
12. Discard the catheter and glove into the bag for incineration. Catheters and gloves should never be used again; fresh ones should be used for each suctioning of the child.
13. Flush through the suction tubing with water.
14. Wash hands.

INTUBATION

Endotracheal intubation can be performed through three routes; nasal (nasotracheal), oral (orotracheal) and tracheal (tracheostomy). The easiest route is the oral route, which is generally used in the child in emergency situations, for short-term support or as the route of choice for preterm babies. The nasal route is technically more difficult to achieve and is often performed once an oral tube has been successfully passed and the child is stable. Nasotracheal tubes have the overriding advantage of increased stability over orotracheal tubes.

Indications

Intubation may be indicated for:

1. respiratory insufficiency or arrest;
2. general anaesthetic;
3. upper airway obstruction (usually a paediatric emergency);
4. control of ventilation, for example in status epilepticus;
5. inability to protect the airway due to absent reflexes; for example, neurological impairment or drug overdose;
6. aspiration.

Although intubation of a child is frequently an emergency, it remains imperative that the whole procedure is calmly executed.

It should be remembered that the child's respiratory tract is different from that of the adult, and special consideration of these differences must be made. The child has a highly vascular nose, which means that bleeding may occur very readily during nasal intubation. Additionally the C-shaped cartilages that support the trachea are particularly elastic in the child and thus the trachea is very flexible. Introducers may be required during intubation to overcome this.

Equipment

Appropriate equipment for the child's size and weight should be assembled:

1. oral airway;
2. endotracheal tube (polyvinyl tubes which mould to the airway at room temperature are preferred; cuffed tubes are generally not used in paediatrics as local trauma may occur in the region of the narrowest point – the cricoid cartilage);
3. functional laryngoscopes (check daily that batteries and bulb are functioning and screwed in properly); straight blades are preferred for neonates and infants, as the epiglottis is rigid, and in older children curved blades can be used;
4. connectors for the endotracheal tubes to enable attachment to both the rebreathing bag and ventilator;
5. suction: Yankauer suckers and suction catheters for use via the nasopharynx and endotracheal tube;
6. cardiac monitor, oxygen saturation monitor;
7. Magill forceps;
8. tape and any other materials required to stabilize the endotracheal tube;
9. atropine (intubation occasionally causes stimulation of the vagal receptors situated in close proximity to the larynx, resulting in bradycardia; atropine blocks vagal activity);
10. sedation;
11. muscle relaxant.

Table 4.5 Guide for nasotracheal tube lengths

Age	Length (cm)
0–3 months	11.8
4–7 months	12.6
8–11 months	13.6
1 year	14.5
2 years	15.2
3 years	15.6
4 years	16.5
5 years	16.8
6 years	17.1
7 years	17.8
8 years	18.3
9 years	18.8
10 years	19.1
11 years	19.1

Table 4.6 Guide for oral Magill tube size and length

Age	size (mm)	Length (cm)
Preterm	2.5	8.5
Full term	3.0	9.5
3 months	3.5	10.5
6–12 months	4.0	11.5
1–3 years	4.5	13.0
4–5 years	5.0	14.0
5–6 years	5.5	15.0
6 years	6.0	16.5
7 years	6.5	17.0
8 years	7.0	18.0
9 years	7.5*	18.5
10–14 years	7–8*	18.5
14+ years		
Female	8.5*	18.5
Male	9.0–9.5*	18.5

*Cuffed tubes may be used.

This equipment should always be immediately available in high-risk areas such as intensive care. Tables exist to guide the choice of the right size of tube (Table 4.5 and 4.6).

Intubation procedure

The nurse should explain what is going to happen to the child, considering the child's age, development status and individual needs and understanding. Parents are often asked to wait outside the unit during the intubation procedure, and this can in itself increase the trauma for both the parents and the child. Parents require careful preparation to give them a realistic idea of what to expect when they return. Good communication with the parents and regular updating is helpful. Often photographs of other intubated children can help to reduce their anxiety.

The nurse should ensure that the child is comfortable and, if necessary, has had adequate sedation. The child's stomach should be emptied of gastric contents or air via the nasogastric tube. The child's head should be positioned with the jaw thrust forward using a neck roll if necessary. Take care not to over-extend the neck, as this may obstruct the airway and interfere with visualization of the larynx. Observe the child's baseline signs before commencement of the intubation procedure. At this point, the relaxant or neuromuscular blocking agent may be administered. This is administered to relax the abdominal and diaphragmatic muscles and also the vocal cords, allowing the passage of the endotracheal tube. In light of the effects of muscle relaxants, efficient manual ventilation must be performed and the child's vital signs carefully observed.

In most cases, oral intubation is intitiated first; this allows for accurate measurement of the endotracheal tube before nasal intubation. During this time the nurse should observe for signs of deterioration in the child's condition or reversal of the anaesthetic agent, reporting any changes to the person who is intubating the child.

Once oral intubation has been achieved and the child's condition is stable, nasal intubation may follow, depending on the unit's policy. The intubation procedure may prove to be difficult for a number of reasons:

1. inability to extend the neck adequately because of cervical spine injury or surgery;
2. inability to open the mouth fully, for example, because of a broken jaw;
3. broken or loose teeth;
4. short neck;
5. small jaw;
6. cleft palate;
7. large tongue;
8. croup or a mass in the airway;
9. epiglottis (intubation is usually performed in theatre, with an ENT surgeon standing by in case a tracheostomy is required);
10. bleeding into the mouth or nose;
11. child not fully sedated.

It is therefore important that a detailed nursing assessment is taken to pre-empt many of these problems. In cases of difficult intubation, pressure may be applied over the area of the cricoid cartilage to assist with visualization of the larynx. An intubating fibreoptic laryngoscope may be required for difficult cases.

Securing the tube

Accidental movement of the tube or extubation may cause damage such as epistaxis, tracheal granulation or stenosis. Therefore, the nurse must ensure that the endotracheal tube remains adequately secured. There are many methods of securing endotracheal tubes and each hospital develops the most suitable method for its patients. However, some general principles apply;

1. minimal movement of the endotracheal tube;
2. minimal trauma to the nose and mouth;
3. use of a tape that does not cause damage to the skin or hair;
4. ensuring that the child's vision and hearing are not impeded.

Many children with an artificial airway *in situ* will also need artificial ventilation, and in these cases a secure means of connecting the tube to the ventilator tubing must be considered. A variety of methods of connecting the endotracheal tube to the ventilator tubing are available, and choice often reflects unit preference. Metal Tunstall connectors or disposable, straight, right-angled or swivel plastic connectors can be used. Increasingly, disposable ventilator tubing is being introduced and used, and this reduces the problems associated with sterilization of reusable circuits. A variety of methods are available for securing either nasal or oral endotracheal tubes; again, very often each unit has its own policy reflecting preferences of the nursing and medical staff. The systems usually incorporate a headband and tape to the cheeks to minimize sideways movements of the tube and to prevent it from being displaced. Regardless of the system used to secure the tube, the nurse should take care to ensure that the tape is renewed as required, and that skin integrity is maintained, especially in the region of the nares (in the case of nasal tubes) and the side of the mouth (in the case of oral tubes).

After intubation

Once the child has been intubated, manual ventilation, if required, is commenced via the rebreathing circuit. Ensure that the child's observations remain stable, and observe that chest movements are bilateral and equal breath sounds can be heard. Uneven chest movements may indicate intubation of the main stem bronchus, usually the right. In this case, the tube must be withdrawn slightly. A lack of breathing sounds accompanied by excess air in the stomach indicates intubation of the oesophagus.

The endotracheal tube must be removed immediately if there is any sign that the tube is in an incorrect position. Manual bag and mask ventilation must then be commenced until the child's condition is stabilized and intubation may be recommenced. Care should be taken when repositioning the child not to cause accidential extubation, and also to try whenever possible to move the head, neck and shoulders simultaneously to prevent trauma caused by movement of the endotracheal tube. In some cases, if the child's condition allows, this could involve disconnecting the child from the ventilator, repositioning and then reconnecting. During this procedure the child's vital signs must be observed and the child reconnected to the ventilator or hand ventilation if problems arise. After every disconnection from the ventilator, the child and the ventilator must be checked.

When the endotracheal tube is correctly positioned, this must be confirmed by chest radiography. An air leak, if present, may be heard around the tube. If the endotracheal tube is too large, there is a risk of postextubation oedema and subglottic stenosis; if it is too small, any spontaneous breathing is hampered by increased resistance due to the small lumen of the tube. It may also be difficult to obtain sufficient peak airway pressure via the ventilator or to suction the child.

Care of the child with an artifical airway

The endotracheal tube bypasses the normal mechanical mechanisms of filtration, protection and humidification, and therefore nursing care must compensate for this, to reduce the risks of complications. Gas delivered via the endotracheal tube must be humidified and warmed to a temperature of 35–36°C. This can be facilitated via a heated water bath such as Fischer, Pakell or Bennet Cascade attached to the ventilator unit. Older children weighing above 12 kg can usually be adequately humidified using a humidifier placed within the ventilator tubing. Humidity combined with adequate suctioning will help to prevent blockage of the endotracheal tube. However, careful observation is required in case the tube becomes obstructed.

Accidental extubation and blocked tube

Although accidental extubation can never be completely eliminated, the nurse should endeavour to minimize the chance of this occurring. Witham-Wilson (1991) proposes areas that nurses should consider to reduce the risk of accidental extubation: 'exercising caution during intentional disconnections, requesting appropriate equipment, using connections with a push twist action, using anti disconnect devices, being knowledgeable and competent in the use of monitoring equipment and avoiding complacency'.

In case of accidental extubation, the size and length of the endotracheal tube should be recorded in the care plan and a replacement tube kept in an easily accessible place, with an appropriate-sized mask and rebreathing circuit with an oral airway for use until reintubation can be facilitated.

If oxygen saturations begin to drop suddenly and the child is satisfactorily connected to the ventilator, a blocked tube must be suspected. Firstly call for help, then try to hand ventilate the child. If this proves difficult, irrigate the endotracheal tube with sterile saline 0.9%, hand ventilate for a few breaths, then apply suction. This procedure may remove the obstruction. However, if the child's condition continues to deteriorate rapidly and ventilation is not possible, the endotracheal tube must be removed immediately, and the child must be hand ventilated using an oral airway and mask until reintubation is facilitated.

In conclusion, suctioning the child with an endotracheal tube *in situ* is a necessary procedure which is not without adverse effects or complication. It is therefore important that the technique used takes into account the relevant research and that the staff are adequately trained and assessed.

Psychological support

Any child with an endotracheal tube *in situ* has limited mobility and field of vision. Whenever possible, sit the child upright so he or she can look around. If an upright position is not manageable because of the child's condition, sedation or paralysis, provide mobiles, bright pictures and toys within the child's line of vision. Talk to the child and encourage the parents to talk to and touch him or her. Play music and nursery rhymes, via a personal stereo if necessary so that other children are not disturbed.

Tube hygiene

Tube hygiene is an important consideration not only to minimize the risk of infection but also to ensure the comfort of the child.

Oral tubes are generally less stable and may stimulate increased salivation, sucking and biting. The child's skin can quickly become excoriated if appropriate action is not taken. The child's mouth should have gentle suction applied using either a large suction catheter or a Yankauer sucker. Regular inspection of the child's mouth, lips and palate should be made to observe for ulceration. Nasotracheal tubes are more stable but create pressure problems at the nares.

The tube should always be positioned so that it is not creating traction on the nostrils or mouth. If the child is ventilated, the tube should be positioned so that any trapped water cannot flow freely into the airway.

Complications

Intubation is not without complications, both during and after the procedure. During the procedure there is a risk of damage to the teeth and gums, epistaxis, tracheal or oesophageal perforation, and laryngeal spasm. Bradycardia, arrhythmias and hypoxia are also associated with intubation. In the longer term there is the risk of subglottic stenosis and infection.

EXTUBATION

The care given in the period during after extubation is vital. The child should be carefully assessed before extubation; observations should be stable and the child's chest should be as clear as possible. The necessary equipment should be available in case reintubation becomes necessary, and often the end of the endotracheal tube will be sent to the microbiology laboratory for culture and sensitivity tests.

If the child has been receiving supplemental oxygen via the endotracheal tube, this will normally continue to be supplied via a headbox, face mask or nasal cannula. Humification of this oxygen is important as this helps to prevent any secretions from becoming tacky and difficult for the child to cope with. Careful and ongoing assessment of the child's colour, chest movements and ability to cope without the artificial airway is vital. Any signs of distress should be noted and monitored, and appropriate action taken. The child will require careful observation for 24 h after extubation.

TRACHEOSTOMY

Tracheostomy is the life-saving surgical formation of an opening into the trachea, performed as either an elective or an emergency procedure. In paediatric respiratory management, tracheostomy formation is not a common occurrence. More sophisticated oral and nasotracheal tubes and ventilation weaning modes have enabled children to be ventilated for longer periods without the formation of tracheostomy.

Advantages

Despite its drawbacks, tracheostomy is the most suitable method of long-term airway management and has other advantages:

1. psychological benefit for the child of easier movement than with an oral or nasal tube;
2. increased field of vision for the child, who is therefore able to play, look at toys or read more easily;
3. easier and more comfortable positioning of the child;
4. reduction of anatomical dead space;
5. easier access for removal of secretions.
6. more secure fixation and therefore less likelihood of trauma to the trachea than with an oral tube;
7. cuffed tube facilitates oral diet;
8. enhanced communication.
9. no damage to the larynx;
10. better toleration than with oral and endotracheal tubes;
11. ease of maintaining good oral hygiene.

The tracheostomy tube differs from the endotracheal tube in that it is shorter, wider and less curved. As a result, resistance to airflow is diminished, facilitating breathing (McKenzie, 1983).

Problems and complications

Stock *et al.* (1986) list the following problems experienced following formation of tracheostomy: displaced tubes, bleeding, obstruction, subcutaneous emphysema, pneumothorax and aspiration.

Complications associated with tracheostomy include the following:

1. infection;
2. crusting;
3. pressure necrosis of the trachea;
4. cuff herniation causing narrowing of the airway;
5. displacement of the tube;
6. scarring at the site of the stoma, with the possibility of a persistent tracheocutaneous fistula after healing.

Types of tracheostomy tube

Three main types of tracheostomy tube are suitable for paediatric patients:

1. plastic (polyvinyl chloride or silastic) tubes, usually without an inner cannula;
2. silver tubes consisting of three parts: obturator, inner cannula and outer cannula;
3. an inflatable cuffed tube used to achieve an airtight seal when prolonged positive ventilation is required to maintain life (Weller, 1991).

The plastic tubes are most commonly used. If a cuffed tube is used, a low-pressure, high-volume (soft) tube should be the one of choice. Soft cuffs have been specifically designed to ensure that capillary refill is not impeded at the site of the inflated cuff. A major advantage of using a tracheostomy tube is that it results in a 50% reduction in anatomical deadspace (Allen, 1987).

Indications

Children with a tracheostomy may be able to breathe spontaneously or may require mechanical ventilatory support. A variety of reasons may lead to the children needing the formation of a tracheostomy:

1. congenital abnormality such as choanal atresia or laryngeal stenosis;
2. subglottic stenosis or other upper airway obstruction and/or abnormalities;
3. prolonged oral or nasotracheal intubation and further long-term ventilation requirement, such as are seen in infants following phrenic nerve damage after cardiac surgery;
4. improved secretion management;
5. acute inflammation, such as epiglottitis;

6. severe chest trauma;
7. laryngeal oedema and possible persistent loss of air leak following intubation;
8. Ondine's curse (sleep apnoea).

Formation of tracheostomy

Where a tracheostomy is indicated, it should if possible be performed as a planned procedure in the operating theatre where there are optimal aseptic conditions (Shepherd, 1986). Emergency tracheostomy can be performed on the unit but this increases the associated risks for the child. As with all surgical procedures, parental informed consent should be obtained. Consent may also be obtained from the child whenever appropriate.

As with all operative procedures, postoperative observation of vital signs should be recorded and any changes reported to anticipate and prevent haemorrhage, infection and complications of anaesthesia. Initially, the newly formed tracheostomy tube will require frequent suction and efficient humidification to ensure that the patency of the airway is maintained.

The tube size will be decided by the surgeon and will be in the region of 1.5 mm smaller than the diameter of the trachea. As with oral and nasotracheal tubes, the aseptic principles of suction are practised with a tracheostomy. In case of emergency, a spare tube of the same size and one size smaller should be kept at the child's bedside, with a tracheal dilator, suction equipment and spare tapes. A stitch cutter is also needed in the initial days after formation of the stoma if the tube is sutured to the skin.

Nursing care of the child with a tracheostomy

The nursing implications are as with any artifical airway: maintenance of patency and prevention of infection. The tube needs to be secure both to ensure that the vital airway is maintained and to promote the comfort of the child.

Securing the tube

The tube is secured by its flanges with cotton tapes. The tapes themselves may be foam padded to prevent irritation of the child's neck and prevent pressure sores. Once the tapes have been fastened, tied and knotted securely, the nurse should check that a finger can be placed between the tape and child's neck with a only little difficulty.

Changing the tube

Once the stoma has healed the tube should be changed on a regular basis to maintain patency and minimize the risk of infection. Normally tubes are left *in situ* for at least the first 48 h after surgery because it can be difficult to reinsert the tube into a newly formed stoma. After this, the tube can be changed according to unit protocol. The first tube change is usually performed by a doctor or anaesthetist in case difficulties in reintubation arise. Thereafter, an experienced paediatric intensive care nurse who has received suitable training, knows the child well and has gained the child's trust, is usually the most appropriate person to do this. However, it is not unreasonable to perform tube changes on the unstable child when a member of the medical team is available in case the stoma closes or collapse or difficulty is experienced in maintaining the airway while the tube is changed.

The procedure for changing the tracheostomy tube will vary slightly according to local policy. However, some general principles apply which universally ensure that the tube change is safe. Before changing the child's tracheostomy tube the nurse should consider the following principles:

1. Check that all the equipment is ready and fully functional. Check the child's history, especially as regards reinsertion of the tube; if difficulties have been experienced in the past, ensure that help is available.
2. The child should be calm, relaxed and adequately sedated, if necessary, and positioned with the neck extended. A neck roll may be used to support this position. However, care should be taken to ensure that the neck is not overextended. The child should be adequately prepared psychologically for the tube change.
3. An aseptic technique is used throughout the procedure. Unit policy with respect to cleaning agents should be followed, but lint-free swabs must be used to prevent fibres from entering the trachea. If the site looks infected, red or swollen, a swab should be taken for culture and sensitivity screen.
4. Throughout the procedure, the child's vital signs should be observed for any signs of deterioration.
5. Generally, two people are required to ensure the safe change of tube, especially if the child is distressed by the procedure.

Tube hygiene and stabilizing the tube

Internal hygiene is maintained by applying suction as required. The stoma itself will require cleaning to prevent the skin from breaking down and becoming infected and crusted by secretions. Additionally, the tapes will need changing on a regular basis, usually daily, although more frequent changes will be needed if they become wet or dirty. It is good practice to ensure that new tapes are fitted and secured before the old ones are removed.

Decannulation

When the decision that the child is ready to be weaned is made, the tracheostomy tube should be changed for one of a smaller size (0.5 mm at a time) until it can be removed. Once the tube has been removed, a sterile dressing should be applied firmly to the tracheostomy site and adhered with non-porous tape. This is again a stage at which nurses will need to spend time reassuring the children and informing them that they will be safe without 'their tube'.

Spigoting of the tracheostomy tube is considered to be inadvisable, especially in the smaller child, as this narrows the airway considerably. Even the use of a fenestrated tube in this way considerably restricts the patent airway.

In the first 48 h after successful decannulation, the child must be closely observed and nursed in an area with easy access to airway support if required (Johnson *et al.*, 1985).

ASSISTED VENTILATION

Artificial ventilation is a means of controlling or supporting ventilation by providing the necessary effort to move gas into the lungs. It aims to treat and correct hypoxaemia and tissue hypoxia, and allows a positive pressure to be maintained in the airways during the ventilator cycle.

This assistance can be delivered by a variety of methods; manually via a rebreathing bag or a self-inflating ventilation bag, or by mechanical ventilation.

A child may require either partial or total ventilatory support depending on the underlying problem. A variety of problems may indicate the elective or emergency need for ventilatory assistance.

Indications

The indications for ventilation are:

1. acute/chronic respiratory failure, as in bronchopulmonary dysplasia or asthma; abnormal blood gases which show either a decrease in PO_2 or a decrease in PO_2 with an increase in PCO_2;
2. absence of spontaneous breathing, e.g. apnoea, drug overdose, central nervous system abnormalities, respiratory muscle weakness;

3. infection, e.g. respiratory syncytial virus pneumonia, croup, epiglottitis;
4. asphyxia, e.g. drowning, smoke inhalation;
5. trauma;
6. congenital abnormalities of the airways;
7. surgery, e.g. prolonged operative times, intraoperative trauma to chest wall or lung.

Hand ventilation

Hand ventilation is a vital skill at which any nurse working in intensive care must be competent. It is necessary in an emergency and is often used during physiotherapy and suctioning.

Two main systems are available; the ambu bag and the anaesthetic rebreathing bag. Both systems can work with either a face mask or directly attached to the artifical airway, and can deliver air or a more concentrated mix of gas. In intensive care, the anaesthetic rebreathing bag is often the preferred choice because the operator can be more sensitive in the delivery of gas and interpretation of the compliance and state of the child's lungs. However, this system is technically more difficult to operate, requiring skill on the nurse's part to create and sensitively operate the valve and respond to changes in the child's lungs. It should be remembered that hand ventilation delivered through a rebreathing circuit connected to pressure monitoring of the system will deliver relatively higher pressures than those delivered by the ventilator at those settings because some pressure is lost in the ventilator's circuit.

Types of mechanical ventilator

Mechanical ventilation can be delivered through either a positive pressure or a negative pressure system. There are two commonly used types of positive pressure ventilator generally available: pressure controlled and volume controlled. The choice of which type of ventilator will depend on criteria such as the age of the child, the underlying reason for requiring respiratory assistance, the type of ventilatory support required and the availability of the equipment in the hospital.

Negative pressure ventilators

Negative pressure ventilators were the earliest means of mechanically supporting ventilation and played a 'particular role in the technological revolution' (Cule, 1989). This form of ventilatory support avoids the need for an artifical airway, can be used for intermittent therapy, and decreases the need for sedation and muscle relaxants. However, it requires a tight-fitting seal to be effective and reduces access to the child. Samuels and Southall (1989) report the efficacy of this form of ventilatory support.

Positive pressure ventilators

There are two main ways of delivering positive pressure ventilation; pressure-controlled/cycled and volume-controlled/cycled.

Pressure-controlled time-cycled ventilators deliver a flow to the lungs until a predetermined peak inspiratory pressure is reached. Therefore the volume delivered to the lungs varies with changes in lung compliance, or obstruction of the endotracheal tube or ventilator (e.g. Babylog, SLE, Sechrist, Bournes and Bear Cub). Small babies and children under 8 kg can be successfully managed on this type of ventilator.

Volume-controlled time-cycled ventilators deliver a preset volume to the lungs with variable pressures attained according to lung compliance or obstruction within the tubing. Pressure limits will almost always be set to prevent hyperexpansion of the lungs. If the pressure limit is exceeded, the pressure limit device 'spills' the excess volume of gas out of the system, thus safeguarding the child from possible barotrauma. The advantage of this type of ventilation is that it will deliver a consistent predetermined volume of gas. There is also usually the facility to measure expired minute volume (EMV). In children, where cuffed endotracheal tubes are not commonly used, allowances must be made for leaks both around the tube and within the ventilator tubing. Examples of this type of ventilator are the Servo B and Servo C.

Ventilator terminology

1. *Complying/synchronizing* with the ventilator means that the patient and the ventilator are breathing together in harmony. Muscle relaxants and/or sedation may be required to achieve synchrony.
2. *Triggering* the ventilator occurs when the child initiates a breath that is registered by the ventilator, which allows the patient to take gas from the system.
3. *Trigger sensitivity* is the sensitivity of the ventilator to the child's attempts to trigger a breath. The sensitivity can be increased or decreased depending on whether the medical staff wish to have complete control over the child's respiration.
4. *Fighting* the ventilator occurs when the child and the ventilator are not in synchrony. This can be frightening and uncomfortable for the child, and ventilation is less effective. It can be caused by the child receiving insufficient ventilation, improving to the point of making effective spontaneous breaths, or being frightened, distressed or in pain.

5. *Deadspace* refers to volume of tubing between the child and the exhalation valve. Deadspace can be added so that the child is essentially rebreathing expired carbon dioxide as a means of correcting respiratory alkalosis.
6. *Weaning off* refers to decreasing the amount of assisted ventilation.

Safety

For a ventilator to meet the needs of both the child and the staff caring for the child, it should possess certain important features:

1. alarms, which function to warn of disconnection from the patient, loss of power, low and high pressures, and failure to cycle, and which should never be silenced while the child is connected to the ventilator;
2. accurate mixing of gases piped from the wall;
3. a system that provides warmed and humidified gases;
4. accurate measurement of pressures in the airways and a reliable maximum pressure control;
5. flexibility of controls to set rate, inspiratory and expiratory ratio and a selection of weaning modes;
6. facility to deliver continuous positive airway pressure (CPAP) and positive end expiratory pressure (PEEP).

Modes of ventilation

It is important to remember that children will almost inevitably require different amounts of ventilatory support during their admission to the intensive care unit. They may be able to contribute in some way to their own ventilation. The mode of ventilation will reflect their underlying condition, drug therapy, level of sedation or consciousness, and often the personal preferences of the team caring for them.

There are two major modes of ventilation, the control mode and the assist mode, although a combination of the two can also be used. The major difference between the two is that in the controlled mode the patient is unable to trigger the ventilator.

Continuous mandatory ventilation and intermittent positive pressure ventilation

In continous mandatory ventilation (CMV) and intermittent positive pressure ventilation (IPPV), a preset number of breaths per minute are delivered at a preset rate and the child is unable to trigger a breath. This mode means that the child is completely dependent on the ventilator. This mode is suitable for use with a child receiving muscle relaxants such a pancuronium bromide and tubocurare, large doses of respiratory depressants such as morphine, anaesthetic agents or sedation.

The rate of CMV or IPPV will not necessarily be the same as the child's expected 'healthy' respiratory rate. It is generally more efficient and therefore ventilation rates in this mode are generally lower.

Intermittent mandatory ventilation (IMV) and synchronized IMV

IMV is a form of ventilation where the patient is either expected or allowed to make some spontaneous respiratory effort. This form of ventilation gives the child a preset number of breaths per minute, but allows space between the breaths for the child to breathe independently. In this mode the expired minute volume (EMV) of the child should be monitored closely, as a drop in EMV may be associated with the child tiring and making insufficient spontaneous effort.

Synchronized IMV (SIMV) is a more sophisticated form of IMV available on some machines whereby the machine is capable of recognizing that the child is initiating a breath and is able to 'hold back'. This mode is more comfortable for the child than the IMV mode.

Continuous positive airways pressure

This is the least amount of ventilatory support available. The child must be able to make spontaneous respiratory effort adequate for their needs. It is often considered to be a weaning mode. CPAP supplies the patient with warmed, humidified, mixed gas at a predetermined pressure. A preset pressure is left in the lungs, thus reducing the initial 'tug' of each respiration. The level of CPAP may be reduced as the patient improves before extubation.

Care of the child receiving artificial ventilation

Although these children are dependent on technology to maintain life, it must be remembered that they and their family need a huge amount of psychological support from the nursing staff. Close observation, primarily of the child but also of the ventilator, is a vital part of the care that keeps the children safe and detects complications:

1. *Child-centred observations*:
   (a) colour and perfusion;
   (b) chest wall movements;
   (c) breathing sounds;
   (d) oxygen saturation;
   (e) cardiac rate and rhythm;

(f) blood pressure;
(g) central venous pressure;
(h) urine output;
(i) level of consciousness;
2. *Ventilator observations*:
   (a) ventilator rate;
   (b) oxygen concentration;
   (c) oxygen flow rate;
   (d) peak inspiratory pressure;
   (e) peak end : expiratory pressure;
   (f) inspiratory-expiratory ratio;
   (g) expired minute volume.

These observations should be carefully documented. Each unit will have a protocol for the frequency of recording observations, but every child should be continually observed and assessed. The child and the family must always be the focus of the nurse's care rather than the technology.

Child-centred observations

Colour and *perfusion* are vital observations, and particular attention should be paid to the mucous membranes and nail beds. It is necessary to check the child's extremities for temperature. Deterioration in any of these parameters may indicate inadequate ventilation, low cardiac output or hypovolaemia.

There should be a symmetric *rise and fall of the chest wall* with each cycle of the ventilator. Asymmetrical chest movement may indicate a displacement of the endotracheal tube (usually down the right main bronchus), pneumothorax, atelectasis or pneumonia. The child's respiratory rate and compliance with the ventilator should be recorded and acted upon as appropriate.

An increase in secretions, collapse or inadequate ventilation may result in either abnormal or deteriorating *breathing sounds*.

A cardiac monitor to check *cardiac rate* and *rhythm* is a vital means of allowing continuous monitoring of the child's cardiac response to ventilation. Tachycardia may indicate hypoxaemia, the child 'fighting' the ventilator, inadequate sedation in conjunction with a paralysing agent, and pain or anxiety. Bradycardia may indicate hypoxaemia, low cardiac state, bleeding, hypovolaemia (a late sign), cardiac arrhythmias unrelated to ventilation, raised intracranial pressure, infection, pyrexia, convulsions in the paralysed child or pneumothorax.

An increase in *blood pressure* may suggest pain, confusion or raised intracranial pressure. Hypotension tends to indicate hypoxaemia, acidosis, overinflation of the lungs and hypovolaemia.

The introduction of positive pressure to the thoracic cavity affects the circulation by increasing *central venous pressure* even if the child is hypovolaemic. Blood returning to the heart from the head may also be impeded, which in turn increases intracranial pressure.

A decrease in *urine output* may denote poor perfusion and therefore deterioration in the child's condition. Any level of less than 1 ml/kg per h should be reported.

It is difficult to determine a child's *level of consciousness* if paralysis and sedation are being administered. However, irritability or fitting must be investigated further to rule out hypoxia or hypercapnia as well as many other causes. Any abnormal limb movements should also be reported.

Ventilator observations

The *ventilator rate* should be recorded as well as the mode by which that rate is being delivered. The ventilatory rate should be compared with the breathing rate of the child. If the child is triggering or fighting the ventilator, the rate will be increased.

If the child is fighting the ventilator, the nurse should attempt to determine whether the child is hypoxic by checking oxygen saturation and blood gases. The result of the blood gas analysis may indicate inadequate ventilation. If these observations prove to be within normal limits, more sedation or analgesia may be required.

Generally, the *oxygen concentration* should be at the lowest concentration required to maintain an oxygen saturation above 95%.

Oxygen flow rates of 5–10 litres now allow small tidal volumes to be delivered without creating high peak pressures.

Peak inspiratory pressure is the highest pressure delivered during a cycle in order to deliver an adequate tidal volume to the lungs. The peak pressure varies according to lung compliance and changes in the endotracheal tube and ventilator tubing. High peak inspiratory pressures cause damage to the lungs, resulting in reduced elasticity of lung tissue, pneumothorax and ultimately irreversible damage. It is therefore important to monitor the peak inspiratory pressure closely and report any changes. Peak inspiratory pressure can be increased by a variety of factors, including the child breathing against the ventilator, coughing, crying or experiencing hiccups, excessive water collecting in the ventilator tubing, and obstruction of the endotracheal tube.

Peak end-expiratory pressure maintains a light distension of the smaller airways during expiration. In children under the age of 6 years there is a deficiency in the elastic structures forming support for peripheral airways. The intrapleural pressure in parts of the lung is only slightly more negative than atmospheric pressure and may at times become positive. This compresses small airways, trapping gas behind the obstruction and causing an inequality in ventilation. Also, the larynx normally supplies 3 cm of PEEP; if this is bypassed by an endotracheal tube, alveoli can collapse completely in expiration and because of surface tension forces will be very difficult to re-expand.

It is therefore important to maintain a higher than normal functional residual capacity by using PEEP, preventing small airways from closing. PEEP also increases the amount of alveolar space available for gaseous exchange.

However, over-distension of the alveoli results in an increase in pulmonary vascular resistance, the high pleural pressures causing a fall in venous return and therefore a decrease in cardiac output. This is more marked in children with cardiac failure or hypovolaemia. Therefore PEEP should be closely observed in conjunction with the child's central venous pressure and blood pressure.

Inspiratory : expiratory (I : E) *ratio* is the ratio of the time spent during the cycle in inspiration and expiration. The I : E ratio is manipulated by the doctor or anaethetist, varying according to the disease process; for example, in ventilating a child with areas of collapse within the lung, a longer inspiration time allows gas to reach the atelectic areas. A child with asthma may require and I : E ratio of 1 : 4 or 1 : 5, allowing greater time for expiration. In hyaline membrane disease, where the lungs are very stiff, an I : E ratio of 1 : 1 or 1 : 1.5 may be preferred.

EMV measures the amount of gas exhaled from the lungs every minute. It is lower than the volume of gas preset to be delivered to the child because of leaks around the endotracheal tube and within the system. A significant fall in EMV may indicate an increased leak around the tube due to a reduction in oedema or disconnection from the ventilator.

Complications of artificial ventilation

Five main categories of complication exist in respect to artifical ventilation; upper airway trauma caused by intubation, increased work of breathing, infection, barotrauma and reduced cardiac output.

Many complications can be averted by skilled nursing care. Scrupulous care of the endotracheal tube can reduce the risk of nasal and oral damage; maintaining the stability of the tube minimizes the possibility of tracheal ulceration, kinking of the tube and intubation of the right main bronchus. Infection can be avoided if care in handling the circuit is seen as a priority; regular changing of the circuit, humidifier hygiene and good suction technique can reduce the risks associated with infection. Aspiration is best avoided, especially in children who are not commonly intubated with cuffed tubes, by maintaining gastric decompression by the use of the nasogastric tube.

Vigilance in observing the effectiveness of the ventilation can indicate either hypoventilation or hyperventilation and the real possibility of a tension pneumothorax. Artificial ventilation can also result in a reduced cardiac output, which can be caused by decreased venous return as a result of PEEP or CPAP.

Stress ulcers and paralytic ileus are also associated with artificial vent-ilation.

PHYSIOTHERAPY AND THE VENTILATED CHILD

Physiotherapy is performed to mobilize secretions, and minimize imbalances in ventilation and perfusion in the child. It is particularly important in the ventilated child, and practice will vary from unit to unit. Physiotherapy may be used therapeutically or prophylactically. Among the many factors that can contribute to the production of excessive secretions in the ventilated child are the underlying disease process, inability to cough, the endotracheal tube irritating the mucous membrane, reduced mucociliary clearance due to the presence of an endotracheal tube, increased susceptibility to infection and the drying of secretions due to inadequate humidity.

Assessment of the child before physiotherapy

Assessment is vital before, during and after physiotherapy to determine whether the treatment is necessary, whether the child is able to withstand the treatment, the effectiveness of the treatment. The child's overall condition should be considered and observation of vital signs should be made before commencement of physiotherapy. The child's general colour, oxygen saturation, arterial blood gases and cardiac stability should be noted. The nurse should also observe the child's chest movements and listen to their breathing sounds. The most recent chest radiograph should be consulted for areas of collapse or other focal problems; this information, and consultation with other members of the multidisciplinary team will indicate the need for specific treatment. The colour, consistency and quantity of secretions obtained should also be noted.

It is important to note how well the child has tolerated physiotherapy on previous occasions and whether the child needs (additional) sedation or analgesia to cope with the treatment.

The nurse should also consider both the type of ventilation that the child is receiving and whether or not this has been altered recently. It is prudent to allow a period of approximately 2 h for stabilization after any changes.

Note should also be made of any associated problems that may either contraindicate or increase the problems associated with physiotherapy, such as abdominal distension, fractured ribs, raised intracranial pressure or whether the child has been fed in the last hour.

All these factors must be considered before performing chest physiotherapy to avoid complications. In some circumstances physiotherapy may still need to be performed despite the poor condition of the child because the risks of not doing so are greater. However, this type of decision should not be taken lightly and will normally need to be made in consultation with other members of the team.

Positioning the child

To complement chest physiotherapy and reduce the risk of stasis of secretions, the child must be turned regularly. The frequency of turning and the most desirable position will depend on which parts of the lungs are being treated. Depending on unit practice, physiotherapy may be performed by a trained physiotherapist, by the nursing staff, or both. However, it is important that nurses are trained adequately and their technique checked regularly.

Firstly, explain to the child and the parents what the procedure entails, and ensure that the child is relaxed and comfortable and well supported by pillows and in the appropriate treatment position.

Approaches to physiotherapy

One method of chest physiotherapy commonly used is that of manual hyperinflation of the lung using a rebreathing circuit and chest vibration. The bag is inflated slowly and deeply during inspiration and then released quickly during expiration to facilitate a high expiratory flow rate. The physiotherapist's or nurse's hands are spread over the area of the lower part of the rib cage and begin to compress the chest at the end of expiration. The chest compression and vibration, along with the quick expiration of the air, helps to move secretions into the larger airways. This procedure is repeated as needed to mobilize the secretions and suction is performed. The child who is able to cooperate is encouraged to cough during suction to further mobilize secretions.

This method may not be practical because of the child's condition, as hyperinflation with vibration can cause a fall in cardiac output and therefore a reduction in oxygen reaching the tissues. It should be avoided, unless essential, in patients with unstable condition, arrhythmia, hypoxaemia, undrained pneumothorax, bronchospasm or haemoptysis.

An alternative is to perform chest vibration during the expiratory cycle of the ventilator. Position the patient to achieve optimal postural drainage. Normal saline 0.9% may be instilled to the endotracheal tube before and during the procedure. However, if this is necessary, the effectiveness of humidification via the ventilation circuit should be questioned.

If there is collapse of lung tissue without retained secretions or once the secretions have been removed, a slow inspiration and expiration is appropriate.

Chest percussion is another method that may be employed in some units. The hand is cupped and the wrist is flexed and tapped against the child's rib cage. A cushion of air should be present to prevent trauma, and a characteristic sound is produced. A sheet or towel should also be used to further protect the child. In small infants a small mask for hand ventilation can produce a similar effect. Percussion also helps to shake free and mobilize secretions.

If at any time during chest physiotherapy the child's condition deteriorates, physiotherapy should be stopped immediately and appropriate action taken.

Preterm infants

It is now recognized that fragile preterm babies often respond badly to handling and traumatic episodes (Long *et al.*, 1980). Physiotherapy falls into the category of potentially traumatic handling, and so special consideration of both the need for therapy and the techniques used should be given before commencement of the therapy itself (Parker, 1990). Studies have been performed assessing the effect of physiotherapy on the baby's transcutaneous oxygen levels (Crane, 1981; Parker, 1985). Parker (1985) suggests parameters for transcutaneous oxygen with readings of 8 kPa or above considered the safe level for the commencement of physiotherapy and readings of 7.3 kPa or below the point at which therapy should not continue.

Downs and Parker (1991) cite three studies (Crane, 1981; Parker, 1985; Bertone, 1988) which suggest that 'chest physiotherapy is necessary when tracheobronchial secretions are not adequately cleared by suction alone and should continue until the infant's chest is clinically clear'. Emphasis is placed on the need for individual assessment of each baby in respect to physiotherapy and suggest that contraindications for physiotherapy are the 'very unstable baby, severe hypothermia, undrained pneumothorax, and pulmonary haemorrhage' (Downs and Parker, 1991).

A variety of techniques are employed in neonatal physiotherapy: face mask percussion, vibration using an electric toothbrush, contact-heel percussion (rhythmic compressions of the infant's chest wall using the thenar and hypothenar eminences) and postural drainage. Studies have demonstrated that, generally, percussion techniques result in an improvement in arterial oxygen levels although the electric toothbrush method is not seen to be beneficial to arterial oxygenation (Tudehope and Bagley, 1980).

The severely ill neonate is particularly at risk from hypoxaemia triggered by suctioning (Cunningham *et al.*, 1984). Shorten (1989) particularly stresses the significance of handling as part of the whole suction procedure in contributing to hypoxaemia. Hyperinflation and hyperoxygenation of neonates is generally not considered necessary practice before suction because of the real risks developing retrolental fibroplasia (Friendly, 1981) and pneumothorax.

Conclusion

The number of times chest physiotherapy is performed is determined by the child's need for treatment and condition, and the nature of the secretions.

After extubation, chest physiotherapy may be continued with breathing and blowing exercises and mobilization as soon as possible for older children.

Along with chest physiotherapy, passive limb movements and regular turning must be carried out on all children who are electively paralysed, sedated or unable to move. This will help to maintain the range of joint movements and soft-tissue extensibility, avoiding foot drop and pressure sores.

DRUGS USED IN RESPIRATORY INTENSIVE CARE

The number and types of drugs used in children with respiratory disease are many and varied and each unit has its own practice. For ease of discussion and simplicity, the following drugs have been classified according to their action or administration. The paediatric pharmacist works closely with the paediatrician in the prescribing of drugs. Table 4.7 gives a guide to dosages in use.

Table 4.7 Drug dosages

Drug		
Morphine	Intravenous bolus/ continuous infusion	Bolus 100–200 μg/kg per h Infusion 10–50 μg/kg per h
Sodium bicarbonate 8.4%	Intravenous bolus/ continuous infusion	Base excess weight one-third will fully correct
Midazolam	Intravenous bolus/ continuous infusion	Bolus 0.1–0.3 mg/kg Infusion 0.1–0.3 mg/kg per h
THAM 7.2%	Intravenous bolus	1 ml = 0.5–1 ml $NaHCO_3$ depending on calculation
Vecuronium Pancuronium	Intravenous bolus/ continuous infusion	Bolus 50–100 μg/kg Infusion 50–80 μg/kg per h
Aminophylline	Intravenous bolus/ continuous infusion	Bolus 4–6 mg/kg Infusion 0.5–1 mg/kg per h
Epoprostenol	Continuous infusion	2–20 ng/kg per min in isotonic saline, infused alone
Atropine	Intravenous bolus/ intramuscular	20–40 μg/kg

Sedation and analgesia

These are grouped together as one can complement the other. Adequate analgesia often helps a child to be comfortable and relaxed while receiving ventilatory support.

Morphine is often used as an analgesic agent either by IV bolus or as a continous infusion. Paracetamol elixir can be given as an oral/nasogastric preparation or rectally as suppositories. For adequate sedation, a useful drug is midazolam, again either as an IV bolus or as a continuous infusion. Chloral hydrate and tricolfos elixir are also used for their sedating properties and have the advantage of not depressing the respiratory drive. They can be given as an oral or nasogastric preparation or as suppositories per rectum. In practice, the administration of both oral and intravenous preparations achieves an optimal effect. When the child is critically ill a paralysing agent may also be added, such as atracurium, vecuronium or pancuronium. However, it should be ensured that the paralysed child is also adequately sedated.

Respiratory specific drugs

These include the β-antagonists such as salbutamol and aminophylline. Also included in this category will be steroid preparations and sodium cromoglycate, which can be used prophylactically. High-dose septrin is now used for the treatment of *Pneumocystis carinii*. In the preterm neonate, drugs such as caffeine and surfactant can be used.

Nebulized drugs

These include the bronchodilators such as salbutamol and ipratropium. Nebulized adrenaline can be used to treat postextubation stridor. Treatment for respiratory syncitial virus (RSV) for the child who is already at risk of being critically ill, such as with immunosuppression or a congenital cardiac defect, now includes ribavirin.

Intravenous drugs

In addition to drugs previously discussed, others used in the respiratory setting include antibiotics which can be used either prophylactically or as a treatment for primary or systemic sepsis. Aminophylline is used for the treatment of asthma, and epoprostenol (prostacyclin) for the treatment of persistent pulmonary hypertension. Where there is vagal stimulation on intubation, atropine can be administered because it acts as a parasympathetic blocking agent.

Acid–base correcting agents

Where there is profound acidosis and/or bicarbonate deficit that is not correctable by increasing artificial ventilation, two preparations are in common use. Sodium bicarbonate ($NaHCO_3$) 8.4% should be administered with an appropriate dose to half-correct the base deficit. Trometalol (THAM) should be used as a second line choice only when bicarbonate is not suitable, such as when there is a raised serum sodium level or PCO_2.

Diuretics

Where there is evidence of pulmonary oedema, intravenous administration of diuretics such as frusemide may be necessary. Where this no longer achieves an adequate result it can be supplemented with human albumin 20% as an osmotic diuretic. Frusemide may also be supplemented by spironolactone either orally or nasogastrically to reduce hypokalaemia.

Practice points

As with all drug administration, it is the individual practitioner's responsibility to be informed about any possible adverse effects of the prescribed medication. Additionally, a paediatric practitioner should have access to an appropriate formulary to validate prescription doses and as an information base. The local drug administration policy should be adhered to as should the guidelines from the UKCC (UKCC, 1989).

EPIGLOTTITIS

Acute epiglottitis constitutes a potential respiratory emergency and should always be considered in those terms. Epiglottitis is the result of bacterial infection, which causes inflammation and oedema of the epiglottis, false cords and aryepiglottic folds. The most common cause of epiglottitis is *Haemophilus influenzae* type B, although *Pneumococci*, *Staphylococcus aureus*, and β-haemolytic *Streptococcus* can be causative agents. Children between the ages of 3 and 10 years are at risk, with a peak incidence at 3–4 years.

Epiglottitis can result in the total occlusion of the child's airway by the oedamatous epiglottis, making emergency intubation and in some cases tracheostomy formation necessary.

Clinical manifestations

The child with epiglottitis presents with three classic symptoms; the presence of drooling, agitation, and the absence of a spontaneous cough (Figure 4.4). The child usually has only a very short history of symptoms and this sudden onset makes the severity of the disorder very frightening for the child and the family.

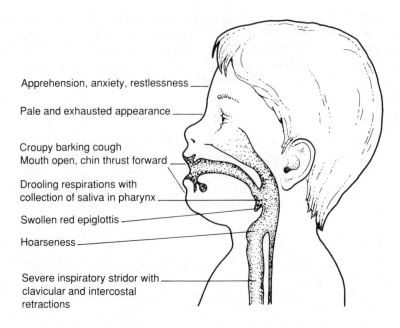

Apprehension, anxiety, restlessness

Pale and exhausted appearance

Croupy barking cough
Mouth open, chin thrust forward

Drooling respirations with
collection of saliva in pharynx

Swollen red epiglottis

Hoarseness

Severe inspiratory stridor with
clavicular and intercostal
retractions

Figure 4.4 The child with epiglottitis.

Classically the child will wake during the night with a sore throat and dysphagia, accompanied by a pyrexia of 39–40°C. The child's pulse is rapid and respirations are often shallow and sound hoarse although the chest movements may appear exaggerated. The child rapidly becomes pale and looks exhausted as a result of the great effort needed to breath. The child is most comfortable when sitting upright, leaning forward, chin thrust forward and with mouth open and tongue out (Figure 4.4). The child's sore throat and fear of swallowing produce a tendency to drool continuously and this in itself can be upsetting for the child. Bearing in mind the anxiety that both the child and the family are experiencing, the most reassuring and safest place for the child to be is on a parent's knee. The child should not be laid flat as this exacerbates the problem by reducing the effectiveness of the diaphragm.

On inspection, which should only be carried out in theatre, the epiglottis appears enlarged, oedematous and cherry red. Extreme care should be exercised when visualizing the epiglottis because gagging can easily precipitate occlusion. The most important thing to bear in mind when caring for the child with epiglottitis is that the epiglottis may occlude at any time. Staff with expertise in intubation and an ear, nose and throat surgeon (in case a tracheostomy is required) should be available to ensure that the child's airway is maintained.

As the epiglottis becomes increasingly oedematous, the child becomes increasingly hypoxic, hypercapneic and acidotic. The child's level of consciousness also deteriorates. Elective intubation under controlled conditions is infinitely preferable to allowing the child to struggle for too long.

The nurse's main responsibilities to the child are those of close observation and continuing reassurance. Before intubation, the nurse should try to ensure that the child remains calm and is not subjected to unnecessary handling or trauma. Some physicians may request that the child is given humidified oxygen to facilitate respiration and reduce hypoxia. However, this can sometimes act as another stressor for the child; in these cases, the child needs to be considered sympathetically.

Intravenous antibiotic therapy is commenced once the child is intubated and the drugs of choice are ampicillin and cefotaxime. Additionally, corticosteroid therapy may be prescribed for the first 24–48 h.

It should be remembered that the child may need to be intubated with an endotracheal tube that is one or two sizes smaller than usual. The child is therefore dependent on a narrow, artificial airway. Tube hygiene should be scrupulous, suction should be applied as required, and warmed humidified gas should be given as prescribed. In practice, the child who requires intubation with a smaller size tube than usual can present some difficulties because the smaller tube may not be very long. Once the tube is in place it should be secured efficiently as reintubation is often associated with increased difficulties, again due to oedema.

The care of the child will depend on the severity of the condition. Intravenous fluids may be required initially and then oral fluids can be introduced (usually once the child has been extubated).

The approach to extubation should be cautious and continued close observation after extubation is essential. Normally the endotracheal tube can be removed within 48–72 h and artificial ventilation is not generally required. Some physicians will listen for leaks around the tube as an indication that the oedema is reducing and that the child can be extubated.

In conclusion, epiglottitis is a respiratory emergency in which the nurse plays a major role in observing and assessing the child and ensuring that care is delivered in a reassuring and relaxed atmosphere.

BRONCHIOLITIS

Bronchiolitis is a common, acute (usually viral) infection of the lower respiratory tract that can result in mild to severe respiratory distress. The pathogen invades bronchiole epithelial cells resulting in those cells sloughing away, oedema and increased mucous secretions. This leads to blockage of varying degrees of the small air passages. Air trapping and overdistension of the lungs can occur which may result in a ventilation–perfusion mismatch, hypoxaemia and hypercapnea. Respiratory failure and apnoea may result from respiratory muscle fatigue and immature ventilatory control. Apnoea attacks, circulatory collapse and exhaustion may result. Bronchiolitis has been reported to increase the predisposition to asthma (Schweich, 1990). Bronchiolitis lasts between 7–10 days and the prognosis is normally good.

The most common infective organism is the respiratory syncytial virus (RSV); other infective agents include adenoviruses, parainfluenza viruses, influenza viruses, rhinoviruses, mumps and mycoplasma pneumoniae (Ramsay, 1989; Guerra et al., 1990).

The child presenting with bronchiolitis will have a moderate pyrexia, paroxysmal cough, rhinitis, wheezing and dyspnoea. The infant/child is often irritable and tired. Those with more severe symptoms will also have intercostal and subcostal retractions, nasal flaring, lethargy, hypoxia and cyanosis.

Bronchiolitis occurs mostly in the winter and spring months and affects children under the age of two years with a peak incidence at six months old. RSV is reported to affect approximately 60% of infants in the first twelve months of life. Although the majority of children/infants do not require medical care, one in fifty require hospitalization and a small percentage (3–7%) develop respiratory failure. Thus those who require intensive care represent only a small proportion of those infected. However, these children may have other disorders or health deficits such as cardiopulmonary disease, prematurity, immunodeficiency, cystic fibrosis, bronchopulmonary dysplasia or anaemia and are therefore more 'at risk'. A significant amount of ICU morbidity and mortality has been reported in the 'at risk' group (Moler et al., 1992).

The treatment for the infant/child with bronchiolitis is normally supportive although ribavirin, an antiviral agent, can be used in the treatment of selected members of the 'at risk' group. Supportive care includes fluid therapy, humidification, oxygen therapy (via head box, face mask or mechanical ventilation) and the use of antipyretics. Suction to the oro- and nasopharynx is vital in ensuring that the nasal passages are kept clear of excessive secretions. This promotes improved respiratory effort and is especially important to the infant who is an obligatory nose breather. The baby with moderate to severe respiratory distress who is tachypnoeic and exhausted will require intravenous fluids during the crisis period of the illness. Intragastric feeds may be appropriate as their condition improves. Antibiotics are only used if a secondary infection is present or develops.

Elective intubation and mechanical ventilation may be required for several days in order to support the child through the very acute stage of the infection. It is important to keep the lungs free from excessive secretions and to prevent the possibility of developing a secondary infection, thus suction must be performed as appropriate to the oro- and nasopharynx and via the endotracheal tube. Close assessment and monitoring of the child's condition must be maintained throughout the illness. Obviously the prime area of monitoring will be related to respiratory and cardiac assessment, including the response to ventilation and the progress of the illness. The intubated and ventilated infant is at risk from pneumothorax and pneumomediastinum. The nurse should be aware that respiratory acidosis may develop and any signs of dehydration should be carefully monitored. Normally the infant/child is weaned off the ventilator as soon as their condition indicates it is safe to do so. Some units may choose to use continuous positive airways pressure (CPAP) for 12–24 hours prior to extubation. It is normal practice for the child to be nursed with an appropriate source (such as a head box or face mask) of humidified air or oxygen after extubation, and until the dyspnoea, and any accompanying hypoxia, is resolved.

Ribavirin therapy is controversial and is used only for selected 'at risk' children. Ribavirin is an agent specific to RSV and although it is considered to be effective it is important to remember that is may have toxic effects on health workers. It is administered using a small particle aerosol generator for 12–18 hours a day for a period of three to five days via a headbox, mask or the ventilator circuit. Inevitably some of the particles may 'escape' into the atmosphere and there is concern that this may place other patients, staff and visitors at risk. There are also reports that the particles precipitate out into the ventilator tubing which creates ventilation problems.

REFERENCES

Allan, D. (1987) Making sense of tracheostomy. *Nursing Times*, **83**(45), 36–8.

Allan, D. (1988) Making sense of suctioning. *Nursing Times*, **84**(10), 46–7.

American Heart Association (1988) *American Heart Association and American Academy of Pediatrics Instructors Manual for Pediatric Advanced Life Support*. American Heart Association, Dallas.

Behrman, R.E. and Vaughan, V.C. (1987) *Nelson Textbook of Paediatrics*, 13th edn, W.B. Saunders, London.

Bertone, B. (1988) The role of physiotherapy in a neonatal intensive care unit. *Australian Journal of Physiotherapy*, **34**(1), 27–34.

Brandstater, B. and Muallem, M. (1969) Atelectasis following tracheal suctioning in infants. *Anesthesiology*, **31**, 468–73.

Boutros, A.R. (1970) Arterial blood oxygenation during and after suctioning in the apnoeic patient. *Anesthesiology*, **32**, 114–18.

Crane, L. (1981) Physical therapy for neonates with respiratory dysfunction. *Physical Therapy*, **61**(12), 1764–73.

Cule, J. (1989) A historical view of intensive care. ITCM, November, 288, 290, 292–3.

Cunningham, M.L., Baun, M.M and Nelson, R.M. (1984) Endotracheal suctioning of premature neonates. *Journal of the California Perinatal Association*, **4**(1), 45–8.

Fanconi, S. and Duc, G. (1987) Intratracheal suctioning in sick preterm infants;

prevention of intracranial hypertension and cerebral hypoperfusion by muscle paralysis. *Pediatrics*, **79**(47, 538–43.

Friendly, D.S. (1981) Eye disorders in neonates, in *Neonatal Pathophysiology and Management of the Newborn*, 2nd edn, (ed. G.B. Avery), J.B. Lippincott, Philadelphia.

Fox, W.W., Schwartz, J.G. and Schaffer, T.H. (1978) Pulmonary physiotherapy in neonates: physiological changes and respiratory management. *Journal of Pediatrics*, **92**, 977–81.

Guerra, C., Kemp, J.S. and Shearer, W.T. (1990) Bronchiolitis, in *Principles and Practice of Pediatrics*, (eds. F.A. Oski), J.B. Lippincott, Philadelphia.

Hazinski, M.F. (1984) *Nursing Care of the Critically Ill Child*. C.V. Mosby, St Louis.

Hudak, C.M., Gallo, B.M. and Lohr, T.A. (1986) *Critical Care Nursing: A Holistic Approach*, 4th edn, J.B. Lippincott, Philadelphia.

Johnson, J.T., Reilly, J.S. and Mallory, G.B. (1985) Decannulation, in *Tracheostomy*, (eds E.N. Myers, S.E. Stool and J.T. Johnson) Churchill Livingstone, New York.

Long, J.G. Philip, A.G.S. and Lucey, J.F. (1980) Excessive healing as a cause of hypoxaemia. *Pediatrics*, **65**(2), 203–7.

McKenzie, C., (1983) Compromises in the choice of orotracheal or nasotracheal intubation and tracheostomy. *Heart Lung*, **12**(5), 485.

Moler, F., Khan, A. and Custer, J. (1992) Mechanical ventilation for RSV infection: does ribavirin improve patient morbidity? *Critical Care Medicine*, **29**(4), S87.

Nagariaj, H.S. Fellows, R., Shott, R. and Yacoub, U. (1980) Recurrent lobar atelectasis due to acquired stenosis in neonates. *Journal of Paediatric Surgery*, **15**, 411–15.

Naigow, D. and Powaser, M.M. (1977) The effect of different endotracheal suction on arterial blood gases in a controlled experimental model. *Heart Lung*, **6**, 808–16.

Oski, F.A. (1990) (ed.) *Principles and Practice of Pediatrics*, J.B. Lippincott, Philadelphia.

Parker, E. (1985) Chest physiotherapy in the neonatal intensive care unit. *Physiotherapy*, **71**(2), 63–5.

Parker, A. (1990) Expert handling. *Nursing Times*, **86**(12), 35–7.

Perlman, J.M. and Volpe, J.J. (1983) Suctioning in the preterm infant: effects on cerebral blood flow velocity, intracranial pressure, and arterial blood pressure. *Pediatrics*, **72**(3), 329–34.

Ramsay, J. (1989) *Nursing the Child with Respiratory Problems*. Chapman and Hall, London.

Samuels, M.P. and Southall, D.P. (1989) Negative extrathoracic pressure in the treatment of respiratory failure in infants and young children. *British Medical Journal*, **299**, 1253–7.

Schweich, P.J. (1990) Emergency medicine except poisoning, in *Principle and Practice of Pediatrics*, (ed. F.A. Oski), J.B. Lippincott, Philadelphia.

Shorten, D.R. (1989) Effects of tracheal suctioning on neonates: a review of the literature. *Intensive Care Nursing*, **5**, 167–70.

Simbruner, E., Coradello, H., Fodor, M., Havelec, L., Lubec, G. and Pollafe, A. (1981) Effect of tracheal suction on oxygenation and circulation and lung mechanisms in newborn infants. *Archives of Disease in Childhood*, **56**,326–30.

Tudehope, D.I. and Bagley, C. (1980) Techniques of physiotherapy in intubated babies with respiratory distress syndrome. *Australian Medical Journal*, **16**, 226–8.

Tyler, M.L. (1982) Complication of positioning and chest physiotherapy. *Respiratory Care*, **27**, 458–66.

UKCC (1989) *Code of Conduct*. UKCC, London.

Weller, B.F. (1991) *The Lippincott Manual of Paediatric Nursing*, 3rd edn, Harper-Collins, London.

Whaley, L.F. and Wong, D.L. (1989) *Essentials of Pediatric Nursing*. CV Mosby, St Louis.

Witham-Wilson, M.J. (1991) Accidental breathing circuit disconnection in the neonatal or pediatric critical care setting. *Pediatric Nursing*, **17**(3), 283–6, 293.

Young, C.S. (1984) A review of the adverse effects of airway suction. *Physiotherapy*, **70**(3), 104–6.

5

Care of the child with cardiovascular problems

Adelaide Tunstill and Cathy McCarthy

About 60% of children with congenital heart disease require surgery and most of this will be needed within the first 2 years of life. 'Closed' heart surgery is performed for extracardiac problems such as patent ductus arteriosus or coarctation of the aorta, and 'open' heart surgery is performed for intracardiac problems and requires the use of cardiopulmonary by-pass.

Operations may be either palliative or corrective. Palliative surgery may be undertaken to improve the child's oxygenation and quality of life if corrective surgery is not possible or if the child is not big enough. Transplantation is now another alternative for severe problems, but the prognosis following cardiac or cardiopulmonary transplanation is still somewhat guarded.

CARDIAC TERMINOLOGY

1. *Stroke volume* is the difference between the end-diastolic volume and the end-systolic volume.
2. *Cardiac output* is the product of the stroke volume and the heart rate.
3. *End-diastolic volume* is the volume of blood in the ventricle at the beginning of systole.
4. *End-systolic volume* is the volume of blood remaining at the end of systole when the valves are closed.
5. *Preload* is the filling pressure.
6. *Contractility* is the shortening of the myocardial muscle fibres.
7. *Afterload* is the resistance or pressure against which the ventricle must eject its contents.

CARDIAC OUTPUT AND RELATED ISSUES

It is important that the nurse understands the normal anatomy and physiology of the heart and lungs and the consequences of cardiac defects that the child may present with.

The heart is in effect two pumps working in parallel, with their associated valves and two systems of connecting vessels, to supply the tissues with sufficient oxygenated blood to meet all the metabolic needs of the cells. As with any pump, the output is calculated by multiplying the volume ejected per stroke by the number of ejections per minute.

Cardiac output depends on stroke volume and heart rate and can therefore vary in response to changes in either, or both. If the stroke volume remains constant, an increase in heart rate will increase the cardiac output. However, if the heart rate increases too much the filling time of the ventricles is greatly reduced so that the end-diastolic volume, and therefore the stroke volume, is reduced and thus the cardiac output is decreased.

Heart rate is influenced by many factors, including metabolic rate, hypovolaemia, hypoxaemia, acidaemia, hypercapnia, age, exertion and emotional upset. The preload or filling pressure determines the stroke volume and the left and right atrial pressures are used as guides.

If the filling pressure is adequate and cardiac output remains low, contractility has to be improved. If contractility is increased, systole takes less time because the fibres shorten and relax rapidly. Therefore, if the heart rate remains stable, the diastolic filling time and the coronary artery perfusion time are increased and thus the stroke volume will increase. Contractility can be improved by the use of catecholamines such as dopamine. Other drugs that may be used are adrenaline, dobutamine and enoximone.

If the cardiac output remains low despite these measures, attempts at reducing the afterload have to be made. This can be achieved by reducing peripheral vascular resistance by administering a vasodilator such as sodium nitroprusside or nitroglycerin.

Careful titration against response of the inotropes and vasodilators is essential in the management of cardiac output.

TYPES OF CONGENITAL HEART DISEASE

There have been nearly a hundred types of abnormality reported. However, it is important to remember that eight common defects make up 85% of the cases of congenital heart disease: patent ductus arteriosus, ventricular septal defect, atrial septal defect, aortic stenosis, coarctation of the aorta, pulmonary stenosis, tetralogy of Fallot and transposition of the great arteries (Jordan, 1979).

The defects can be divided into groups according to the physiological abnormality they produce; cyanotic lesions with decreased pulmonary blood flow, cyanotic lesions with increased pulmonary blood flow, acynanotic lesions with a left-to-right shunt, left heart obstruction, and right heart obstruction (Jordan and Scott, 1989; Jordan, 1979). Some examples of the lesions associated with the physiological abnormalities are very briefly discussed below. Tetralogy of Fallot will be discussed in more detail as it is a good example of a defect with both duct-dependent circulation and low pulmonary blood flow.

Cyanotic lesions with decreased pulmonary blood flow

Cyanosis occurs only when there is a right-to-left shunt through a septal defect and an obstruction in the right heart beyond the site of the defect. Most commonly, the obstruction is at the pulmonary valve, but it can be at the tricuspid valve or at pulmonary vascular level.

1. tetralogy of Fallot (ventricular septal defect (VSD), pulmonary stenosis, overriding aorta and right ventricular hypertrophy);
2. pulmonary atresia with VSD;
3. pulmonary atresia without VSD;
4. tricuspid atresia.

Tetralogy of Fallot

Originally described in 1888, the tetralogy of Fallot has four defects (see Figure 5.1): pulmonary infundibular stenosis, VSD, overriding aorta and

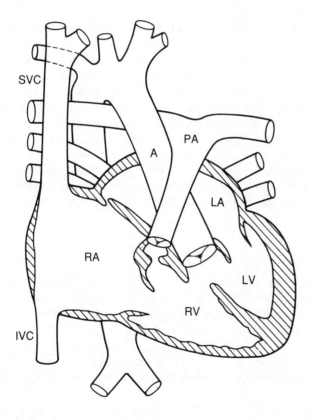

Figure 5.1 Tetralogy of Fallot. A, aorta; IVC, inferior vena cava; LA, left atrium; LV, left ventricle; PA, pulmonary artery; RA, right atrium; RV, right ventricle; SVC, superior vena cava. Reproduced from Kelvar, C.J.H. and Harvey, D. (1987) *The Sick Newborn Baby*, 2nd edn. Baillière Tindall, London.

right ventricular hypertrophy (RVH). Two main physiological consequences result from the tetralogy of Fallot:

Circulatory changes following birth

Tetralogy of Fallot is an example of a duct-dependent lesion. One of the principal aims when caring for a neonate with this defect must be to prevent ductal closure.

Shortly after the birth, when the umbilical cord is clamped, the pressures in the right side of the heart fall, allowing an increase in pulmonary bloodflow. This is further enhanced by a reduction in the pulmonary vascular resistance (PVR) as a result of rising oxygen levels and pH. The resulting increase in the left atrial pressure (LAP) above right atrial pressure (RAP) causes the foramen ovale to close.

Rising oxygen levels also inhibit the production of prostaglandin PGE_2, which, together with PGE_1, is responsible for maintaining ductal patency. As a consequence, the smooth muscle in the wall of the ductus contracts. Physiological closure is usually achieved within the first 24 h although permanent closure will not be achieved for at least 3 weeks.

Maintenance of a patent ductus in the neonate with severe tetralogy of Fallot is necessary to overcome the inhibition to pulmonary blood flow caused by pulmonary stenosis. This is most commonly achieved by administering prostaglandin E_1 (0.005 μ g/kg per min) as an intravenous infusion. Apnoea is a well recognized side-effect and therefore facilities for hand ventilation and emergency intubation should be near at hand. All patients should be closely monitored for apnoea attacks. Tachycardia and pyrexia are also sometimes seen.

Low pulmonary blood flow

Perhaps the most characteristic feature is the variability in resistance to right ventricular outflow. Any right-to-left shunting is said to be dependent on that resistance. A rise in right ventricular outflow tract resistance will produce a cyanotic attack. This is most commonly seen by nurses when the infant is feeding or crying. Shunting will also occur during cardiac catheterization or induction of anaesthesia. 'Squatting', which is so often described in the literature, is rarely seen now because of early surgical repair.

Reduced oxygen delivery to the tissues is the end result of a low pulmonary blood flow. The infant gradually tries to compensate for and adapt to this abnormal state. Total blood volume is known to increase. This is accompanied by a rise in haemoglobin level to increase oxygen-carrying capacity. A rightward shift in the oxygen dissociation curve improves delivery to the tissues as the haemoglobin will give up its oxygen load more easily. The systemic venous bed also increases in size. These mechanisms, aimed at compensation, are important to the paediatric intensive care nurse as they act as pointers to the most likely complications in the postoperative period.

Cyanotic lesions with increased pulmonary blood flow

1. *Transposition of the great arteries.* The aorta arises from the right ventricle and the pulmonary artery from the left ventricle, thus producing two separate circulations. Severe cyanosis becomes apparent when the ductus closes.
2. *Double-outlet right ventricle.* This is an uncommon condition in which both the great arteries arise from the right ventricle.
3. *Truncus arteriosus.* The primitive truncus has failed to divide into the pulmonary artery and aorta. There is always a high VSD and a single truncal valve. There are three types:
   (a) the pulmonary arteries arise from the truncus with a common stem (this is the most suitable for surgery);
   (b) the pulmonary arteries arise separately from the back of the truncus;
   (c) the pulmonary arteries arise separately from the side of the truncus.
4. *Total anomalous pulmonary venous connection.* All the pulmonary veins drain directly or indirectly into the right atrium. Classification is made according to the site of the connection:
   (a) supracardiac: connected to the ascending vein and then to the left innominate vein (commonest) or directly to the superior vena cava;
   (b) cardiac: connected to the right atrium or the coronary sinus;
   (c) infracardiac: connected to the inferior vena cava or the portal vein.

Acyanotic lesions with left-to-right shunt

1. *Patent ductus arteriosus.* The ductus joins the bifurcation of the main pulmonary artery to the aorta just beyond the subclavian artery. In the fetus it carries blood from the pulmonary artery to the descending aorta, bypassing the lungs. It normally closes functionally within 10–15 h of birth, due to constriction of specialized tissue (confined to the ductus) by stimulation from the high oxygen content of the blood passing through it.

2. *Ventricular septal defect*. This is the commonest heart lesion diagnosed in childhood. The defect is usually single, but multiple lesions can be found. The majority of defects are found in the membranous septum just below the aortic valve, but as they often involve some of the surrounding muscular septum it is more accurate to call them perimembranous lesions.

3. *Atrial septal defect*. This is the second commonest cardiac defect and can be classified into two groups:
   (a) simple ASD (or ostium secundum defect);
   (b) complex ASD (or atrioventricular defect). *Ostium primum* is an example of the complex ASD where the defect lies in the lowest part of the atrial septum and includes a cleft in the anterior leaflet of the mitral valve.

Left-heart obstruction

1. *Coarctation of the aorta*. This defect involves a narrowing at the junction of the arch and descending aorta. The preductal type often causes breathlessness and heart failure leading to death in the first month of life. Symptoms can occur in the first 10 days of life when the ductus arteriosus closes. Symptoms are dramatic and urgent resuscitation is essential. It is one of the most important emergencies in babies. Coarctation in older children is usually picked up at a routine medical examination when absent or weak femoral pulses are discovered. Complications result from hypertension and include heart failure and dissecting aneurysm. Premature coronary artery disease can occur in later life.

2. *Aortic valve stenosis*. This accounts for about 5% of all congenital heart disease presenting in infancy and childhood. An isolated aortic valve stenosis is about four times as common in boys as in girls. Severe aortic stenosis may be seen in infancy, causing heart failure or sudden death. In older children it can be discovered on a routine examination and many have no symptoms.

3. *Aortic atresia*. This presents within the first 24 h of life and is evidenced by severe dyspnoea and heart failure.

4. *Hypoplastic left heart syndrome*. This syndrome is characterized by underdevelopment of the left heart. The severe form comprises atresia of the aortic valve and atresia or hypoplasia of the mitral valve with a rudimentary left ventricle.

Right-heart obstruction

1. *Pulmonary valve stenosis*. This is a common defect affecting more females

than males. It may cause severe cyanosis in the neonatal period, requiring urgent surgery.
2. Pulmonary atresia.

PSYCHOLOGICAL CARE OF THE CHILD

Psychological care of the child needs to start as soon as the parents learn the diagnosis. To find that their baby has a heart defect comes as a tremendous shock to most parents. Repeated explanations are necessary and if possible written information should be available. Parent support organizations may give some parents comfort and information.

If the child is old enough, he or she should be prepared for hospital admission. There are many suitable books available. All questions asked by the child should be answered simply but truthfully. A preadmission visit to the hospital may be possible so that both the child and the parents may have some idea of what to expect. If this is not feasible, preparatory booklets should be sent out to the parents before admission. Details of parents' accommodation and facilities should also be made available beforehand so that the parents have one less thing to worry about later.

On admission to the ward, the child should be given the opportunity to settle in before any procedures are carried out. The play leaders can be helpful in providing equipment and dolls to prepare the child for the operation while in a safe playroom setting. It is important that all the staff involved in caring for the child and the family give comprehensive, appropriate and compassionate explanations of the treatment and care that the child will need. The family should be informed of the possible risks and side-effects and be encouraged to ask questions.

A visit to the intensive care unit the day before the operation is helpful for the parents so that they can be oriented to the unit, see all the equipment and hear all the background noises without their child being involved. The child should also be taken to see the unit, if old enough. Parents need to be warned that as long as their child is intubated he will not be able to speak or cry out loud. The fact that, while lying on the bed, the child is unable to see much of the equipment is helpful for many parents and explains why many ceilings in intensive care units are decorated with pictures and mobiles. Nursing and medical routines as far as they exist need to be explained and the parents may be given a timetable of events expected for the operative day. Usually, it is helpful for the nurse who is to take care of the child after operation to meet the parents and get to know the child. During the time that the child is undergoing surgery, the parents should be encouraged to do something to pass the time; sitting waiting for 4–5 h may seem interminable.

If they are waiting, progress reports from theatre may be helpful and continuity of information is vital.

Once the child is back in the intensive care unit after surgery and is attached to all the necessary equipment, the parents may be brought in. Once again, they will need explanations about the surgery and 'attachments', and it is helpful if the surgeon sees them and explains what has been done. Simple but comprehensive explanations are important at this stage and the families will require a large amount of support and reassurance. Many parents will experience an initial euphoria when they hear that their child has survived the surgery, and this will last for about 48 h. However, when the child is extubated, feeling pretty miserable and crotchety, the parents will also be tired and at a low ebb. It is at this point that nurses need to be especially patient and encouraging to both the patient and the parents.

Hospitalization may have a temporary effect on a child's development. There may be some altered behaviour, differences in sleep patterns, regression and so on, but if there has been adequate preparation beforehand and support during and after surgery, these effects are reduced to a minimum.

PERIOPERATIVE ISSUES

Some 45–90 min before the child is due to go to theatre, heavy premedication will be administered. Following induction, intubation and placement of lines, it is now accepted that cardiopulmonary bypass can itself be used to lower the nasopharyngeal temperature to 26°C. Surgical repair begins when the temperature has fallen to 24°C. A systole usually occurs between 24 and 20°C. Infusion of cool cardioplegic solution into the aortic root will cool the myocardium and arrest the heart.

Extracorporeal warming commences when the repair is complete. Peripheral vasoconstriction is corrected to allow refilling of the peripheral circulation while the patient is on bypass. When the nasopharyngeal temperature reaches 35°C and the peripheries are warm, bypass is discontinued.

Protamine (6 mg/kg IV) is administered to reverse the heparin given immediately before the institution of bypass. Frusemide (0.25 mg/kg IV) may be given if there is no diuresis. Serum potassium levels which can fall by 1.5 mmol/l when the body temperature is lowered below 30°C, are checked frequently and corrected.

Despite adequate reversal of heparinization, the cyanosed child may experience bleeding problems after operation. This can be further compounded by rapid transfusion of large quantities of blood products.

RECEIVING A CHILD FROM THEATRE

It is important to ensure that the child's bed space is prepared and that the nurses who will look after him understand their role in receiving the child onto the unit.

Equipment required is likely to include:

1. cardiac monitor capable of recording electrocardiogram, three pressures and two temperatures; rhythm strip recorder; transducers and flush bags or syringe pumps;
2. ventilator plus a rebreathing circuit with suitable connectors;
3. vacuum points both for chest drain attachment and for endotracheal aspiration; suitably sized suction catheters;
4. intravenous infusion pumps plus stands;
5. stethoscope and dynamap or sphygmomanometer;
6. charts, preferably to cover 24 h vital signs and fluid balance; prescription and nursing sheets;
7. general nursing equipment;
8. a bed or Baby-Therm made up with suitable linen and, if it is to be taken to the theatre, a portable oxygen cylinder and infusion stand.

On the patient's admission to the unit, the nurses should immediately assess the child's colour, feel if the child is warm to the touch, and make an initial assessment of blood loss via the chest drains. If this is satisfactory, the child can be connected to monitoring equipment and the fluid lines should be organized. All the information relating to the actual surgery, duration of bypass, presence and position of drains, fluid and monitoring lines, and size and length of the endotracheal tube should be documented by the surgeon and anaesthetist.

PRINCIPLES OF POSTOPERATIVE CARE

In the postoperative period, much of the nurse's time will be spent anticipating and correcting problems induced by hypothermia and cardiopulmonary bypass. It is therefore necessary to understand the physiological sequelae of cardiopulmonary bypass in order to be able to initiate care effectively.

After open heart surgery, the aim should be to have as near normal cardiac function as possible. Cardiac output may be adversely affected by alterations in rhythm, preload, afterload and the accumulation of pericardial fluid. The preoperative anatomy and the adequacy of the corrective operation are obvious factors affecting cardiac output after operation.

Cardiac output is assessed immediately the patient returns to the intensive care unit and treatment is commenced as necessary. Preload may be assessed by looking at the patient and feeling the limbs for warmth as well as by checking the central venous or right atrial pressure. Blood and fluid losses must be accurately measured and a balance kept; initially, it will be found that patients require a large amount of colloids. This is due to rewarming and resultant vasodilation. Continued blood loss of more than 5 ml/kg per h may indicate the need for re-exploration of the chest.

Respiratory care

It is common to describe the need for respiratory support as extending until the child is haemodynamically stable, peripherally warm and well perfused, urinary output is adequate and bleeding has stopped. However, this more accurately describes the criteria for weaning from intermittent positive pressure ventilation (IPPV). The chest radiograph taken immediately after return to the unit allows a check on the position of the endotracheal tube, the expansion of both lungs, the placement of lines and the position of the nasogastric tube.

To achieve effective control of ventilation, sedation and analgesia will be required. These may be given as bolus doses but it is now widespread practice to administer continuous infusions, thereby achieving background sedation and analgesia, and avoiding peaks and troughs in plasma concentration associated with bolus administration.

Morphine is the most popular drug (0.01–0.02 mg/kg IV, four hourly), but as sensitivity is sometimes increased after cardiopulmonary bypass it is advisable to give only 0.1 mg/kg initially.

The following infusions are frequently used:

1. morphine 0.5 mg/kg in 50 ml dextrose 5% at 2 ml/h (20 μg/kg per h);
2. midazolam 6 mg/kg in 50 ml dextrose 5% at 1 ml/h (2 μg/kg per min);
3. fentanyl 100 μg/kg in 50 ml dextrose 5% at 2 ml/h (4 μg/kg per h); dose range is 4–10 μg/kg per h;
4. vecuronium 0.1 mg/kg; dose is 1–3 μg/kg per min.

Should ventilation be required for longer than 24 h, chloral hydrate or a suitable alternative should be given. This is a particularly useful drug for children with Down syndrome with altered sensorium, who often appear resistant to morphine sulphate.

Tracheal suction should be performed within the first hour of return from theatre. The quantity and character of the secretions should be noted and vital signs and air entry should be checked after completion. Thereafter, suction should be performed as the secretions dictate.

The application of positive end expiratory pressure (PEEP) will aid oxygenation. It is particularly helpful in children who develop pulmonary oedema or intrapulmonary shunting, or who show evidence of collapse on chest radiography. Children with tetralogy of Fallot are known to have a thickened right ventricle and will have had a systemic pulmonary shunt before corrective surgery, increasing the likelihood of respiratory problems in the postoperative period. PEEP may also prove to be useful after prolonged bypass and extensive transfusion. Higher levels of PEEP may be used to slow intrathoracic bleeding. However, it should be applied with caution as it will diminish both venous return and cardiac output.

It is appropriate to wean the child from the ventilator when haemodynamic stability has been achieved without large doses of inotropic agents, if there is minimal blood loss from the chest drains and the arterial blood gases are adequate. It is usual to use a period of constant positive airways pressure (CPAP) before extubation. This allows the application of a constant distending pressure during spontaneous ventilation, thus reducing the work of breathing.

Extubation is performed when adequate blood gases are maintained with an F_{iO_2} of 0.5% or less and the chest radiograph shows that both lungs are well expanded. Copious secretions are a contraindication. After extubation, a humidified oxygen-enriched gas mixture should be delivered to the child via a headbox or mask. The child's position should be changed every 2 h to encourage drainage of secretions from the peripheral airways. Gentle pharyngeal suction performed at the same time encourages the child to cough and expand the lungs.

The child who becomes drowsy and unresponsive after extubation may be developing a rising P_{CO_2}; conversely, irritability and distress may indicate developing hypoxaemia. Arterial blood gas levels should be checked and the anaesthetist informed if the result is unsatisfactory.

Chest physiotherapy usually commences on the first morning after operation. Individual unit policy varies widely in this, with some preferring to start within a few hours of the child's arrival in the unit. Sessions should be short and frequent using appropriate techniques such as percussion, vibration, hand ventilation, instillation of 0.5 ml sterile isotonic sodium chloride (0.9%) and suction of both the trachea and pharynx.

The physiotherapist will usually consult the nurse caring for the child as to whether it is appropriate to treat. To perform physiotherapy safely, a knowledge of both the child's preoperative condition and surgery is required. Assessment of the child's current status should be carried out before physiotherapy, and if there is haemodynamic instability the medical staff should be consulted.

Fluid balance

Retention of sodium (Na^+), increased excretion of potassium (K^+) and diminution of urine flow are all characteristic of the postoperative period. Insensible fluid loss is influenced by body temperature, ambient temperature and the humidity of the inspired gas.

The principles underlying the postoperative period fluid regimen are therefore to restrict sodium and water intake and to give supplemental potassium. On day 1, 50% of maintenance fluid requirement is given, and full requirements are achieved over a 2–3 day period. Liberalization of fluids is guided by the child's fluid balance. A typical postoperative fluid regimen is shown in Table 5.1. Fluid may be given as 5 or 10% dextrose.

Table 5.1 Example of a postoperative fluid regimen

Weight (kg)	Maintenance
< 10	Up to 100 ml/kg per 24 h
10–20	1000 ml/24 h + 50 ml/kg for every kg above 10
> 20	1500 ml/24 h + 20 ml/kg for every kg above 20

Blood sugar levels should be estimated every 2–4 h; this will act as a guide to the amount of dextrose required.

It is usual to administer potassium chloride (KCl) intravenously to maintain serum levels of 4–4.5 mmol/1. Unit protocols vary from adding potassium to maintenance fluids to preparing a very concentrated solution which is administered separately and titrated according to serum levels. Hypokalaemia may cause unifocal ventricular ectopics, which should be treated if they occur at frequent intervals. (Before administering digoxin, the nurse should check the latest serum potassium level. If it is low, the medical staff should be consulted before digoxin is administered.)

The early introduction of enteral feeding makes sense both nutritionally and as a means of easing problems of electrolyte balance. It obviates the need to administer H_2 antagonists as antacids. Gastric pH should be maintained above pH 4. A nasogastric tube will have been inserted in theatre and if it is left to drain freely it will help to prevent sudden gastric dilatation. It is a commonly held belief that the mere presence of a nasogastric tube will help to prevent gastric reflux, but it should be remembered that it renders the gastro–oesophageal sphincter incompetent.

Clear fluid should be tried first, and this is usually given as 5% dextrose. If the tube is unclamped 10 min before the next feed, the amount absorbed can be estimated. The majority of small children can be fed with appropriate commercially prepared formula. However, if this is poorly tolerated, as evidenced by a large aspirate, feeding should be temporarily suspended and then gradually reintroduced. If gastric feeding is poorly tolerated, nasojejunal feeding may be an appropriate alternative. In the unstable critically sick child, absorption from the gut may be poor and in these circumstances total parenteral nutrition should be given to avoid protein catabolism.

Urine output is expected to be 0.5–1 ml/kg per h, and failure to achieve this should be discussed with medical staff. Hypovolaemia can be corrected by administering blood or plasma 5 ml/kg as a bolus in addition to the replacement of chest drain losses. In the adequately hydrated patient with optimal filling pressures, frusemide 1 ml/kg IV is given and it may need to be repeated several times during the postoperative course. A negative fluid balance should be achieved for at least the first 48 h.

Chest drain loss is replaced millilitre for millilitre with either blood or plasma as indicated by the child's packed cell volume (PCV). As indicated above, boluses of colloid will be needed at intervals to maintain an adequate circulating volume. The blood loss in ml/kg should be estimated at frequent intervals. Emergency surgical intervention may be indicated if the loss exceeds 5 ml/kg per h, particularly when it is accompanied by hypotension and peripheral vasoconstriction. In calculating hourly and daily fluid balance, all sources of intake and output should be included. Some units prefer to separate fluid and colloid balance, but an overall picture can be of great value.

Analgesia and sedation

Recovery will be enhanced in a child who is relaxed and pain free. Morphine is a popular and widely used opiate in the paediatric intensive care unit. It can be administered as a bolus or continuous infusion. An initial bolus dose of 0.1 ml/kg IV followed by an infusion of 0.5 mg/kg in 50 ml dextrose 5% at 2 ml/h is an example of a regimen which provides adequate analgesia without respiratory depression. The side-effects of morphine include analgesia, sedation, respiratory depression, decreased gastrointestinal motility, nausea and vomiting (Booker, 1989). It is advisable to reduce the dosage by half when weaning the child from ventilatory support, but to continue administration until the chest drains have been removed.

The use of fentanyl as an intravenous infusion has become more common in paediatric intensive care units in recent years. Like morphine, it can cause hypotension and severe respiratory depression, but it is useful for children who are known to have an elevated pulmonary vascular resistance or who are expected to have an unstable postoperative period. Fentanyl may be administered in a dose range of 4–10 µg/kg per h. An intravenous infusion of 100 µg/kg in 50 ml at 2 ml/h will give 4 µg/kg per h.

In addition to morphine a benzodiazepine is usually selected for its tranquillizing property. Midazolam (2–5µg/kg per min) by infusion is widely used. In this dose range it does not have clinically significant cardiovascular or respiratory effects. The amnesic effect is particularly welcome for a child in the intensive care unit (Booker *et al.*, 1986; Lloyd Thomas and Booker, 1986).

Muscle relaxants may be indicated in the presence of an elevated pulmonary vascular resistance (PVR) or generalized instability. Atracurium and vecuronium are both examples of agents in common use which can be administered by continuous infusion. As both are acidic compounds (pH 3–4), they can be inactivated if administered through the same intravenous line as an alkali (Goudsouzian, 1989).

Of the neuromuscular blocking agents in the long-acting group, pancuronium (0.1 mg/kg IV) is undoubtedly the most popular in paediatric intensive care. Associated tachycardia and the consequent concern for increased myocardial oxygen consumption have led to the use of atracurium and vecuronium in preference to pancuronium.

POTENTIAL POSTOPERATIVE COMPLICATIONS

A variety of complications may occur in the postoperative period and these can be minimized by the careful assessment of the child. The nurse must obviously be aware of potential complications, which may include cardiac tamponade, pleural infusions, arrhythmias, renal failure, infection, phrenic nerve palsy, gastrointestinal problems and neurological complications.

Cardiac tamponade

Cardiac tamponade is the most important acute factor that may interfere with filling of the heart. Tamponade is usually the result of occluded chest drains and should always be suspected if there is sudden cessation of chest drainage with associated deterioration in the condition of the patient. The clinical signs are a rising central venous pressure, decreasing arterial pressure, tachycardia and peripheral constriction. On the chest radiograph, a widened mediastinum will be evident. Treatment consists of prompt volume replacement to maintain cardiac output, and the theatre should be informed of the need for further surgery. If necessary, the sternal wound should be opened on the ward and the clots evacuated. Myocardial contractility may be decreased transiently and the use of an inotropic agent may be necessary after volume replacement has been tried to improve the cardiac output. Right heart failure may occur if there is still a degree of right ventricular outflow tract obstruction, but this will probably be due to operative swelling and will lessen as the oedema subsides. Residual shunt across the ventricular septum may also be seen.

Pleural effusions

Pleural effusions can occur as a result of congestive cardiac failure or post-cardiotomy syndrome. If the child is still ventilated the peak inspiratory pressures may rise. The chest radiograph will show an opacity on the affected side. Treatment normally requires insertion of a chest tube to drain the fluid. Occasionally, chyle (lymph fluid) may collect in the pleural cavity as a result of injury to the thoracic duct during surgery. It may also occur in children with a high central venous pressure, especially in children who have had a total cavopulmonary connection. It is difficult to diagnose until the child has started an oral diet or is taking normal milk, when the fluid draining will become cloudy white in colour. Treatment consists of draining the fluid and giving the child a low-fat diet, which will limit the production of chyle. If it persists surgery may be necessary to repair the thoracic duct.

Arrhythmias

Arrhythmias that compromise cardiac output or perfusion must be treated immediately. The most common arrhythmias seen following cardiac surgery include supraventricular tachycardia, various forms of heart block and right bundle branch block. Significant ventricular arrhythmias such as ventricular tachycardia or fibrillation are relatively rare, but if present usually indicate serious deterioration in the child's condition.

If the child's surgery has involved any manipulation of the natural pacing mechanisms of the heart, oedema of those areas may cause temporary arrhythmias. For this reason, two temporary pacing wires are left *in situ* after surgery and these may be attached to an external pacing system if necessary. If the wires are not required, they can be rolled up and stuck to the chest until their removal several days later.

Electrolyte imbalance may cause arrhythmias. Potassium, sodium and calcium levels should be checked regularly and corrected as necessary. Nurses should be aware of the child's potassium levels before giving digoxin or diuretics. Bolus doses of potassium may need to be given to correct the serum levels.

If a large amount of blood has been transfused the citrate will cause calcium binding, and small amounts of calcium gluconate (usual dose 1 ml calcium gluconate per 100 ml blood transfused) should be given.

Hypoxaemia, acidosis and excessive use of catecholamines can all be reasons for arrhythmias and should be treated quickly.

If compromising arrhythmias persist, cooling the patient to 33–34 °C may have a beneficial effect.

In some circumstances, control of a tachycardia may be achieved by over-pacing the heart at a rate exceeding the ectopic rate and then slowly reducing the rate. Defibrillation or cardioversion will occasionally be necessary to interrupt 'disorganized' electrical activity. This may well cause asystole, and the necessary drugs should be available.

Renal failure

This may occur after bypass surgery owing to reduced renal perfusion. It may also occur before surgery in the sick neonate with preductal coarctation of the aorta. After bypass surgery it is essential to measure the urinary output accurately. A minimum output of 0.5 ml/kg is acceptable but, if the output drops below this, diuretics should be given. If there is no response, peritoneal dialysis will be considered. Peritoneal dialysis may be commenced if there is fluid overload, which may occur in the neonate requiring extra drugs and therefore more fluid.

Metabolic acidosis develops in the patient with acute renal failure as a result of the inability of the kidneys to excrete endogenously produced acid. Metabolic acidosis may be treated with intravenous sodium bicarbonate but, if serum sodium levels are increasing, peritoneal dialysis will be required.

Haemofiltration and haemodialysis are alternatives, but are rarely necessary after cardiac surgery.

Infection

The risk of infection is high in the postoperative cardiac patient. Most centres are in favour of at least 24 h of prophylactic antibiotics to cover the surgery. Because of the lengthy procedures, the introduction of various tubes and equipment and very often the poor nutritional state of the patient, the danger is real.

Obviously, the need for sterility during the introduction of arterial and venous lines, urinary catheters and the endotracheal tube is recognized. However, handwashing in the intensive care unit by all personnel is equally important, and it may well be up to the nurse at the bedside to ensure that this is practised.

The nurse must be alert for signs of infection: redness at insertion points of the line, inflammation of the wound, unexplained swellings, changes in the tracheal secretions, cloudiness of the urine, persistent hyperpyrexia or hypothermia and greyness in the neonate, etc. Relevant specimens should be sent to the microbiology department and appropriate antibiotics prescribed. Because of the side-effects of some of these antibiotics, blood levels of these may need to be estimated and dosages changed.

Regular chest physiotherapy will help to clear chest secretions and lead to earlier extubation.

Gastrointestinal complications

These are not often seen after cardiac surgery, but care should be taken to prevent certain problems. Oral fluids should not be introduced until bowel sounds are heard, as there may be a transient paralytic ileus following bypass surgery. Narcotics, hypokalaemia or drugs such as nitroprusside, which affects smooth muscle, may affect gastric function. Acute gastric dilatation is often seen after cardiac surgery, especially in infants, and a reasonably large-bore nasogastric tube should be left on free drainage. Another problem occasionally seen in infants following cardiac surgery is necrotizing enterocolitis. This is treated by discontinuing gastric feeds and replacing them with total parenteral nutrition, administering systemic antibiotics and an antifungal agent, and monitoring for signs of perforation of the bowel.

Phrenic nerve palsy

Occasionally during cardiac surgery the phrenic nerve is damaged, causing paralysis of the hemidiaphragm. It should be suspected if the child proves difficult to wean from the ventilator. On radiography, the affected diaphragm will be higher. Most children manage with one properly functioning diaphragm, but in the baby it may be necessary to plicate the diaphragm surgically to wean the baby from the ventilator.

Neurological complications

Neurological complications may follow cardiac surgery and are usually as a consequence of severe hypoxaemia and/or hypotension. Metabolic acidosis and hypoglycaemia may cause neurological damage, and fluid overload and electrolyte inbalance may cause cerebral oedema. During the course of open-heart surgery there is always the risk of air embolization. Clotting disturbances may cause intracerebral bleeding and in rare instances thrombosis may occur in the severely polycythaemic child. Hypocalcaemia may cause convulsions, as may hyperpyrexia. The nurse should assess the child neurologically as soon as possible after surgery and be aware of any change in cerebral state.

To diagnose the cause of the problem, an electroencephalogram, lumbar puncture or brain scan may be needed. Symptoms should be treated accordingly.

RESUSCITATION

Hypoxia is the most common cause of cardiac arrest in infants and children. Other major causes include congenital heart disease, hypovolaemia (which is poorly tolerated by infants and children), hypothermia (which causes stress on the cardiovascular system) and hypoglycaemia due to low glycogen stores.

For teaching purposes, the management of resuscitation is divided into basic and advanced life support. The skills required for advanced life support are emphasized, as this is most appropriate for the paediatric intensive care unit; however, basic life support (Table 5.2) is equally important.

Table 5.2 Guidelines for basic life support

	Method	Rate (compressions/min)	Ratio of chest compressions to ventilations
Baby	Encircle the chest with both hands; interlink the fingers behind the spine; use thumbs	120	5 : 1
Small child	Two fingers	100	5 : 1
Older child	Heel of one hand	80–100	15 : 2

The ABC of resuscitation is familiar, basic, vitally important and easily remembered as Airway, Breathing and Circulation. An open and clear airway is essential if the infant or child is to be resuscitated successfully. In the smallest infants this will be assisted by placing a support under the shoulders. The nasal passages should also be checked for any obstruction, as infants are obligatory nose breathers.

Assessment of the adequacy of the infant's respiratory effort should begin by looking for normal chest movement. The presence of intercostal recession and flaring of the nares is indicative of distress. See-saw movements of the chest and abdomen indicate some degree of airway obstruction. In the absence of congenital heart disease, hypoxic infants do not appear cyanosed; they are more accurately described as pale, ashen or grey.

Arrest that is primarily cardiac in origin is rare, which contrasts with extreme bradycardia. The heart rate and pulse volume can most easily be assessed by palpating either the brachial or the femoral artery. Causes of absent or weakened pulses should be considered, and operative scars are sometimes a clue. Coarctation of the aorta will cause a weakened pulse in the left brachial and both femoral arteries. Cardiac catherization may also be implicated.

Hypoxia-induced bradycardia usually responds well to adequate ventilation. However, an inadequate pulse indicates low cardiac output which necessitates external cardiac compressions. The lower half of the sternum, one finger breadth below the internipple line, is considered the most appropriate site in infants and children.

Advanced life support

Advanced life support involves the use of equipment and, like basic life support, applies the ABC sequence. Either an oropharyngeal or nasopharyngeal airway can be used to maintain the patency of the airway. During resuscitation an oropharyngeal airway, which fits comfortably over the back of the tongue, will be used.

Before intubation is attempted the child should be preoxygenated; this is best achieved by using a facemask that fits snugly, resulting in minimal leakage. The use of a clear plastic mask allows continuous observation of the airway and the colour of the child's face. Ventilation can be achieved using either a self-inflating rescucitation bag with a pressure-limiting device or a gas-filled Jackson–Rees modification of Ayre's T-piece. Use of the latter demands more skill. In either case, the use of 100% oxygen is mandatory.

To secure a stable airway as rapidly as possible, it is usual to intubate orally, only changing to a nasal tube when the child's condition has stabilized. A laryngoscope together with both curved and straight blades will be needed. A straight blade is preferred for infants, as it allows direct elevation of the epiglottis. Both cuffed and uncuffed tubes together with appropriate connections should be available. A pair of small and large Magill forceps will be required for nasal intubation. Most units have a table for determining the size and length of the tube. Air entry should be checked with a stethoscope to detect accidental intubation of the right main bronchus. The tube is then firmly secured according to unit policy.

Support of the circulation is dependent on intravenous access. If this is not available, adrenaline, atropine and lignocaine (Table 5.3) may be given via the tracheal tube. Doubling the intravenous dose should ensure that sufficient will be absorbed through the pulmonary vascular bed to achieve

Table 5.3 Drugs used in resuscitation

Drug formulation	Action	Dose
Adrenaline 1 in 10 000	Inotrope Chronotrope	0.1 ml/kg

Atropine
    0.1 mg/ml
	Parasympathetic blocking agent
	    Use for severe bradycardia
	    particularly associated with
	    tracheal intubation.
		0.02 mg/kg

Sodium bicarbonate
    <6 months 4.2%
    >6 months 8.4%
	Corrects acidosis
	Increases CO_2 production
	Reacts with calcium
	Inactivates adrenaline
		1 mmol/kg,
		e.g. 2 ml/kg of
		    4.2% solution,
		    1 ml/kg of
		    8.4% solution

Lignocaine 1%	Use to treat multifocal
	    ectopics, ventricular
	    tachycardia, bigeminy
		0.1 ml/kg

Calcium chloride
    10% solution
	Increases myocardial
	    contractility
		0.1 ml/kg

Glucose 25% solution	Corrects hypoglycaemia	0.5–1.0 g/kg 2–4 ml/kg

therapeutic blood levels. The use of the intra-osseous route is now recognized as effective.

Poor peripheral circulation during resuscitation makes central venous access the method of choice. The use of the external jugular and femoral routes is most convenient.

Monitoring of the electrocardiogram and the blood pressure should be continuous, as should the recording of all fluids and drugs administered. Pulse oximetry is an added bonus.

2 g dextrose to 1 unit insulin may be used to return potassium to the cells.

When nursing a child who is considered to be at risk of collapse, precalculating the dose of drugs needed, in mg/kg and ml solution, is time well spent.

Hypovolaemia should be corrected with 10 mlg/kg colloid and this may need to be repeated.

Ventricular tachycardia and ventricular fibrillation are relatively uncommon, but require treatment by defibrillation 2 J/kg. This can be repeated before increasing the charge to 4 J/kg. Paediatric paddles of 4 or 8 cm size should be used.

During and after the resuscitation process, care should be taken to prevent hypothermia. Monitoring the arterial blood gases will guide the management of ventilation and provide clues to the possible cause of collapse. Plasma electrolytes and blood sugar should be checked regularly. Chest radiography should be performed as soon as possible.

Parents should be kept informed of their child's progress throughout resuscitation. Decisions concerning parental presence should be made by the staff involved together with the parents. Parents often need reassurance that their child is still alive. This can best be achieved by allowing them to see the child straight away. They should be prepared for the child's altered appearance. As soon as possible a member of the medical and nursing staff with whom the parents are familiar should discuss the possible cause of collapse and the likely events over the next few hours. The availability of a parents' interview room is of great benefit.

REFERENCES AND FURTHER READING

American Heart Association (1986) Standards and guidelines for cardiopulmonary resuscitation (CPR) and emergency cardiac care (ECC). *Journal of the American Medical Association*, **255**, 2905–92.

Booker, P,D., Beechey, A. and Lloyd-Thomas, A.R. (1986) Sedation of children requiring artificial ventilation using an infusion of midazolam. *British Journal of Anaesthesia*, **58**, 1104–8.

Booker, P. (1989) Intravenous agents in paediatric anaesthesia, in *Textbook of Paediatric Anaesthesia Practice*, (eds E. Sumner and D.J. Hatch), Baillière Tindall, London, pp. 61–90.

Goudsouzian, N.G. (1989) Relaxants in paediatric anaesthesia, in *Textbook of Paediatric Anaesthesia Practice*, (eds E. Sumner and D.J. Hatch) Baillière Tindall, London, pp. 91–112.

Hatch , D.J. and Sumner E. (1986) *Neonatal Anaesthesia and Perioperative Care*, 2nd ed., Arnold, London.

Hazinski, M.F. (1984) *Nursing Care of the Critically Ill Child*, C.V. Mosby, St Louis, Missouri.

Jordan, S.C. (1979) *A Synopsis of Cardiology*, 2nd edn, John Wright, Bristol.

Jordan, S.C. and Scott, O. (1989) *Heart Disease in Paediatrics*, Butterworths, London.

Kelnar, J.H. and Harvey, D. (1987) *The Sick Newborn Baby*. Baillière Tindall, London.

Llynn, A.M., Opheim, K.E. and Tyler, D.C. (1984) Morphine infusion after paediatric cardiac surgery. *Critical Care Medicine*, **12**, 863–7.

Resuscitation Council (UK) (1989) Revised recommendations. *British Medical Journal*, **299**, 442–8.

Rogers, M.C. (1987) *Textbook of Paediatric Intensive Care*, Williams and Wilkins, Baltimore.

Royal College of Physicians (1987) Resuscitation from cardiopulmonary arrest: training and organisation. *Journal of the Royal College of Physicians*, **21**(3), 175–82.

Stark, J. and de Leval, M.R. (1983) *Surgery of Congenital Heart Defects*, Grune and Stratton, London.

Sumner, E. (1989) Anaesthesia for patients with cardiac disease, in *Textbook of Paediatric Anaesthesia Practice*, (eds E. Sumner and D.J. Hatch), Baillière Tindall, London, pp. 305–38.

Zideman, D.A. (1986) ABC of resuscitation: resuscitation of infants and children. *British Medical Journal*, **292**, 1584–8.

Zideman, D.A. (1989) Resuscitation in paediatrics, in *Textbook of Paediatric Anaesthetic Practice*, (eds E. Sumner and D.J. Hatch), Baillière Tindall, London, pp. 555–77.

Care of the child with neurological needs

6

Carolyn Davies

The management of the child requiring neurological intensive care offers a great challenge to the paediatric nurse. Prompt action supported by adequate knowledge of the condition will ensure optimal recovery for the child. Slow, inappropriate action by inexperienced staff may have disastrous results, and consequently there is no place for such a nurse within the paediatric intensive care unit caring for the neurologically sick child.

Care of the neurologically sick child requires nurses to be expert in many things. First, they must be experienced in nursing children, able to distinguish between the differing cries of a baby, knowing what developmental stage a child should have reached physically and cognitively for his or her age, and able to talk honestly and empathetically with the parents of a sick child.

Secondly, they must have excellent nursing skills. A child with a major neurological deficit requires comprehensive nursing support and this must be undertaken with the greatest of care and efficiency to prevent unnecessary disturbance to the child.

Finally, they must be well informed about the child and the family they are caring for, aware of the altered physiology caused by the disease process and its management, and experienced in operating the extensive and complicated equipment used within the unit.

CENTRAL NERVOUS SYSTEM ANATOMY

To interpret the signs and symptoms of injury or disease to the brain, it is important to have a basic understanding of the complex structures of the brain and their function.

The brain is encased by the skull, the outer layer of which is the periosteum. Connecting the skull to the periosteum is a layer of loose connective tissue forming a potential space. The brain is enveloped by three distinct membranes or meninges: the pia mater, the arachnoid mater and the dura mater. Two structures formed from the dura mater extend into the brain fissures; the falx cerebri and the tentorium. These structures help to protect the delicate tissues of the brain from shock and infection. The space between the arachnoid mater and the pia mater is referred to as the subarachnoid space and contains cerebrospinal fluid (CSF). The largest part of the brain is the cerebrum, which is divided into two hemispheres separated by the falx cerebri, which lies in the longitudinal fissure. The cerebellum lies at the back of the skull, separated from the cerebrum by the tentorium, which lies in the transverse fissure. The brain stem, consisting of the pons and medulla oblongata, lie beneath the cerebrum and in front of the cerebellum.

The cerebral ventricles and the subarachnoid space are filled with CSF, which is produced by the choroid plexus found in the four ventricles. It is reabsorbed by villi found on the arachnoid mater.

CSF acts as a buffer to the brain, cushioning it from injury, and also as an important means of transporting nutrients and removal of waste products.

Blood vessels, nerves and CSF pass through openings in the skull known as foramina. Two of the largest foramina are the tentorial notch, found just above the cerebellum, and the foramen magnum just below the brain stem, through which the spinal cord passes.

CENTRAL NERVOUS SYSTEM PHYSIOLOGY

The central nervous system is a complex organ not only maintaining its own components in balance, but coordinating the function of other organs within the body. It is constantly receiving, interpreting and acting on vital messages. This versatility makes it essential to life. Imbalance, due to disease or trauma, may have far-reaching consequences to the function of an individual as a whole.

The central nervous system consists of two parts: the brain and the spinal cord. The brain is encompassed by the skull which, except in the very young child, is a fixed and rigid structure. The major components of the brain are CSF, brain tissue and blood. Consisting of approximately 90% water, the brain is incompressible. As a result, a rise in volume of one of the components must be compensated for by a fall in volume of the others, to ensure tissue perfusion and to prevent ischaemic damage to the brain tissue (Ganong, 1985).

Autoregulation

This equilibrium is controlled by a process known as autoregulation, whereby tissues have the capacity to regulate their own blood flow by altering vascular resistance, and so compensate for alterations in perfusion pressure.

Arterioles in the brain are sensitive to change in metabolism. Local changes in oxygen and carbon dioxide levels and pH will result in an immediate response.

In normal health, individuals are able to compensate for minor changes in intracranial pressure (ICP); a rise in systemic blood pressure is proportional to the rise in ICP over a considerable range ensuring adequate cerebral perfusion pressures (CPP) at all times. The normal range of ICP is 0–15 mmHg, but this may vary greatly depending on the activity being undertaken by the individual. Strenuous exercise, straining and coughing may all cause temporary spikes in ICP.

In the young child whose skull sutures are not fused, a constantly rising ICP will result in the sutures separating and the skull expanding to accommodate and protect the swelling brain (hydrocephalus). In the older child, the sutures are fixed and only a certain amount of volume increase can be tolerated.

If the autoregulation mechanism becomes stressed, other compensatory systems come into play. These include:

1. reabsorption of CSF;
2. movement of CSF to the spinal compartment, where a reduction of blood in the extradural venous plexus prevents local increase in pressure;
3. ventricular collapse, with diversion of CSF to the spinal theca;
4. collapse of the major venous sinuses.

If treatment is delayed, a point will eventually be reached where the brain can no longer compensate for the increase in pressure and where the ICP exceeds the mean arterial pressure and cerebral blood flow falls, resulting in minor rises of ICP having catastrophic results on cerebral perfusion (Figure 6.1).

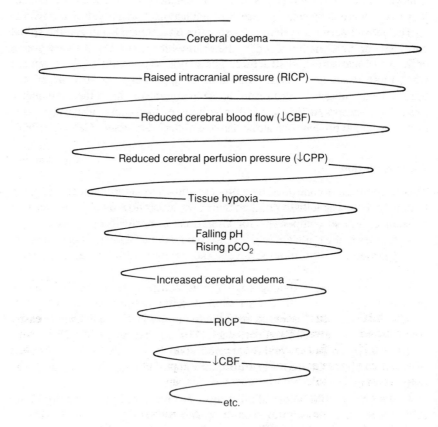

Figure 6.1 Effect of failure of compensatory mechanisms on cerebral perfusion. It is essential that this downhill spiral is broken if treatment is to be effective and death prevented.

The continuing rise in pressure will cause compression of the brain, resulting in poor or absent cerebral perfusion, hypoxia and tissue ischaemia. In the most severe cases, it may lead to herniation of the brain stem and ultimately death.

RAISED INTRACRANIAL PRESSURE

Causes

The causes of raised intracranial pressure can be summarized as follows:

1. *Space-occupying lesions*:
   (a) cerebral abscess;
   (b) primary tumours: medulloblastoma, cerebellar astrocytoma, brain stem glioma, choroid plexus papilloma, optic glioma, craniopharyngioma;
   (c) intracranial haemorrhage;
   (d) metastatic tumours;
   (e) invasive tumours (from outside the skull);
   (f) cysts;
2. *Hydrocephalus*:
   (a) obstruction of CSF flow due to tumour or adhesions;
   (b) thrombosis of venous sinuses;
   (c) thickening/adhesions of meninges (following meningitis);
   (d) congenital abnormalities of the brain;
3. *Acute encephalopathies*:
   (a) infections: viral, bacterial, fungal;
   (b) Ischaemic/anoxic states; near-miss cot death, cardiac arrest, drowning, strangulation, suffocation;
   (c) metabolic/toxic states: hypoglycaemia, renal failure, hepatic failure, hyperbilirubinaemia, hypercalcaemia, hypo/hypernatraemia, thyroid crisis, adrenal insufficiency, Reye's syndrome, scalds and burns, inborn errors of metabolism;
4. *Head injury*:
   (a) trauma,
   (b) non-accidental injury.

Signs and symptoms

The signs and symptoms of raised ICP are given in Table 6.1.

Testing for doll's eye reflex

1. Hold the patient's eyes open.

Table 6.1 Signs and symptoms of raised intracranial pressure

Sign/symptom	Area of brain affected	Comments
Papilloedema	Optic nerve (II)	Caused by: Engorgement of retinal veins Reddening of the optic disc Blurring of the disc margins Retinal haemorrhage
Convergent strabismus	Abducens nerve (VI), midbrain	Caused by direct pressure on the abducens nerve
Dilated non-reactive pupils	Oculomotor nerve (III), midbrain	Caused by compression at the tentorial hiatus results in paralysis of the occulomotor nerve
Doll's eye reflex	Lower pons, vestibular nuclei (VIII)	Positive doll's eye reflex determines the status of the VIII, VI and III cranial nerves and their brain stem pathways
Vomiting	Vomiting centre, reticular formation, medulla oblongata	Direct pressure on the medulla stimulates the vomiting centre
Headache	Whole	General pressure of the whole of the brain causes headache, which is exacerbated by lying down, coughing and bending
Altered respiratory patterns	Cerebral cortex voluntary system, pons/medulla automatic system	
Cheyne–Stokes respiration	Cerebral hemispheres	Cheyne–Stokes respiration: periodic breathing alternating deep breathing with apnoeic episodes

Table 6.1 *(cont'd)*

Sign/symptom	Area of brain affected	Comments
Central neurogenic respiration	Low midbrain, upper pons	Central neurogenic hyperventilation: regular deep rhythm
Apneustic respiration	Mid/low pons	Apneustic breathing: characterized by pauses between full inspiration and expiration
Cluster breathing	Low pons, high medulla	Cluster breathing: irregular gasping breaths
Ataxic breathing	Medulla	Irregular pattern with periods of apnoea and shallow breathing
Poor temperature control Anterior response to heat Posterior response to cold	Hypothalamus	Large swings between hypothermia and hyperthermia may occur if the hypothalamus is directly affected
Posturing Decorticate	Areas above the brain stem	Decorticate means 'without cortex' and is demonstrated by flexion of the upper limbs and extension of the lower limbs
Decerebrate	Areas below the brain stem	Decerebrate means 'without cerebrum' and is demonstrated by stiff extension of the upper limbs with the palms turned outwards and extension of the lower limbs

Table 6.2 Intracranial pressure monitoring devices

Type	Advantages	Disadvantages
Intraventricular catheter	Most accurate measurement of ICP CSF can be drained or sampled easily Easy access for drug administration Volume/pressure response estimation Passage through open anterior fontanelle in young infants, therefore negating need for burr hole	Invasive technique, risk of infection increases with length of monitoring Slight risk of intracranial haemorrhage following catheter insertion Location of lateral ventricle may be difficult if there is ventricular collapse or midline shift due to swelling Catheter blockage due to blood, CSF, brain tissue
	Measurement of ICP direct from CSF	Iatrogenic drainage of CSF may cause herniation if three-way taps are placed incorrectly Requires frequent calibration
Subarachnoid screw	Does not require penetration of the cerebral tissue	Invasive technique, risk of infection increases with length of monitoring Difficult to drain large volumes of CSF Screw may become occluded with blood or tissue Requires frequent calibration Not possible in children under 6 months as the vault of the skull is too thin to support the screw
	CSF can be drained and samples taken Comparatively easy to insert; can be done at the bedside	
Epidural sensor	Less invasive, therefore reduced risk of infection Sensor cannot be occluded with blood or tissue Comparatively easy to insert	Cannot drain or sample CSF Does not measure pressure directly from CSF space Not possible to recalibrate system after insertion, making readings unreliable
Intraparenchymal fibreoptic transducer	Very accurate Comparatively easy to insert Transducer cannot be occluded with blood or tissue Self-calibrating Does not require fluid-filled system, therefore artefact is reduced Reduced risk of infection	Catheter is very fragile Dedicated equipment is necessary Invasive technique, small risk of bleeding or infection Cannot drain or sample CSF (kit available for ventriculostomy with transducer-tipped catheter)
Transfontanelle monitoring (fontanometer)	Non-invasive Simple to apply Good correlation with CSF pressures	Cannot drain or sample CSF May interfere with ultrasonography

2. Watching the eyes carefully, turn the patient's head quickly but gently to one side and then the other.
3. If the patient's eyes do not move in their sockets, the doll's eye reflex is absent.
4. If the patient's eyes move conjugately toward the inner and outer canthi, the doll's eye reflex is present.

Intracranial pressure monitoring

ICP monitoring devices (Table 6.2) provide valuable information in the management of patients with raised ICP. This information is accurate only if the equipment used is calibrated appropriately and when necessary altered with changes of the patient's position. The type of device chosen will also dictate whether or not the patient needs transfer to the operating theatre for insertion, which is an important consideration in the very unstable patient.

Once *in situ*, calibrated and working effectively, the system will give continuous information about the patient's ICP and cerebral perfusion. Normal ICP ranges from 0 to 15 mmHg.

Healthy individuals may have 'spikes' in ICP as a result of normal activities such as coughing, sneezing and straining; as long as these spikes are transient, no ill effects will be incurred. When ICP rises and is sustained above normal limits, regulatory mechanisms fail and cerebral blood flow becomes directly dependent on CPP. Rising ICP and falling systemic blood pressure result in a fall in CPP and, if prolonged, cerebral ischaemia. Studies in children have demonstrated that CPP must be maintained above 40 mmHg to prevent neurological sequelae (Tasker *et al.*, 1988).

Cerebral perfusion pressure is calculated as follows:

$$CPP = MAP - ICP$$

where MAP = mean arterial pressure.

Nursing responsibilities

In monitoring a patient's ICP, the trend of pressure readings may be more important than individual readings: therefore, regular recording of ICP, MAP, CPP and central venous pressure (CVP) are essential. Early recognition of rising pressures will enable clinicians to institute more aggressive management. Other responsibilities will include regular checks of the catheter insertion site to ensure that there is no local infection or leakage of CSF, and maintenance of connecting tubing to prevent it from becoming kinked, trapped or taut.

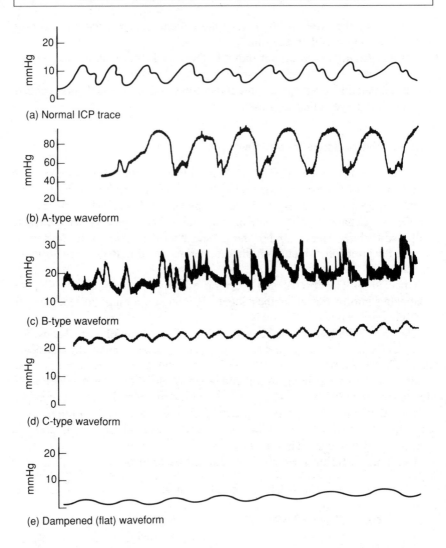

(a) Normal ICP trace

(b) A-type waveform

(c) B-type waveform

(d) C-type waveform

(e) Dampened (flat) waveform

Figure 6.2 Intracranial pressure waveforms.

Interpreting intracranial pressure waveforms

The ICP waveform should be clear and well defined. It may reflect the respiratory and haemodynamic patterns within its trace; this is normal (Figure 6.2). The waveform demonstrates a steep upward slope (systole) followed by a downward slope (diastole), which may be interrupted by a small pulse wave (dicrotic notch). Dampened waveforms will occur if the catheter becomes occluded in any way. Common problems are blockage due to blood or swelling brain tissue and kinking of the catheter. Alarm limits should be set to respond if the pressure exceeds 20 mmHg.

The intracranial waveform will be affected by changes in intrathoracic pressure as well as changes in intracranial pressure. Transient changes in ICP can generally be tolerated provided the circulating blood volume is adequate to support cerebral perfusion. Sustained spikes in pressure must be treated immediately. If a continuous trace of the ICP is being recorded, it is useful to indicate on it when procedures are undertaken so that the patient's response can be evaluated retrospectively.

A waves demonstrate a sharp rise, plateau and fall in ICP. Pressures may rise as high as 50–100 mmHg. They are often seen as a temporary response to noxious stimuli, e.g. airway suctioning or pain. If they are sustained, they may be associated with a decreasing cerebral compliance and increasing neurological deficit. They must be treated without delay.

B waves demonstrate sharp rises in ICP occurring every 0.5–2 min. The rises are not sustained, but occasionally precede A waves.

C Waves are rapid, small and rhythmic. They fluctuate with changing haemodynamics and respiration, and indicate limited ability for further compensation.

Intensive nursing care of the child with raised intracranial pressure

To establish a baseline for observations and progress, it is important to take a detailed nursing history of the child's physical and cognitive development from the parents or other close relatives. In the case of younger children, this should include details such as sounds or words the child is able to verbalize, whether the child can sit, stand or walk, and what fine motor skills have been mastered. It is often wise to warn parents at this stage that their child may regress following illness, but that with stimulation and encouragement may quickly reachieve their milestones. This period of history taking gives the nurse a unique opportunity to form a relationship with parents and family and to identify any predisposing factors of the child's illness that may be of use in the planning of care. The nurse should briefly explain to the parents what they might expect to occur over the next few days, what their role may be in the care of their child, and what accommodation and facilities are available for them and their family. It will also give the parents an opportunity to ask questions regarding the management of the child and to clarify any points they may have misunderstood in previous interviews.

When planning care for a critically ill child, it is usual to organize therapies and care to coincide, minimizing disturbance of the child and maximizing periods of rest. This clustering of care is appropriate for the child with raised ICP, but consideration must be taken of the type and frequency of the procedures being undertaken as, in the unstable patient, the most routine of procedures may result in a sharp rise in ICP and consequent cerebral ischaemia.

Before the formation of a plan of care, an overall assessment of the child should be made and baseline observations of vital signs measured and recorded. These should include pulse rate, blood pressure, respiratory rate, and peripheral and core temperature. Neurological observations will include the child's level of consciousness, orientation, alertness, ability to remember, coordination, strength of limbs, pupil size and reaction to light.

Glasgow coma scale

The Glasgow coma scale, which is simple to learn, is a quick way to assess and evaluate a person's level of consciousness. Its use is limited in children, whose cognitive development and language skills are limited by age, and it therefore requires adaptation.

The Glasgow coma scale (Table 6.3) measures three neurological reactions: motor control, verbal response and eye opening. Each response assumes a score, the total of which can be used as a guide to the level of consciousness. The higher the score, the greater the level of consciousness. Changes in score indicate deterioration or improvement in condition and can be used as a method of on-going evaluation of a patient's neurological status (Teasdale and Jennett, 1974).

A child's maturity must be taken into account when calculating Glasgow coma scores. A sick child admitted to a strange environment, surrounded by

Table 6.3 Glasgow coma scale

	Adult scale (> 10 years)	Score	Paediatric scale (0–10 years)
Best eye-opening response	Spontaneously	4	Spontaneously
	To speech	3	To speech
	To pain	2	To pain
	None	1	None
Best verbal response	Orientated	5	Orientated
	Confused conversation	4	Words
	Inappropriate speech	3	Vocal sounds
	Incomprehensible sounds	2	Cries
	None	1	None
Best motor response	Obeys commands	5	Obeys commands
	Localizes pain	4	Localizes pain
	Flexion to pain	3	Flexion to pain
	Extension to pain	2	Extension to pain
	None	1	None

Table 6.4 Normal aggregate scores for children

Age	Maximum score
Birth to 6 months	9
6 months to 1 year	11
1–2 years	12
2–5 years	13
5 years upwards	14

unfamiliar people, may be unwilling to cooperate, although there may be no neurological deficit. Neonates and infants cannot speak or obey commands. Table 6.4 indicates the maximum score to be expected at differing ages (Simpson and Reilly, 1982)

Management of raised intracranial pressure

Guidelines for the managment of raised ICP are summarized in Figure 6.3. A nursing care plan is given in Table 6.5.

The objective of management is to increase the ratio of cerebral oxygen supply to cerebral oxygen demand. By reducing the ICP below 20 mmHg and maintaining CPP above 50 mmHg (Frewen *et al.*, 1985) this can be achieved. In the case of neonates and infants, where the mean arterial blood pressure is an average of 60 mmHg, parameters of 10 mmHg for ICP and 40 mmHg for CPP should be used (Levene and Evans, 1985; Rogers *et al.*, 1980).

Hyperventilation

Elective intubation and ventilatory support inducing the state of hyperventilation helps to lower raised ICP by reducing alveolar carbon dioxide levels. Reducing circulating carbon dioxide levels causes vasoconstriction and a resultant decrease in cerebral blood flow. Hyperventilation must be carefully controlled and monitored by frequent arterial blood gas estimations. The aim of hyperventilation is to maintain the P_{aCO_2} between 3.3 and 4.0 kPa and the P_{aO_2} between 12 and 13.3 kPa. Assuming the child has a normal haemoglobin concentration and an adequate mean arterial pressure, this will provide an adequate oxygen supply to vital organs. The P_{aCO_2} should not be brought below 2.7 kPa as this will cause severe vasoconstriction leading to cerebral lactic acidosis and cerebral ischaemia. In hand-ventilation of a patient with raised ICP, the circuit should include a capnograph monitor so that the operator is able to control the amount of carbon dioxide displaced. A reduction in P_{aCO_2} may also be achieved by ensuring that the dead space of the ventilatory tubing is kept to a minimum.

Table 6.5 Nursing care plan for raised intracranial pressure

Child problem/need	Aim	Nursing care	Rationale
Inappropriate breathing pattern due to raised ICP	Maintain a patent airway to ensure adequate gaseous exchange	Endotracheal suction as required Instillation of saline before suction as required Humidify ventilator gases to temperature of 35–36°C Ensure endotracheal tube is secure and fixed comfortably	Humidity and saline instillation will dilute secretions, easing aspiration Endotracheal aspiration will remove secretions, ensuring patency of tube A secure endotracheal tube will prevent accidental extubation and prevent trauma to the airway
	Hyperventilate to maintain arterial blood gases at P_aO_2 12–13.3 kPa P_aCO_2 3.3–4.0 kPa	Check that ventilator settings are set as prescribed Observe and record oxygen saturation Assist with blood gas sampling Observe and record capnograph readings Use capnograph in hand-ventilation circuit	Regular checks of the ventilator settings will prevent accidental change Regular checks of blood gas status ensures that hyperventilation is maintained at appropriate levels The capnograph should be used in the hand-ventilation circuit to prevent P_aCO_2 levels falling too low
Reduced cerebral perfusion due to raised ICP	Maintain intracranial pressure at 0–15 mm Hg Maintain cerebral perfusion pressure above 50 mmHg Prevent spikes in ICP Improve patient's level of consciousness	Observe and record ICP/CPP Immediately report any significant change in pressures Evaluate ICP monitor trace for accuracy and calibrate monitor when necessary Evaluate child's level of consciousness using an agreed formula, e.g. paediatric Glasgow coma scale	Rapid response to rising ICP and falling CPP will afford maximal protection of brain tissue integrity Trends in observations are as important as sudden changes and may indicate a need for change of management Calibration of all equipment is essential in providing accurate information

Table 6.5 *(cont'd)*

Child problem/need	Aim	Nursing care	Rationale
		Observe and record as required: response to sedation, pupil size/reaction, spontaneous movement, response to noxious stimuli, seizures, cerebral function monitoring	Constant evaluation of the child's condition against agreed parameters will enable nurses to measure the effectiveness of care and note any improvement or deterioration in the child's condition
		Observe and record as required all haemodynamic parameters, noting response to stimuli	
Sudden rise in ICP associated with a fall in CPP	Prevent cerebral ischaemia	Hand-ventilate patient maintaining end-tidal CO_2 above 3.3 kPa	Hyperventilation 'blows off' excess carbon dioxide causing vasoconstriction and a reduction of ICP; if too much is blown off, cerebral perfusion can be compromised
		Check patient's level of consciousness and if necessary administer additional sedation	Increased level of consciousness will increase cerebral metabolism increasing the oxygen demand and resulting in increased cerebral blood flow causing a rise in ICP
		Inform medical practitioner Check child's airway is not obstructed	
		Check the child's head is in the midline position and that the neck vessels are not obstructed	
		Assist in the administration of mannitol if prescribed	Mannitol is a hypertonic solution, which creates an osmotic gradient causing water to move from the brain tissue into capillaries; its action is rapid and the resultant loss of fluid reduces ICP
		Note the CPP and the time it is below an acceptable level (Figure 6.3)	Low CPP is associated with poor prognosis

Table 6.5 *(cont'd)*

Child problem/need	Aim	Nursing care	Rationale
Inability to cough due to intubation and ventilation	Prevent stasis of secretions Prevent secondary infection	Assist physiotherapist with chest therapy Ensure that patient is sedated before the procedure Observe child for marked rises in vital signs during procedure Take remedial action on any rise in ICP Endotracheal aspiration to be performed quickly and efficiently	Because of the patient's immobility and inability to cough, secretions will pool in dependent parts of the lungs, creating a reservoir for bacteria and increasing the risk of infection Because of the noxious stimulation of physiotherapy and the resultant endotracheal aspiration, it is essential that the patient is heavily sedated to prevent spikes in ICP Aspiration of secretions results in a fall in P_aO_2 and rise in P_aCO_2 resulting in cerebral vasodilation and a rise in ICP
Inability to move due to brain injury and use of muscle relaxants	Prevent obstruction of neck vessels Prevent contracture deformities Prevent pressure sores	Elevate head of bed to an angle of 30° Nurse in midline position Support head in midline with sandbags Nurse limbs in neutral position Log roll patient when turning using at least two nurses Undertake a full range of passive exercises as tolerated Assess pressure points and turn as necessary Utilize pressure-relieving aids as required, e.g. mattress overlays	Elevation of the bedhead enhances gravitational venous outflow from the head Nursing the patient with the head midline ensures that cerebral venous outflow is not obstructed by jugular compression leading to a rise in ICP Passive exercise will prevent contraction deformity by maintaining the full range of joint/limb movement Relief of pressure points will prevent tissue ischaemia by ensuring adequate perfusion of the tissue; relief of pressure results in rebound hyperaemia

Table 6.5 (cont'd)

Child problem/need	Aim	Nursing care	Rationale
Altered haemodynamic status due to fluid restriction	Maintain fluid balance as prescribed by clinician Maintain adequate cardiac output Preserve renal function Diagnose inappropriate antidiuretic hormone secretion promptly	Monitor all fluid input hourly, ensuring that input remains within prescribed volume Include all drug volumes in hourly input Monitor all output hourly, include blood samples in output Ensure that a minimum of 1 ml/kg per hr of urine is produced Perform urinanalysis 4-hourly Monitor and record as required the heart rate and rhythm, blood pressure, CVP and respiratory effort 4-hourly measurement of blood glucose	Fluid restriction reduces the overall circulating volume of the body, helping to reduce cerebral blood volume and reducing ICP 50–75% of normal maintenance is the usual fluid restriction imposed; this may be reduced further if the situation requires it Urine output less than 1 ml/kg per h may indicate underperfusion of the kidneys and impending renal failure; increased fluids or the introduction of an inotrope or diuretic to the drug regimen may alleviate this Continuous monitoring of the child's haemodynamic status is essential for rapid assessment of condition
Inability to control temperature due to brain tissue injury	Maintain normothermia: 36–37°C Maintain 1°C difference between peripheral and central temperature	Measure and record peripheral and central temperatures Utilise heating or cooling blanket when necessary Use tepid sponge to reduce pyrexia Administer antipyretic agents if prescribed	Hyperthermia causes vasodilation of cerebral vessels and a consequent rise in ICP Hyperthermia causes a rise in cerebral metabolism with a consequent rise in oxygen requirement Large differences in core and peripheral temperature indicate peripheral vascular shutdown

Table 6.5 *(cont'd)*

Child problem/need	Aim	Nursing care	Rationale
Inability to care for own hygiene needs	Promote hygiene Prevent secondary infection	Bed bath daily or as necessary Change nappy as necessary Include parents in child's hygiene care Clean teeth and mouth 4–6 hourly Clean urinary catheter site 4–6 hourly Observe intravenous arterial and ICP monitoring sites for signs of infection; change dressings according to unit policy	Regular attention to the hygiene needs of the patient will prevent the build-up of bacteria and reduce risk of opportunistic infection Participation of family members in the child's care will help to reduce their feelings of isolation
Disorientation due to reduced level of consciousness	Maintain orientation as far as possible	Establish relationship with child by talking to him or her especially before procedures Provide a controlled environment for the child, preventing unnecessary disturbance Define different times of the day, e.g. darken the room at night Include parents in care	Continuity of care and orientation of the patient will help to prevent intensive care psychosis and speed the patient's convalescence Parents will provide ongoing continuity and security for the child
Inability to blink due to effect of muscle relaxants	Prevent corneal ulceration Prevent secondary infection	Clean eyes 4–6 hourly Ensure eyes are closed and protected	Damage to the cornea will be prevented if the eyes are kept moist and free from infection

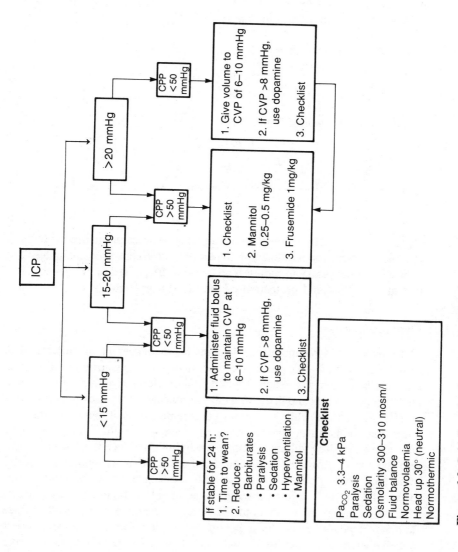

Figure 6.3 Guidelines for the management of raised intracranial pressure.

Carbon dioxide excess and oxygen deprivation will cause cerebral vasodilation and a resultant increase in cerebral blood flow, and should be avoided at all costs (Figure 6.4). Nursing care will include the maintenance of a clear airway and monitoring of end-tidal volume, carbon dioxide levels, oxygen saturation and transcutaneous P_{aCO_2} and P_{aO_2}.

Increased cerebral blood flow $\uparrow P_{CO_2}$

$\downarrow P_{O_2}$

$\downarrow$ pH

Decreased cerebral blood flow $\downarrow P_{CO_2}$

$\uparrow P_{O_2}$

$\uparrow$ pH

Figure 6.4 Effect of changing blood gas pressures on cerebral blood flow

Hyperventilation before airway suctioning may be necessary to prevent hypoxic episodes. Patient cooperation with hyperventilation cannot be guaranteed and so it will be necessary to paralyse and sedate the patient to guarantee effective management and protection of the respiratory field.

Fluid management

The correct fluid balance is critical in the management of children with raised ICP. Small changes in volume may have catastrophic effects on the child's cerebral perfusion. Calculations of fluids required will be based on the child's weight and in the first days of management be severely restricted to 50–75% of the child's normal requirements. It is essential that the nurse maintains strict control over the infusions, which may be many and varied. All drug volumes, maintenance fluids and feed must be calculated into the daily allowance and recorded hourly. Urinary output is equally important, and output should be at least 1 ml/kg per h. Continuous monitoring of CVP will give an accurate assessment of the child's fluid status. The use of intravenous mannitol 2C% and frusemide will help to reduce fluid overload. Mannitol is a potent hypertonic solution, causing water to move from the brain tissue into the capilliaries to be excreted. If the blood–brain barrier is compromised, there is a risk that mannitol will enter the brain, causing rebound cerebral oedema. It is essential that patients receiving mannitol are carefully monitored and that the drug is not used indiscriminately (Levene and Evans, 1985). Both mannitol and frusemide have been shown to reduce the formation of CSF. Serum and urine osmolality will be checked regularly by clinicians. The serum osmolality should be maintained at 300–310 mmol/l. Inappropriate antidiuretic hormone secretion is a common complication of patients with raised ICP and should be suspected in the hyponatraemic patient if urine osmolality is higher than serum osmolality.

Intravenous colloid or inotropes may be used where the mean systemic arterial blood pressure falls and adequate cerebral perfusion cannot be guaranteed.

Barbiturate coma

If hyperventilation and osmotherapy fail, rising ICP may be controlled by inducing a barbiturate coma. Barbiturates are known to reduce cerebral metabolic rate with a resultant reduction in cerebral blood flow and ICP:

Barbiturate coma

↓

Lowers cerebral metabolic rate

↓

Lowers cerebral blood flow

↓

Lowers intracranial pressure

Phenobarbitone and thiopentone are the most common drugs of choice.

Because maximum cerebral swelling may not occur for up to 72 h (depending on the child's condition), barbiturate therapy is continued for 3–4 days. During this time, serum drug levels should be checked to ensure that they have reached the appropriate therapeutic range. The long-term action of phenobarbitone hinders the process of neurological assessment and must be taken into account for 2–3 days after administration has been stopped or reduced.

NEUROLOGICAL TESTS

Brain scan

Brain scanning involves the administration of a radioactive isotope to the child. A gamma camera scans the head, measuring the X-rays emitted by the circulating isotope, recording their distribution. Dark contrast indicates a high uptake of radioactivity. The brain is normally an area of low isotope uptake, with the scalp and venous sinuses being highly defined.

Interpreting results

Areas of contrast, where uptake of the isotope is high, may indicate cerebral haemorrhage, haematoma, arteriovenous malformations or a tumour. Low-contrast areas may indicate decreased perfusion, infarcted brain tissue or lesions such as an abscess.

Nursing care

Brain scanning requires the child to be moved to a scanning room, and it is therefore essential that appropriate transportable monitoring equipment is available. The child must be accompanied by a qualified nurse trained in the care and observation of neurologically ill children. A complete explanation of the procedure should be given to the child and the family. The procedure may be lengthy and so the child's complete cooperation should be sought. Where compliance cannot be guaranteed, sedation may be necessary. If sedation is contraindicated, elective intubation and ventilation is instituted.

Radiation hazard is minimal. Normal precautions used on the ward, such as the wearing of gloves for the handling of excreta, are usually all that is necessary.

Computed tomography

An X-ray scanner takes serial images around an axial plane of the child's head. The computer then calculates the density to X-rays of points inside the cranium. Results are presented as pictures similar to radiographs. High-density structures such as bone show as white images, and low-density structures such as CSF as black images. Tissue is demonstrated in varying shades of grey. White matter is less dense than grey matter and can therefore be distinguished from it.

Interpreting results

Computed tomography (CT) scanning can be used for whole body imaging. It gives clear outlines of body structures such as bones and organs. Head scans give only information about the structures within the cranium. They can indicate shifts in structures due to swelling, haemorrhage and tumours, but do not afford information about the functional capacity of those structures. CT is an important tool in the diagnosis of cerebral oedema and in differentiating between cerebral contusion and haematoma following head injury.

Nursing care

This procedure requires transfer to a specialist unit and the same care must be exercised in the movement and observation of the patient as for brain scanning.

The procedure requires the patient to be completely still for a long time; it is not painful, but requires the head to be secured. The movement of the large scanning equipment around the patient may be distressing and frightening, making the child uncooperative. Sedation and/or intubation, depending on the child's condition, may be necessary to ensure a well defined scan.

Metal objects that fix intubation headgear or ventilating tubes must be avoided as metal deflects X-rays and affects the quality of the scan.

The nurse supervising the child and any others present during scanning should be protected in the normal way for X-ray imaging.

Electroencephalography

Information on the brain is transmitted by means of electrical currents. Although these electrical impulses are small, they can be detected by electro-encephalography (EEG).

EEG is a non-invasive means of recording brain activity. Electrical impulses generated by the cerebral cortex are sensed by electrodes fixed to the scalp of the patient. Each electrode produces a line trace representing activity in part of the cerebral cortex. This trace is then interpreted by trained personnel.

Interpreting results

The EEG is most commonly used in the diagnosis of epilepsy. It may also be used in the diagnosis and prognosis formation in other disease processes affecting cortical function.

Anoxia or *encephalopathy* will result in gross slow activity. It is necessary to complete a series of recordings over a period of time to identify a trend. An increase in frequency may be the result of a return of cortical function. Decrease in frequency indicates further loss of cortical function. No improvement over a 24 h period is strongly indicative of a poor prognosis (Boyd, 1989).

Intracerebral pathology, e.g. multiple emboli, disseminated intravascular coagulopathy or herpes simplex encephalitis, may result in focal or multifocal abnormalities. If these discharges persist over a period of days it is strongly indicative of permanent local damage. A series of follow-up EEGs may be helpful in assessing the child's potential (Boyd and Harden, 1991).

Loss of cerebral function will be demonstrated by isoelectric or near isoelectric (flat) tracings. Large doses of CNS depressants may produce a near-isoelectric trace and it is essential that drug levels are monitored before performing an EEG. EEG may be used in association with other tests to confirm brain death (Cole, 1991). Isoelectric traces recorded for 20–30 min on two occasions at least 12 h apart indicate irreversible loss of cerebral function.

Nursing care

The procedure should be explained to the child and the parents. It is important that the child is still during the test. The EEG technician must be made aware of any medication that the child has received as it may affect the results.

The nurse may be required to provide stimulus to the child, and this may be in the form of a noise or more noxious stimuli depending on the child's level of consciousness.

Electrical equipment being used to monitor the child occasionally causes artefacts on the trace; in such cases it will be necessary to turn some equipment off. Essential monitoring devices should not be disturbed.

After the procedure, cleaning of the scalp and hair will be required.

Cortical evoked potentials

Stimulation of sensory organs results in the transmission of electrical messages to the cerebral cortex. These electrical events have characteristic patterns, which can be measured in positive and negative waveforms. They are described as primary evoked potentials.

The following techniques can be performed, when necessary, at the child's bedside.

Cortical evoked potentials (CEP) include brain stem auditory evoked potentials (BAEP), somatosensory evoked potentials (SEP) and visual evoked potentials (VEP).

CEP provide information about neuron transmission along specific pathways of the brain. CEPs are not affected by drugs such as barbiturates.

Brain stem auditory evoked potentials

Auditory stimuli are delivered to each ear. The potentials resulting from transmission of the sound to the brain via the auditory pathway are recorded. It is essential that the physician is aware of the patient's normal auditory function and checks that the auditory canals are clear before commencement of the test.

This test demonstrates function in the posterior portion of the brain stem. It may be used to aid diagnosis of brain stem death (Steinhart and Weiss, 1985).

Somatosensory evoked potentials

This technique is used to supplement other tests. It provides information about a limited area of the cerebral cortex. The technique involves stimulation of the upper and lower limbs. Recordings demonstrate neuron transmission from the spinal cord to the brain. Results are useful in providing information about lesions of the spinal cord and brain stem (Boyd and Harden, 1991).

Visually evoked potentials

Visual stimuli are delivered to the patient in the form of flashing lights. Electrical activity from the occipital cortex is measured in response to the retinal stimuli. Flash VEP provide information about the visual cortical areas and the specific sensory pathway. This is most often used after the acute stage of illness to assess visual function.

GUILLAIN–BARRÉ SYNDROME (infective or idiopathic polyneuritis)

Guillain–Barré syndrome is a rapidly progressing neuropathy characterized by the absence of tendon reflexes, motor weakness and an increase in CSF protein levels without an associated rise in cell count (Winer, 1987). The syndrome may occur at any age and its incidence shows a male to female ratio of 2:1. Guillain–Barré syndrome is the commonest form of peripheral neuropathy affecting children (Brett, 1991).

A high percentage of patients (50–75%) will have a history of a mild febrile illness preceding the onset of symptoms, and it is thought that the disease process may be the result of an autoimmune reaction (Levy et al., 1979).

Pathophysiology

In polyneuritis, the myelin sheath that surrounds the nerve axon (Figure 6.5) is damaged by an inflammatory response. The myelin sheath is formed from complex layers of the Schwann cell membrane which envelope the axon of the motor neurone acting as insulation to the nerve impulses passing along it. Nerve tissue is a relatively poor conductor, and demyelination of the axon results in failure of normal conduction, muscle weakness and paralysis.

The diagnosis of Guillain–Barré syndrome is made by a process of elimination. Paralysis caused by toxins, infection and metabolic imbalance must all be ruled out. The child with Guillain–Barré syndrome will present with some or all of the following (Winer, 1987):

1. Essential criteria:
   (a) Progressive weakness of two or more limbs (usually lower limbs and symmetrical),
   (b) Loss of tendon reflexes: areflexia,
   (c) Progression of illness with plateau by 4 weeks;

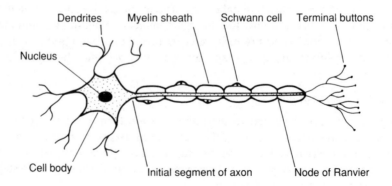

Figure 6.5 Structure of a neurone.

2. Supportive criteria:
   (a) Paraesthesia: pins and needles, numbness,
   (b) Cranial nerve involvement, most commonly the seventh nerve causing facial weakness; this may progress to the muscles controlling swallowing,
   (c) Autonomic system dysfunction resulting in tachycardia and unstable blood pressure,
   (d) Absence of fever at onset of neurological symptoms
   (e) CSF protein elevated after 1 week of symptoms with normal cell count
   (f) Slow nerve conduction.

Management

The potential for respiratory embarrassment means that a child presenting with features supporting a diagnosis of Guillain–Barré syndrome must be nursed within an environment where elective intubation and ventilation can be carried out promptly and easily.

Regular recording of vital signs should include monitoring of tidal volume and oxygen saturation; a fall in either or both parameters may indicate ascending paralysis with reduced ability to maintain adequate respiratory effort. Chest physiotherapy will help to prevent pooling of secretions in dependent lung fields, which would lead to consolidation and a risk of opportunistic infection. Where respiratory failure is suspected, arterial blood gas estimation will demonstrate a rising carbon dioxide level. If artificial ventilation is required, nasal intubation will be employed in the first instance; tracheostomy may be performed at a later date if a prolonged course of the illness is anticipated.

Nursing care of the child with Guillain–Barré syndrome is generally supportive. It is therefore essential that the nurses caring for the child are experienced and easily able to identify subtle changes in the child's physical and psychological condition.

Inability to move due to muscle weakness will result in the child being at risk of pressure sores, muscle wasting and joint contracture. In an attempt to prevent all of these complications, a regimen of passive and active exercises should be employed. Initial assessment will be undertaken by the physiotherapist, but passive exercises are an excellent way of actively including parents.

Frequent position changing, ensuring that limbs are nursed in neutral positions and the employment of support systems for pressure relief will all help to prevent complications of immobility.

In the initial stages of the child's illness it may be possible to continue with a normal diet. Allowing children to choose their own food includes them in planning their own care and gives them something to look forward to. It may also result in higher compliance with diet. Children should be positioned comfortably in an upright position for meals, as this will aid swallowing and digestion. Supervision during meals and drinks is essential in case of episodes of choking due to a reduced ability to swallow. Accurate knowledge of the child's weight is necessary to calculate drug and calorie requirements and the child should be weighed on a weekly basis.

Increasing bulbar palsy is an indication that oral feeding has to be abandoned and nasogastric or parenteral nutrition instituted. The involvement of a dietitian will ensure that a well balanced diet is provided to meet the child's nutritional requirements.

Autonomic instability is a recognized complication of Guillain–Barré syndrome (Winer, 1987; Cole and Matthew, 1987). For this reason, continuous monitoring of the child's ECG is important so that cardiac arrhythmias are identified early and treatment instituted promptly. Arrhythmias may occur spontaneously or more commonly as a result of stimulation, e.g. change of tracheostomy tube. It is important that an explanation of the function of this equipment is given to the child and the parents to alleviate fears they may have in association with complex monitoring equipment.

Restriction of the child's mobility may result in further complications related to elimination. Allowing the child to go to the toilet, where possible, will prevent embarrassment and preserve dignity, but it is important to have a nurse or other carer in close attendance. Ensuring an adequate fluid intake will prevent stasis of urine and a well balanced diet should provide enough roughage to prevent constipation.

Anxiety and frustration at their inability to move and control the environment will rank highly in children's response to illness and it is important that the nurse takes time to reassure the child on a frequent basis. An explanation in language the child can understand, coupled with encouragement to participate fully in activities where possible may occupy his or her attention and allay fears. As always, honesty is the key to a trusting relationship between child and nurse.

The course of the illness may run an unpredictable pattern. However, the severity of the symptoms will reach a plateau by the end of the second week in 50% of patients, the third week in 80% and the fourth week in 90%. Plasmapheresis has been used with some success in the treatment of Guillain–Barré syndrome, although its use continues to be controversial (Hughes *et al.*, 1981; Levy *et al.*, 1979; Cole and Matthew, 1987).

Intensive nursing and physiotherapy will prevent the complications associated with this debilitating disease and hasten recovery and rehabilitation. The majority of children will make a good functional recovery spontaneously within 12 months of onset of symptoms. Severity of symptoms and need for artificial ventilation are not necessarily an indication for poor prognosis (Cole and Matthew, 1987).

EPILEPSY

Epilepsy can be loosely divided into two groups: idiopathic, where the cause is unknown; and symptomatic, as the result of a disease state or following cerebral injury.

Clinically epilepsy is subdivided into three types: grand mal, petit mal and temporal lobe epilepsy. Each type demonstrates seizures of a characteristic pattern. Seizures are a result of sudden electrical discharge from neurones within the damaged area of the cortex. In managing epilepsy it is important to diagnose the underlying cause.

Where the treatment of epilepsy by conventional therapeutic means has failed and the child has continued seizures without regaining consciousness, or where individual seizures are prolonged, management within a paediatric intensive care setting is indicated, as continuance of such seizures is life threatening (Brown and Hussain, 1991).

Prolonged convulsions will result in the patient becoming shocked. Respiratory failure may be potentiated by the administration of anticonvulsant drugs, which have a direct effect on the respiratory centre of the brain stem.

Management

As with all children with life threatening illnesses, the first rule of management is the assessment of the airway, breathing pattern and circulation. In cases of status epilepticus, elective intubation and ventilation are indicated to protect the airway and ensure adequate oxygenation. Convulsive activity is associated with an increase in cerebral blood flow and metabolic activity which, in turn, leads to lactic acid build up, hypoxia and cerebral oedema leading to cerebral injury (Brown and Hussain, 1991). Until proved otherwise, the child should be managed using an RICP (raised intracranial pressure) protocol.

The use of paralysing agents for ventilation will stop clinical fits, and prevent fatigue and hyperpyrexia. Under such treatment, the only indication of a fit may be a sudden rise in blood pressure or heart rate. The use of continuous EEG or cerebral function monitor is therefore indicated for ease of management. The EEG may also be used to predict decreasing brain function due to cerebral damage (Boyd, 1989).

The nurse's responsibilities in the care of the child with status epilepticus will depend on the underlying cause and course of management. The need for close observation cannot be stressed enough. This should include vital signs, neurological assessment, blood sugar estimation, and observation for signs of raised ICP and convulsive activity, whether clinical or subclinical. Continuous monitoring of oxygen saturation will supplement information given by the regular assessment of arterial blood gases.

Drug therapy

By the time a child reaches intensive care with status epilepticus, it is likely that large doses of paraldehyde, phenytoin and diazepam will have been given. Further therapy will depend on the protocol of individual units. Whatever drug or group of drugs is administered, the need for close monitoring is paramount. Table 6.6 summarizes the anticonvulsant drugs used, their action and desired route of administration.

HEAD INJURY

Head injury continues to be a major cause of death and disability in children (Rosman *et al.*, 1983). In 1989 The Royal Society for the Prevention of Accidents (ROSPA) reported that 9000 children were killed as a result of cycling accidents; of these half were a direct consequence of head injury. Other causes may include road traffic accidents, physical child abuse, sporting accidents and falls.

Brain injury resulting from trauma to the head occurs in two phases. Primary brain injury occurs at the time of the trauma, and secondary injury is the sequelae to the initial damage.

Primary brain injury

Severity of brain damage will depend on the cause of the injury and whether

Table 6.6 Drugs used in the management of status epilepticus

Diazepam	Dose and route	Advantages and disadvantages
Diazepam	0.25–0.3 mg/kg IV 0.5 mg/kg rectally	Rapid effect with short duration Respiratory depressant Local irritation Rectal administration has unpredictable absorption Continuous infusions must be changed 4 hourly as diazepam binds to the plastic of the syringe

Phenytoin	10 mg/kg IV loading dose;
	  bolus must be given slowly
	  over 20 min
	5 mg/kg 1 h later
	Maintenance = 10 mg/kg
	  divided dose per 24 h
		Action in 20–30 min
		High pH requires administration via central line to prevent
		  tissue necrosis
		Rapid administration may result in arrythmias, bradycardias
		  and hypotension
		Levels must be monitored
		Does not cause depression of consciousness

Phenobarbitone	Loading dose 25 mg/kg IV stat dose
	10 mg/kg per 24 h IV
	5 mg/kg 12 hourly
	  adjust dose to maintain
	  plasma levels at 30–35 μg/ml
		Anticonvulsant without excessive sedation with normal dose
		Induction of barbiturate coma at high dose
		Long half-life of 3–5 days
		Causes respiratory depression
		Causes hypotension

Table 6.6 (cont'd)

	Dose and route	Advantages and disadvantages
Diazepam		
Thiopentone (2.5%)	5 mg/kg loading dose 4 mg/kg per h (70µg/kg per min to a maximum 400µg/kg per min)	Rapid action Short action Requires patient to be intubated and ventilated Causes hypotension Reduces cerebral metabolism and therefore reduces oxygen metabolism Reduces cerebral bood flow
Chlormethiazole (Heminevrin)	5–10 mg/kg per h Solution of 8 g/l in 4% dextrose	Reaction with certain plastic infusion sets Thrombophlebitis risk Causes fever and headaches Useful in resistant cases of status epilepticus
Paraldehyde	0.15–0.3 ml/kg intramuscularly or rectally	Causes drowsiness Induces coma Takes 20 min to work when given intramuscularly When given rectally may take up to 2 h to work Rectal doses should be mixed with equal parts of arachis oil Not recommended for intravenous use due to the risk of fat embolism in the lung and pulmonary haemorrhage May cause sterile abscess if given subcutaneously Dissolves plastic syringes

it was penetrating or blunt trauma. Primary brain injury may result in haemorrhage, contusion and neuronal sheering (Punt, 1989).

Haemorrhage may occur at any level within the brain or its surrounding structures. The majority of scalp swellings in older children are the result of subgaleal haematomas (Rosman *et al*., 1983), but in the newborn infant other causes must not be ruled out. These include caput succedaneum, cephalohaematoma and porencephalic cyst. Scalp lacerations should be sutured quickly, especially in the young child, as a significant volume of blood can be lost in a short time.

Contusion or bruising of the cerebral tissue most often occurs in acceleration/deceleration injury, when the force of the incident causes the internal structures of the brain to be forced against the rigid form of the cranial vault. Severe contusion will cause damage to the cortex and may present with focal seizures or neurological deficit. Lesions occurring directly beneath the site of impact are referred to as *coup* injury; those occurring on the opposite side to impact as a result of rebound action are referred to as *contracoup* injury.

Neuronal sheering is by far the most damaging element of primary brain injuries. Distortion of the brain tissues may lead to the creation of sheering forces between grey and white matter. This results in stretching of the nerve fibres which, consequently leads to impaired function. The brain stem reticular formation, which is responsible for consciousness, may also be affected. This condition is referred to as concussion. Where disturbance is minimal, recovery without neurological deficit can be expected; however, in severe cases of concussion, permanent damage may result (Punt, 1989).

Secondary brain injury

Intracranial *bleeding* may occur following a relatively minor head injury. The resultant swelling forms a space-occupying lesion which results in a rise in ICP. If the clot is not removed rapidly, the patient may die from cerebral compression leading to herniation. Urgent burr-hole exploration proceeding to craniotomy is indicated if an extradural clot is identified.

Children with subdural and extradural clots may not develop signs of brain haemorrhage for up to 12 h after injury (Punt, 1989). This is why children with seemingly trivial head injuries are often admitted to hospital and observed closely over 24 h.

Following head injury, intracellular water accumulates as a response to the trauma (cytotoxic *oedema*). Focal swelling may occur where the brain has areas of contusion. Management of the child with closed head injury and resultant cerebral oedema is on the same basis as the medical and nursing management of any child with raised ICP.

Seizures may be associated with head injury and occur within the first week after injury in approximately 5% of children who are admitted to hospital for management (Rosman *et al.*, 1983). Seizures as a result of head injury are treated in the same way as non-traumatic seizures, but drugs with a sedative effect should be avoided.

Skull fracture

Skull fractures can be divided into six main groups:

1. Linear
2. Depressed
3. Compound
4. Basal
5. Diastatic
6. 'Growing'

Approximately 75% of paediatric skull fractures are *linear* (Rosman *et al.*, 1983). They require no treatment but may be associated with intracranial bleeds, which require urgent medical treatment. Linear fractures of the temporal bone, in particular, result in extradural haematoma as the middle meningeal artery lies within this bone and damage to the integrity of the bone may result in the vessel being ruptured.

Depressed fractures occur when a portion of the skull is forced below its normal level. This can happen in two ways: first, as a result of complete fragmentation of a piece of bone and, secondly, if part of the skull is indented. (This is only seen in the newborn.)

Depressed skull fractures can result in contusion and laceration of the brain tissue and generally require surgical repair.

Compound skull fracture is associated with laceration of the scalp and damage to the dura. It requires urgent treatment as the risk of infection is extremely high. Management includes careful debridement of the wound and prophylactic antibiotic and tetanus therapy.

Basal skull fractures are difficult to diagnose by radiography because of the complex features represented on the film. Alternative signs such as peri-oribital or postaural bruising (battle sign) may be more indicative of a basal skull fracture (Rosman *et al.*, 1983). Meningitis is a recognized complication of basal skull fracture (Punt, 1989) due to damage of the dura causing CSF leakage into the nasal sinuses and middle ear (rhinorrhoea, otorrhoea). Radiography of the skull may demonstrate intracranial air (pneumocephaly).

Diastatic skull fracture is defined as traumatic separation of cranial bones at suture sites. It is most commonly seen in children under 4 years of age.

Growing skull fractures are cysts containing CSF at the site of linear or diastatic skull fractures which prevent fusion of the bone. They are most commonly seen in children under 3 years of age and require surgical repair.

Nursing management

The aim of management of a child with a head injury is to prevent secondary damage occurring to an already injured brain. The damaged brain does not tolerate sudden changes in physiological status and any deviation from normal parameters will result in increasing cerebral oedema and decreased cerebral perfusion. Baseline observations must be recorded as early as possible and should include a paediatric Glasgow coma score. Scores below 8 will require urgent intensive therapy (Raphaely et al., 1980) although consideration should be given to the child's age when using the Glasgow coma scale. Examination of the patient should rule out any other potentially serious injuries, and until proved otherwise injury to the cervical spine should be presumed.

Protection of the airway by intubation should be considered if there is any risk of anoxia. Nasal intubation should be avoided if a basal skull fracture is suspected. Once intubated, the child can be hyperventilated to aid reduction of ICP. The nose and ears must be observed for bleeding or CSF leakage.

A detailed history should be obtained from the child's carer and should include details of any loss of consciousness, complaints of dizziness or vomiting and the time and duration of these events.

Further management may include postoperative care and care based on that for a child with raised ICP.

REYE'S SYNDROME

Reye's syndrome is an acute encephalopathy of childhood associated with a high mortality rate. Its cause remains unknown but evidence suggests that a prodromal viral infection associated with the ingestion of salicylates may potentiate this serious illness (Chu et al., 1986).

Reye's syndrome is described as a biphasic illness (Glasgow, 1987), the first stage being a relatively trivial infection most commonly caused by varicella or influenza B virus. The child begins to vomit 3–4 days later. The vomiting becomes protracted and may contain altered blood. It is usually at this point that advice from the general practitioner is sought. The second stage of the illness progresses to neurological involvement, the child becoming drowsy and lethargic with the possible complication of convulsions. From this point it is essential that referral to a specialist unit is prompt and appropriate management instituted to prevent long-term sequelae and death.

Pathophysiology

Electron microscopy of cells shows severe disruption of mitochondrial function in the cells of the liver, resulting in abnormal amino acid and lipid metabolism and production of toxic substances such as ammonia (Glasgow, 1987).

Histology of tissue at autopsy shows fatty acid infiltration of the liver, kidney and myocardium. This disruption to normal hepatic function leads to further complications, including hypoglycaemia, prolonged prothrombin time and cerebral oedema.

Presentation

1. Mild viral illness.
2. Protracted vomiting for 3–4 days.
3. Unexplained convulsion.
4. Reduced level of consciousness.
5. Abnormal posturing in response to stimuli.
6. Collapsed child.
7. Near-miss cot death or sudden infant death syndrome.

Management

Successful management of this illness hinges on prompt diagnosis. The appropriate diagnostic tests are listed in Table 6.7. A number of studies have demonstrated the importance of swift referral to specialist units for management and how delay in diagnosis and transfer are associated with poor outcome (Dezateux *et al.*, 1986).

Table 6.7 Diagnostic tests for Reye's syndrome

	Values in Reye's syndrome	Upper limit of normal range
Blood glucose	Low	3.9–5.6 mmol/l
Blood ammonia	>3 × normal upper limit	50 μmol/l
Alanine aminotransferase (ALT)	>3 × normal upper limit	40 units/l
Aspartate Aminotransferase (AST)	>3 × normal upper limit	50 units/l
Prothrombin time	Extended beyond normal upper limit	3 s beyond control time

Specific management will include controlled hyperventilation, restriction of fluids while preserving an adequate circulating blood volume to maintain mean arterial pressure, and correction of hypoglycaemia and abnormal coagulopathy.

Table 6.8 Lovejoy's coma scale (modified)

Stage	Level of consciousness	Respiration	Response to pain	Pupils
1	Drowsy/lethargic	Normal	Appropriate	Normal
2	Restless/agitated	Rapid	Appropriate	Normal
3	Light coma	Rapid	Decorticate	Normal
4	Deepening coma	Variable	Decerebrate	Fixed/dilated
5	Deep coma	Apnoeic	Flaccid	Fixed/dilated

Expert nursing care will ensure minimal disturbance of the patient and reduce the risk of spikes of ICP and seizures. The nurse should observe for abnormal bleeding from puncture sites or stress ulceration and regularly measure the blood glucose level.

The patient's level of consciousness can be assessed using Lovejoy's coma staging (Table 6.8) (Lovejoy et al., 1975).

Stage 1 coma indicates conservative management, while a child at stage 2 and above will require aggressive management, particularly for raised ICP.

SUMMARY

The care and management of the child requiring neurological intensive care is constantly changing in response to the efforts of experts working and researching in the field. Important as this work is, it is virtually valueless unless those who have direct responsibility for the management of the child keep up to date and guarantee an optimum standard of care. A minimum requirement must be appropriately trained nursing and medical staff working within an environment where adequate support services can be provided (Standards for paediatric intensive care, Paediatric Intensive Care Society, UK, 1991, unpublished).

While planning the management of the neurologically sick child, the role of parents and close family as partners in care must not be underestimated. With time and support they can become active participants in their child's care, providing an element of continuity that, even with the best of efforts, nursing shifts prevent. In time it should give them the confidence to take on the challenge of prolonged rehabilitation, which may be necessary when their child leaves the intensive care unit. Although our work as intensive care nurses may end at this point, theirs is just beginning.

REFERENCES

Boyd, S. (1989) Paediatric clinical neurophysiology in the intensive care unit. *Care of the Critically Ill*, **5**, (6), 238–41.

Boyd, S.G. and Harden, A. (1991) Clinical neurophysiology of the central nervous system, in *Pediatric Neurology*, 2nd edn, Churchill Livingstone, Edinburgh, Chapter 25, pp. 717–95.

Brett, E.M. (1991) Neuromuscular disorders. II. Peripheral neuropathy, in *Paediatric Neurology*, 2nd edn, Churchill Livingstone, Edinburgh, Chapter 4, pp. 117–39.

Brown, J.K. and Hussain, I.H.M.I. (1991) Review article: status epilepticus. II: treatment. *Developmental Medicine and Child Neurology*, **33**, 97–109.

Chu, A.B. Nerurkar, L.S., Witzel, N. *et al.* (1986) Reye's syndrome: salicylate metabolism, viral antibody levels, and other factors in surviving patients and unaffected family members. *American Journal of Diseases in Childhood* **140**, 1009–12.

Cole, G.F. (1991) Acute encephalopathy of childhood, in *Paediatric Neurology*, 2nd edn, Churchill Livingstone, Edinburgh, Chapter 23, pp. 667–99.

Cole, G.F. and Matthew, D.J. (1987) Prognosis in severe Guillain Barré syndrome. *Archives of Disease in Childhood*, **62**, 288–91.

Dezateux, C.A., Dinwiddie, R., Helms, P. and Matthew, D.J. (1986) Recognition and early management of Reye's syndrome. *Archives of Disease in Childhood*, **61**, 647–51.

Frewen, T.C., Sumabat, W.O. and Del Maestro, R.F. (1985) Cerebral blood flow, metbolic rate and cross-brain oxygen consumption in brain injury. *Journal of Paediatrics*, **107**, 510–13.

Ganong, W.F. (1985) *Review of Medical Physiology*, 12th edn, Lange, Los Altos, California, Chapter 32, p. 504.

Glasgow, J.F.T. (1987) Eponymous syndromes – Reye's syndrome: acute encephalopathy. *Update* **34**, (5), 535–42.

Hughes, R.A.C., Kadlubowski, M. and Hufschmidt, A. (1981) A treatment of acute inflammatory polyneuropathy. *Annals of Neurology, Supplement to vol. 9*, 125–31.

Levene, M.I. and Evans, D.H. (1985) Medical management of raised intracranial pressure after severe birth asphyxia. *Archives of Disease in Childhood*, **60**, 12–16.

Levy, R.L., Newkirk, R. and Ochoa, J. (1979) Treatment of chronic relapsing Guillain Barré syndrome by plasma exchange. *Lancet*, **ii**, 741.

Lovejoy, F.H., Bresnan, M.J., Lombrose, C.T. and Smith, A. (1975) Anticerebral oedema therapy in Reye's syndrome. *Archives of Disease in Childhood*, **50**, 933.

Punt, J. Head injury. *Care of the Critically Ill*, **5** (6), 233–7.

Raphaely, R.C., Swedlow, D.B., Downes, J.J. and Bruce, D.A. (1980) Management of severe pediatric head trauma. *Pediatric Clinics of North America*, **27** (3), 715–27.

Rogers, M.C., Nugent, S.K. and Traystman, R.J. (1980) Control of cerebral circulation in the neonate and infant. *Critical Care Medicine*, **8** (10), 570–4.

Rosman, P.N., Oppenheimer, E.Y. and O'Connor, J.F. (1983) Emergency management of pediatric head injuries. *Emergency Medicine Clinics of North America*, **1** (1), 141–74.

Simpson, D.A. and Reilly, P.L. (1982) Paediatric coma scale. *Lancet*, **ii**, 450 (letter).

Steinhart, C.M. and Weiss, I.P. (1985). Use of brain stem auditory evoked potentials in paediatric brain death. *Critical Care Medicine*, **13**, 560–2.

Tasker, R.C., Matthew, D.J., Helms, P., Dinwiddie, R. and Boyd, S. (1988) Monitoring in non-traumatic coma part 1: invasive intracranial measurements. *Archives of Disease in Childhood*, **63**, 888–94.

Teasdale, G. and Jennett, B. (1974) Assessment of coma and impaired consciousness: a practical scale. *Lancet*, **ii**, 81–4.

Winer, J.B. (1987) Eponymous syndromes – Guillain Barré syndrome. *Update 1*, **35** (9), 972–6.

Care of the child with acute renal failure

7

Julie Asquith, Margaret Hicklin and Carmen Griffiths

Acute renal failure develops when renal function is diminished to a point where body fluid homeostasis can no longer be maintained. This is manifested usually by a reduction in urine output and an associated inability to excrete the by-products of metabolism, the loss of regulation of electrolyte concentration, and possible acid–base imbalance. Uraemia then occurs with the accumulation of by-products of nitrogen metabolism. The level of uraemia and the serum level of creatinine are used to establish the level of renal impairment.

Serious derangements of hydration and extracellular fluid chemistry occur more rapidly in infants than in older children and adults owing to the larger ratio of surface area to weight. The water turnover relative to body weight is very much higher in small individuals. A 6-month old baby would require a quantity of water equivalent to 15% of body weight daily. These parameters need to be monitored closely to maintain homeostasis. Table 7.1 gives the normal fluid requirements for infants and children.

Table 7.1 Daily fluid and nutrient requirements for infants and children

Weight	Fluid requirement (ml/kg)	Energy requirement (kcal/kg)
Newborn (up to 72 h after birth)	60–100	100 per 24 h
For each kg < 10 kg	100 per 24 h	
For each kg 11–20 kg	Add 50 per 24 h	Add 50 per 24 h
For each kg > 20 kg	Add 20 per 24 h	Add 20 per 24 h

Body surface area formula for fluid requirements: $1500 \ ml/m^2$ body surface area per 24 h.

AETIOLOGY

There are many causes of acute renal failure. These may be divided into three categories: prerenal, postrenal and intrinsic. Not uncommonly, the cause of acute renal failure is multifactorial.

In *prerenal failure*, decreased perfusion of the kidneys leads to decreased renal function. *Postrenal failure* is primarily due to obstructive disorders of the upper or lower urinary tract. *Intrinsic renal failure* includes diseases of the kidney itself.

PATHOPHYSIOLOGY

Prerenal failure

Prerenal causes of acute renal failure include those where decreased renal perfusion has occurred because of a decrease in the total or 'effective' blood circulating volume. The capacity of the kidney to function is preserved with the restoration of an adequate circulating blood volume.

A decrease in intravascular volume leads to a fall in cardiac output and an increase in renal arteriolar resistance, causing a decline in renal cortical flow and thus glomerular filtration rate. If hypoperfusion is not reversed, parenchymal damage may develop. The causes of prerenal failure include hypovolaemia, hypotension, hypoxia and severe sepsis (Table 7.2).

Table 7.2 Causes of acute renal failure in children and infants

Prerenal	Intrinsic	Postrenal

1. Hypovolaemia
   Burns
   Haemorrhage
   Gastrointestinal losses
   Renal disease with
     salt wasting
2. Hypoxia
   Hyaline membrane
    disease
   Pneumonia
   Aortic clamping
3. Hypotension
   Haemorrhage
   Septicaemia
   Heart failure, often
    associated with major
    cardiac surgery
   Disseminated intra-
    vascular coagulation
	1. Glomerulonephritis
	   After streptococcal
	    infection
	   Systemic lupus
	    erythematosus
	2. Vascular disorders
	   Haemolytic uraemic
	    syndrome
	   Renal vein thrombosis
	3. Acute tubular necrosis
	   Shock
	   Burns
	   Crush injuries
	   Nephrotoxins, e.g.
	    mercury, myoglobin
	4. Acute interstitial nephritis
	   After viral infection
	   Drugs, e.g. methicillin
	5. Tumours
	   Uric acid nephropathy
	   Parenchymal infiltration
	6. Developmental abnormalities
	   Cystic disease
	   Hypoplasia/dysplasia
		1. Vesicoureteric reflux
		2. Obstructive uropathy.
		   Urethral valves
		   Tumour, e.g.
		    Wilms or neuro-
		    blastoma
		3. Acquired
		   Blood clot
		   Calculi

Postrenal failure

Postrenal failure includes obstruction of the urinary tract. As a single normal kidney is capable of maintaining adequate fluid and electrolyte balance, both ureters would have to be obstructed for a decrease in renal function to occur. When urine flow is obstructed, there is an increased pressure in the ureters and this can cause an increase in the hydrostatic pressure in the collecting ducts and renal tubules. With increased hydrostatic pressure in the Bowman's capsule, there is a decrease in glomerular filtration rate, intensifying tubular reabsorption and developing oliguria or anuria. Posterior urethral valves are a common cause of congenital obstructive renal failure in newborn male infants. This may present as acute renal failure and oliguria in the neonatal period. Relief of the obstruction followed by spontaneous diuresis will allow the return of normal renal function provided parenchymal damage has not occurred.

Intrinsic renal failure

This category includes disease of the kidney or injury to the kidney. Unlike in prerenal failure, rehydration is not followed by diuresis. The following examples fall into the category of intrinsic renal failure.

Acute tubular necrosis, or *vasomotor neuropathy*, is the term commonly used in the clinical setting to describe intrinsic renal failure of unknown aetiology. Although the term implies noticeable histological changes, these are not present. Suggested mechanisms used to explain this process include a reduction in renal blood flow and a fall in glomerular filtration rate, tubular obstruction and passive backflow of the filtrate across injured tubular cells into the peritubular capillaries. The causes of acute tubular necrosis are very similar to those responsible for physiological oliguria. Inadequate treatment of the latter would inevitably lead to true acute tubular necrosis.

Intrinsic renal failure in the newborn period and early infancy is usually secondary to sepsis and birth asphyxia. Other causes occasionally seen include unilateral or bilateral renal vein thrombosis, obstructive lesions and dysplasia or hypoplasia of the kidneys. The most common cause of intrinsic renal failure in toddlers and children between the ages of 6 months and 8 years is *haemolytic uraemic syndrome*. Endemic outbreaks occur mainly in the spring and summer. The child may present with a history of gastroenteritis. Bloody diarrhoea persists with acute haemolytic anaemia and a falling platelet count. Acute renal failure ensues with oliguria.

Glomerulonephritis also falls into this category; the rapidly progressive forms are common causes of acute renal failure in older children. The small vessels thrombose due to activation of the coagulation system in the kidney, which can lead to acute renal failure.

An increasing cause of acute renal failure is acute *interstitial nephritis*, usually as a result of hypersensitivity to a therapeutic agent. Some drugs in use are very nephrotoxic, particularly aminoglycosides, cephalosporins and sulphonamides. Renal failure in this instance may recover spontaneously following withdrawal of the toxic agent.

Tumours may also cause intrinsic renal failure by obstruction of the tubules by uric acid crystals or by infiltration of the kidney.

CLINICAL FEATURES

Clinical features vary according to the cause of acute renal failure. A detailed history may indicate a particular cause, for example preceding gastroenteritis, respiratory infection or rash.

In acute tubular necrosis the causative disorder is reflected in the condition of the child who may be shocked and obviously hypovolaemic. The preceding cause becomes apparent from the history.

The history of acute tubular necrosis can be divided into four phases:

1. *oliguric phase* (occasionally anuric) following the originating cause/insult, which may be omitted with a high urine output from the onset;
2. *polyuric phase*: an abnormally high volume of poor quality urine, explained as an appropriate failure of tubular reabsorption of filtrate relative to the fall in glomerular filtration rate.
3. *diuretic phase*;
4. *recovery.*

DIAGNOSIS

It is important to identify the underlying cause of acute renal failure to differentiate between prerenal, postrenal and intrinsic renal failure. The child will present with abnormal blood chemistry including a high blood urea concentration (Table 7.3). First, obstructive causes should be excluded. The following investigations will aid in this diagnosis:

1. plain abdominal radiography;
2. abdominal ultrasonography;
3. micturating cystogram;
4. DTPA (diethyalaminetriaminepentaacetic acid) renal scan to give an indication of the functional state of the kidney and the perfusion of the kidney.

The plasma creatinine concentration is a good indicator of the glomerular filtration rate. A raised level will confirm the presence of renal failure; however, lower levels do not exclude this as they may have been taken before the level has had time to rise.

Urinalysis in acute tubular necrosis displays low urea and creatinine levels and a high sodium level; the relative density of the urine levels at about 1.010. However, in prerenal failure, the opposite would be the case: high urea and creatinine levels, a low sodium and a high osmolarity.

The fractional sodium excretion (FE_{Na}) is a reliable index when differentiating between these two groups. This index is derived by dividing sodium clearance by creatinine clearance:

$$FE_{Na} = \frac{\text{Urine sodium concentration} \times \text{serum creatinine concentration}}{\text{Urine creatinine concentration} \times \text{serum sodium concentration}} \times 100$$

Table 7.3 Differential diagnosis of prerenal and renal failure

	Prerenal failure	*Renal failure*
Composition of urine		
Volume (ml/kg)	< 0.5	Variable
Urine : plasma urea ratio	> 8 (high)	< 3 (low)
Urine : plasma creatinine ratio	> 30 (high)	< 20 (low)
Sodium (mmol/l)	< 10	> 20
Osmolality (mmol/kg)	> 500 (high)	< 300 (low)
Relative density	> 1.025 (high)	< 1.010 (low)
FE_{Na} (%)	< 1%	> 1%
Composition of plasma		
Urea	Raised	Raised
Creatinine	Raised	Raised
Urea : creatinine ratio	> 20 : 1	20 : 1

This describes the proportion of sodium in the glomerular filtrate excreted in the urine, thus representing the renal tubular ability to reabsorb sodium. Random specimens of urine and blood may be sent for analysis. The result is invalid if the child has recently taken diuretics or has a chronic salt-wasting lesion.

If the child's clinical status and serology is inconclusive a renal biopsy may be necessary.

CONSERVATIVE MEDICAL AND NURSING MANAGEMENT

As previously discussed, the renal system maintains homeostasis. Inevitably, disruption of renal function will cause imbalances in body chemistry. Homeostasis is achieved by the adjustment of urinary output in response to input from diet and metabolism. Continuing intake when output has diminished will lead to retention of water and sodium. This is accompanied by hypertension. With an underlying illness preceding acute renal failure, these children are generally catabolic, and therefore the production of urea, creatinine, uric acid, guanidine, hydrogen ions, potassium and phosphate are all increased. The plasma concentration increases owing to an inability to clear these substances adequately.

The management of acute renal failure is focused on reducing the input of these substances into the body and the use of dialysis to remove them artificially. The underlying disorder will require specific treatment and the child must be cared for generally with particular emphasis on nutrition.

FLUID BALANCE

The management of the child's fluid intake before the diagnosis of acute renal failure will determine whether the child is hypovolaemic or hypervolaemic. Hypovolaemia should be corrected promptly using plasma or blood to restore the circulating blood volume. The circulating blood volume can be monitored by measurement of the central venous pressure and the central–peripheral temperature differential. The use of vasodilator drugs may be necessary if the peripheral perfusion continues to be poor in the presence of a high venous pressure. The correction of volume depletion will often be quickly followed by restoration of urine production. If a low circulating blood volume persists, there may be further kidney damage with accompanying hyperkalaemia and metabolic acidosis.

Alternatively, hypervolaemia may develop as a consequence of aggressive fluid administration in an attempt to encourage the kidneys to function again. The child may develop pulmonary and peripheral oedema. This may occur in conditions where acute renal failure is superimposed on pre-existing cardiac failure following cardiac surgery. Positive pressure ventilation may be necessary before dialysis can be instigated to reverse the fluid overload. Induced diuresis may be attempted by using diuretic agents. This may work even in the presence of a low renal blood flow and low glomerular filtration rate. Frusemide is one of the most effective diuretics, prescribed as a single dose of 1–2 mg/kg to 5–10 mg/kg. Dopamine, a positive inotrope, may be used in prerenal failure. In low doses of 2–5 μg/kg per min, given as a continuous infusion, it can produce dilation of the renal artery, increasing renal blood flow and thus producing a diuresis without an effect on the cardiac output or the systemic arterial blood pressure. Higher doses of dopamine (5–10 μg/kg per min) can stimulate cardiac function along with renal vasodilation, thus effectively increasing cardiac output and the systemic arterial blood pressure. High-dose dopamine (15–20 μg/kg per min) causes a reduction in renal blood flow and should therefore be avoided.

Fluid restriction is essential regardless of whether diuresis is achieved in hypervolaemic children. The input is restricted to insensible losses: 400 ml/m^2 per 24 h plus a volume equivalent to measured urinary and nasogastric output. In stable oliguric patients this may be calculated on a daily basis, according to the previous day's output. With polyuric patients, fluid assessment needs to be more frequent, possibly hourly with replacement of urine output on a volume basis, millilitre for millilitre. It is important that all fluid administered is of high nutritional value. This will be discussed later in this chapter in connection with nutritional support.

HYPERKALAEMIA

Hyperkalaemia can develop very rapidly, causing cardiac arrhythmias and death with levels of 6 mmol/l and above. Potassium intake must be severely restricted unless the plasma potassium level is unusually low. The failing kidney is unable to excrete the potassium load increased by a movement of potassium ions from the intracellular to the extracellular compartment caused by metabolic acidosis, tissue hypoxia, infection and catabolism.

Children with hyperkalaemia must be monitored closely, noting changes in their electrocardiogram. Changes include tall peaked T-waves, possibly followed by depression of the S–T segment, prolonged P–R interval and widening QRS complex, ventricular fibrillation and cardiac arrest. Emergency measures may be necessary to prevent cardiac arrhythmias. These include:

1. intravenous sodium bicarbonate 8.4% (1 mmol/kg) to alkalinize the serum and move potassium from the vascular circulation into the intracellular space;
2. intravenous 10% calcium gluconate (0.1–0.2 ml/kg) to counteract the effects of hyperkalaemia on the neuromuscular membranes (bradycardias may occur);
3. oral and/or rectal calcium resonium (1 g/kg) to exchange calcium for potassium;
4. intravenous glucose 50% solution (1 ml/kg with regular insulin (1 unit/5 g glucose) given over 1 h; the insulin drives potassium into the cells and the glucose is given to counteract hypoglycaemia;
5. intravenous salbutamol (4 μg/kg) infused over 5 min to increase the cellular uptake of potassium ions;
6. dialysis.

Of these six measures, only the ion-exchange resin and dialysis remove potassium from the body. The other options temporarily normalize the plasma potassium concentration; the necessity for dialysis remains.

HYPONATRAEMIA

A fall in serum sodium concentration may be attributed to the dilutional effects of water retention. If the extracellular fluid volume is increased, water restriction is the appropriate action for hyponatraemia; the serum sodium concentration will then return to normal. Cautious sodium supplementation may be necessary.

There is a redistribution of body fluid that occurs in hyponatraemia. If the sodium deficit is calculated on the assumption that the sodium space represents 30–35% of body weight in infants under 1 year of age and 20–25% in older children, there may be an underestimation of total body sodium deficit. Reassessment will be necessary, but the possibility of overestimation is minimal.

HYPOCALCAEMIA

Hypocalcaemia is caused by phosphate retention and depression of the plasma concentration of 1,25-dihydroxycholecalciferol (an active form of vitamin D). This in turn induces resistance in bone to the calcium mobilizing effects of the parathyroid hormone.

Hypocalcaemia may need to be corrected. Administration of calcium is not always adequate, further indicating the need for dialysis. Hypocalcaemia should be avoided as it can depress cardiovascular function and exacerbate cardiac arrhythmias resulting from hyperkalaemia.

PHOSPHATE ABSORPTION

Hyperphosphataemia is a common feature in children with acute renal failure. When present in conjunction with a normal serum calcium concentration, the calcium and phosphate may precipitate. Hyperphosphataemia may be prevented by using phosphate-binding agents such as aluminium hydroxide or calcium carbonate, which reduce the absorption of phosphate from the gut. Insoluble aluminium phosphate is formed in the gut and eliminated. The diet given will be low in protein and phosphate.

METABOLIC ACIDOSIS

Metabolic acidosis occurs as a result of failure to excrete hydrogen ions. Sodium bicarbonate is given to correct the acidosis. The dosage is calculated according to the child's base deficit:

$$\text{mEq } NaHCO_3 \text{ administered } = \text{ base deficit } \times \text{ kg body weight } \times 0.3$$

As the buffering action of sodium bicarbonate results in the formation of carbon dioxide, it is essential that the child receiving bicarbonate has adequate ventilatory function; otherwise, respiratory acidosis may develop. It is important to highlight that large doses of sodium bicarbonate are associated with increased risk of intracranial haemorrhage. There may be water retention and oedema accompanying the administration of sodium bicarbonate due to the presence of sodium. Acidosis causes a shift of potassium ions into the vascular space. This increase in serum potassium concentration may further exacerbate the existing hyperkalaemia.

HYPERTENSION

Raised systemic blood pressure is frequently present in acute renal failure.

The reason depends on the underlying cause of acute renal failure. In *haemolytic uraemic syndrome* the hypertension is associated with high plasma renin activity. In *strepococcal glomerulonephritis* it is generally due to fluid retention.

Acute rises of systemic pressure may predispose to abnormal neurological signs, e.g. hypertensive encephalopathy, and cardiovascular compromise can occur. The first line of treatment of hypertension in acute renal failure is usually a vasodilator: intravenous hydralazine (0.2 mg/kg per dose) or an intravenous infusion of sodium nitroprusside (0.5–0.8 µg/kg per min).

Oral preparations can be used for persistent hypertension. These include:

1. *Vasodilators*:
   (a) hydralazine, oral 2 mg/kg per day
   (b) nifedipine, oral/sublingual 0.25 mg/kg per day
   (c) minoxidil, oral: <12 years 0.1–0.2 mg/kg per day, >12 years 5–10 mg/day;
2. *Beta-blockers*:
   (a) propranolol, oral, 2 mg/kg per day,
   (b) atenolol, oral, 0.5–1 mg/kg per day.

HAEMATOLOGICAL COMPLICATIONS

Acute renal failure can produce anaemia and clotting disorders.

Anaemia occurs due to the lack of production of erythropoietin. This is essential for the stimulation of the production of red blood cells in the bone marrow.

Clotting times are prolonged as platelet function is depressed in acute renal failure. Platelet count, prothrombin time and partial thromboplastin time should be checked regularly.

Blood transfusion and platelet transfusion may be necessary. Ranitidine may be prescribed prophylactically to prevent gastrointestinal bleeding, and antacids can be prescribed to reduce the risk of stress ulcers.

NUTRITION

It is important to remember that the metabolic rate and daily energy requirements are approximately two and a half times greater in the first year of life than in adulthood.

Uraemic children also have a greater requirement for energy, because uraemia is a catabolic state. It is essential to consider the child's daily intake in relation to general condition and energy requirements for growth. Brain growth is greatest in the first year of life, and malnutrition can lead to considerable mental retardation generally accompanied by poor body growth.

Nutrition should be commenced as soon as possible for the child with acute renal failure to prevent excess protein catabolism. Enteral feeding should be the first choice. If the child is unable to eat or will not eat, gastric or jejunal feeding should be commenced. If enteral feeding is not tolerated, parenteral nutrition should be instituted. Whatever the route of nutrition, the restrictions of fluid and protein must be considered. Nutrition should provide adequate calories in the form of glucose and essential amino acids to minimize the accumulation of metabolic waste products.

The rationale for prompt intensive nutritional therapy in acute renal failure is primarily fourfold:

1. prevention of cachexia and support of the child's general condition;
2. minimization of catabolism, limiting the increase of potassium, urea, phosphate and hydrogen ions in the extracellular fluid;
3. maximization of healing of the renal lesion;
4. reduction of the occurrence of severe infection.

It is essential to consider the following when giving nutritional therapy to a child in acute renal failure:

1. appropriate water and electrolyte intake;
2. regulated protein intake;
3. adequate calorie intake;
4. regulated phosphate intake;
5. appropriate vitamin and mineral intake.

It is important to reduce the amount of nitrogenous waste to be excreted while maintaining the nitrogen balance. (Nitrogen balance is the relationship between nitrogen taken in, usually in food, and nitrogen excreted in urine and faeces). These children may need more protein and a higher calorie intake because of the physiological stress from their underlying condition.

Restricting protein intake will inevitably reduce nitrogenous waste because there is no excess protein to be metabolized. Excess nitrogen is utilized for other body compounds. The energy source must be adequate to ensure that the intake of protein is not used for energy, to prevent tissue degeneration. The ideal energy intake should be 30% above basal requirements.

ENTERAL FEEDING

When the child is oliguric and before dialysis has been initiated, the limiting factor in nutrition is volume. It is difficult to achieve an adequate calorie intake in a volume of 400 ml/m^2 daily. This is more attainable now with the use of highly concentrated energy supplements; a feed can be produced which is a mixture of carbohydrate and fat. The carbohydrate is formulated as a glucose polymer, for example Caloreen (Roussel). The fat source is available as Prosparol (Duncan) which is an arachis oil emulsion.

A recipe of:
200 g Caloreen + 130 ml Prosparol + 400 ml water provides 465 ml total fluid and 1385 kcal, i.e. 3 kcalories/ml.

Protein can be added to this feed in the form of Clinifeed (Sophargo). Clinifeed contains 4 g protein per 100 ml. For oral consumption this preparation is flavoured with milk shake flavourings. This feed is hyperosmolar relative to plasma and therefore it is better to start with quarter strength feed working up to full strength over a period of 3–4 days.

These children often suffer from nausea and vomiting and/or anorexia. Enteral nutrition may therefore not be appropriate and parenteral nutrition may be required.

PARENTERAL NUTRITION

Parenteral nutrition should be used only if enteral feeding is not tolerated. Parenteral nutrition is not without its risks and these must be considered when choosing this option.

Administration

Many of the solutions used in parenteral nutrition are hyperosmolar, and so a central venous catheter is preferable. Ideally, a double- or triple-lumen catheter should be used to allow for multiple infusions. Subclavian and internal jugular veins are the vessels of choice as they are readily accessible in the neck. An alternative vessel would be the femoral vein, but the risks of infection are far greater.

Parenteral nutrition may continue for weeks, so the use of a silicone or polyurethane catheter is preferable as they provoke less thrombus formation and do not become brittle. Central venous catheters must be inserted under strict aseptic conditions. If possible, the catheter should be tunnelled under the skin before entry into the vessel. This reduces the risks of infection. The insertion site should be dressed aseptically, preferably with a transparent adhesive dressing which allows easy, regular inspection. Parenteral nutrition offers the perfect culture medium for bacteria in children who may already be immunocompromised. The risk of infection is very high. The central venous catheter should not be used for blood sampling or for the measurement of central venous pressure. It is imperative that the line is always treated aseptically with minimal intervention and breaking of the system.

The position of the central venous catheter must be confirmed by chest radiography. The position of the catheter tip and the absence of pneumothorax, haemothorax or hydrothorax must be established.

Table 7.4 indicates the immediate and delayed complications of catherization.

Table 7.4 Complications of catheter insertion

Complication	Clinical sequelae
Arterial puncture	Haematoma
	Carotid artery lacerations
	Subclavian artery puncture
	Ascending cervical artery laceration
	Internal mammary artery laceration
	Pulmonary artery laceration
	Brachiocephalic false aneurysm
	Aortic puncture
	Aortic dissection
	Arteriovenous fistula
Pleural and mediastinal injury	Pneumothorax
	Haemothorax
	Haemomediastinum
Venous cannulation	Air embolism
	Catheter embolism
Lymphatic vessel injury	Thoracic duct laceration
Neurological injury	Phrenic nerve injury
	Brachial plexus injury
	Recurrent laryngeal nerve injury
	Horner's syndrome
	Fatal cerebrovascular episodes
Tracheal injury	Endotracheal tube cuff puncture
Malposition of catheter	Extravascular
	Intravascular
Delayed complications	Air embolism
	Thrombosis
	Vascular or cardiac perforation
	Sepsis

Parenteral nutrition should be administered using a volumetric pump. These ensure that the prescribed fluid is given at the correct rate and also that the patency of the catheter is maintained.

Regimen (Figures 7.1 and 7.2)

The same considerations are necessary when prescribing parenteral nutrition as with enteral feeding for the child in acute renal failure. Total parenteral nutrition should include:

Intravenous feeding prescription form for children > 10 kg body weight

All figures are per kg per 24 h

NAME	:	*WARD* :	
HOSPITAL NO.	:	*DATE* :	
PACT CODE	:	*WEIGHT*:	
REASON FOR TPN:			

Regimens 12 and 13 are used for children 10–30 kg body weight
Regimens 14 and 15 are used for children > 30 kg body weight
Regimens 12 and 14 are used for first 2 days; regimens 13 and 15 thereafter

	Regimen number (day)			
	12	13	14	15
Protein (g)	1	2	1	1.5
Carbohydrate (g)	4.5	7.5	2	5
Total fluid for TPN (ml/kg)				
Addamel (ml)	0.2	0.2	0.2	0.2
Sodium (mmol)	3	3	3	3
Potassium (mmol)	2.5	2.5	2.5	2.5
Calcium (mmol)	0.14	0.17	0.14	0.15
Magnesium (mmol)	0.05	0.07	0.05	0.06
Phosphate (mmol)*	0	0	0	0
Solivito N (ml)	1	1	1	1
Vitlipid N Infant (ml)	1	1	1	1
Fat (g)	1.5	2	1	2

*Addamel contains no phosphate, but the phosphate content of Intralipid is assumed to be bioavailable. However, phosphate should be monitored in patients on long-term feeding and added, particularly where growth has been retarded before nutritional care.

Additives/omissions _____

Please state in terms of mmol/kg _____

DOCTOR'S SIGNATURE: BLEEP NO: ☐☐☐☐☐

Figure 7.1 Intravenous feeding prescription form for children > 10 kg body weight.

Intravenous feeding prescription form for neonates and infants < 10 kg body weight

Any deviation from the standard regimen must be clearly marked
All figures are per kg per 24 h

NAME	:	WARD	:
HOSPITAL NO.	:	DATE	:
PACT CODE	:	BIRTHWEIGHT	:
REASON FOR TPN	:	FEEDING WEIGHT	:
STAGE IF BABY PRETERM	:	DATE OF BIRTH	:

Regimens 1–5 are used for the first 5 days of parenteral nutrition: regimen 6 for day 6 and beyond

	Regimen number (day)					
	1	2	3	4	5	6
Protein (g)*	0.5	0.75	1.0	1.5	2.0	2.5
Carbohydrate (g)	8	10	10	12	12	14
Total fluid for TPN (ml/kg)						
Ped-El (ml)	2	2	3	3	3	4
Sodium (mmol)	5	5	5	5	5	5
Potassium (mmol)	2.5	2.5	2.5	2.5	2.5	2.5
Calcium (mmol)	0.32	0.33	0.49	0.5	0.52	0.69
Magnesium (mmol)	0.06	0.07	0.1	0.11	0.12	0.15
Phosphate (mmol)†	0.15	0.15	0.23	0.23	0.23	0.3
Solivito N (ml)	1	1	1	1	1	1
Vitlipid N Infant (ml)	1	1	1	1	1	1
Fat (g)	1	1	2	2	3	3.5

†Only the phosphate content of Ped-El to be included. This figure becomes 0.7 mmol/kg, including Ped-El, if the patient is preterm.
*Vamin Infant in infants aged < 6 months; Vamin 9 Glucose in infants aged > 6 months.

Additives/omissions _____

Please state in terms of mmol/kg _____

DOCTOR'S SIGNATURE: BLEEP NO: ☐☐☐☐☐

Figure 7.2 Intravenous feeding prescription form for neonates and infants 10 kg body weight.

1.   a fluid source: water;
2.   an energy source:
     (a) carbohydrate,
     (b) lipid,
     (c) protein;
3.   a nitrogen source: amino acids;
4.   metabolites:
     (a) electrolytes and minerals,
     (b) trace elements,
     (c) vitamins.

Fluid source

Water is an essential nutrient which accounts for 85% of body weight in preterm neonates and 60% of body weight in adults. The child in acute renal failure being managed conservatively with a strict fluid restriction makes the prescription of parenteral nutrition a considerable challenge.

Energy source

Calories are provided predominantly by lipids and carbohydrate. An adequate supply of energy from these sources is essential to reduce protein oxidation for energy needs.

Carbohydrates

Glucose is the carbohydrate of choice. Other sources such as fructose may cause a lactic acidosis. Glucose is readily utilised by the red blood cells, cardiac muscle and the brain. Ten per cent glucose has a calorific value of 2.5 kcal/ml. Concentrations greater than 10% should be infused via a central vein. Glucose solution is usually hypertonic to the body fluids; such fluids will not be tolerated by peripheral veins. Extravasation can cause burns, necrosis and the possible need for skin grafting. Glucose intolerance in infants and children is uncommon; it is generally an early indication of sepsis. Insulin is rarely indicated. If it is necessary a starting dose of: 0.05 units insulin/kg per hour should be prescribed.

Lipids

Parenteral lipid emulsions are isotonic, rich in essential fatty acids and provide a concentrated calorie source. Intralipid 20% (Kabivitrum) yields 2.0 kcal/ml. Lipid can be administered peripherally and centrally. Intravenous lipid emulsions are made from soya beans. An energy source comprising a mixture of lipid and glucose results in improved nitrogen retention. It is important that dietary balance is achieved between lipid content (30–50%) and protein content (7–16%) to facilitate protein synthesis and the maintenance of normal metabolism. For each gram of nitrogen infused, there should be 200 kcal of non-protein. Caution should be taken when prescribing lipid for preterm neonates; they have a reduced tolerance to lipid emulsion. Infants with hyperbilirubinaemia have an increased risk of kernicterus when lipid is administered. This is due to the release of free fatty acids during lipid hydrolysis. The free fatty acids can displace bilirubin. Lipid emulsion is given as a separate infusion with added vitamins. Lipid is calculated to be administered over a 20 h period so that the infusion can be stopped for 4 h before daily blood sampling to reduce the distortion of results that may otherwise occur. It is important to remember that lipid can damage the membranes of blood gas analysers; great care should be taken. If the lipid infusion is running behind, no attempt should be made to catch up; this may result in inadequate clearance of lipid from the blood, particularly in neonates. A lipid clearance test should be performed daily.

Nitrogen source

Amino acids are essential for the production of protein. There is at present no ideal amino acid solution available for paediatric parenteral nutrition. Children have special requirements for the amino acid histidine and neonates for cystine, cysteine and taurine, in addition to the eight amino acids required in adults. The eight essential amino acids are leucine, isoleucine, valine, lysine, methionine, phenylalanine, threonine and tryptophan. Neonates have a limited ability to metabolize excessive intakes of phenylalanine and tyrosine. It is suggested that Vamin Infant (Kabivitrum) should be used for infants < 6 months of age. The profile of Vamin Infant is based on breast milk protein, which includes cysteine and tyrosine. Vamin Infant contains 9.3 g nitrogen/l. This corresponds to 58 g protein. It contains 2.4 kcal/ml. Over 6 months of age, Vamin 9 Glucose (Kabivitrum) is advocated; its amino acid profile is based on egg protein with added cysteine. Vamin 9 Glucose contains 9.4 g nitrogen/l, which corresponds to 60 g protein. The energy content is 6.5 kCal/ml, of which 4.0 kCal are provided by the glucose. It is suggested that in renal failure the protein content of parenteral nutrition should be reduced to 500 mg/kg per day.

Metabolites

Electrolytes and minerals
Seven electrolytes and minerals should be considered when administering parenteral nutrition. These include sodium, potassium, chloride, acetate, magnesium, phosphorus and calcium. The quantity of electrolytes and minerals administered varies depending on the child's condition and must be based on laboratory results.

It is important to remember that calcium and phosphate can precipitate in solution, producing crystals. Commercially prepared solutions of electrolytes and mineral solutions can be used. Ped-El (Kabivitrum) is advocated for neonates and infants of <10 kg body weight. In children of >10 kg, Addamel (Kabivitrum) is used.

Trace elements

Ped-El and Addamel also provide the trace elements required. These are present in the body in very small amounts, but are necessary for many of the body's biochemical and physiological processes. Children receiving long-term parenteral nutrition may develop deficiencies, particularly of zinc, copper, magnesium and selenium. These levels should be monitored and corrected accordingly.

Vitamins

Vitamins are essential for the facilitation of amino acid, fat and carbohydrate metabolism. Both fat- and water-soluble vitamins must be included. Vitlipid Infant (Kabivitrum) is used to administer fat-soluble vitamins A, D_2, E and K to children under the age of 11 years. This is added to lipid emulsion solutions. Older children are given Vitlipid Adult (Kabivitrum). Solivito (Kabivitrum) is the freeze-dried preparation used to administer water-soluble vitamin B complex, vitamin C, biotin and folates. This preparation is reconstituted with glucose 10% and can be added to glucose solutions or lipid emulsions.

Investigations

A full biochemical, haematological and nutritional assessment (Table. 7.5) must be undertaken before commencement of parenteral nutrition. Blood and, if possible, urine is sent for analysis. These investigations should continue on a regular basis to monitor the adequacy of the parenteral nutrition.

Complications

It is important that the nurse monitors the effects of parenteral nutrition, recognizing and preventing associated complications.

Sepsis

This is the most serious complication. Strict aseptic technique can prevent infection. Ideally the parenteral nutrition should be made up in pharmacy in the sterile supplies department using laminar flow rooms. The administration set should be changed every 24 h. The catheter site dressing should be

Table 7.5 Haematological, biochemical and nutritional monitoring

	Investigation		
	Daily	*Weekly*	*Monthly*
Haematological		Haemoglobin White cell count Platelets	Coagulation screen
Plasma chemistry	Blood glucose (6 hourly for first week) Sodium Potassium	Albumin Bilirubin Calcium Phosphate Liver function tests Amino acid profile (preterm infants only)	Zinc Copper Magnesium Selenium
Urine chemistry	Urea Elecrolytes Glucose (6 hourly for first week)		
Physical	Weight	Head circumference (infants only) Length (infants only) Anthropometric measurements (long-term patients only) Mid arm muscle circumference Tricep measurements	

changed as necessary. The catheter used for the administration of the parenteral nutrition should be restricted to that function only. The child's vital signs should be recorded frequently to enable detection of sepsis as early as possible. If the catheter is thought to be the source of infection it should be removed. Blood cultures should be taken. Insertion of another catheter should be delayed for at least 12 h until appropriate antibiotic therapy has been commenced.

Glucose imbalance

Blood glucose levels should be monitored initially at least 6 hourly. More frequent monitoring may be indicated for the very young infant and the very sick infant or child. Hyperglycaemia may be due to excessive glucose administration, sepsis or stress. Hypoglycaemia may occur if parenteral nutrition is abruptly stopped.

Thrombosis

This may occur because the catheter, a foreign body, can cause trauma to the inside of the vein, causing platelet aggregation and fibrin formation. The child may develop oedema of the involved arm, neck and face. The catheter should be removed and the affected arm elevated.

When parenteral nutrition has been administered for more than 2 weeks, it must be discontinued over a period of 2 or 3 days as enteral feeding is re-established, thus ensuring that enteral feeding is successful and reducing possible hypoglycaemia.

DIALYSIS

Indications for acute dialysis

The indications for acute dialysis are often multifactorial. Generally, dialysis is indicated for children in acute renal failure where aggressive conservative management has been unable to control hypervolaemia, electrolyte imbalance or acid–base balance.

The indications for dialysis include:

1. fluid overload (uncontrolled hypertension with generalized or pulmonary oedema);
2. hyperkalaemia (serum potassium >6 mmol/l);
3. metabolic acidosis;
4. uraemia;
5. hyperphosphataemia;
6. hypocalcaemia;
7. multiple system organ failure;
8. catabolic patient, e.g. burns;
9. hypernatraemia;
10. poisoning, e.g. iron, aspirin, alcohol, lithium, chloral hydrate, barbiturates, lead, mercury, carbon tetrachloride.

Peritoneal dialysis and haemodialysis are both relatively low risk. Both are effective methods of managing acute renal failure, and the choice often depends on local practice. Peritoneal dialysis is most easily used for babies as there may be problems in establishing adequate circulatory access for haemodialysis.

It is important to stress that once the need for dialysis has been established it should be instituted immediately. Fatalities associated with acute renal failure are often due to delay in starting dialysis.

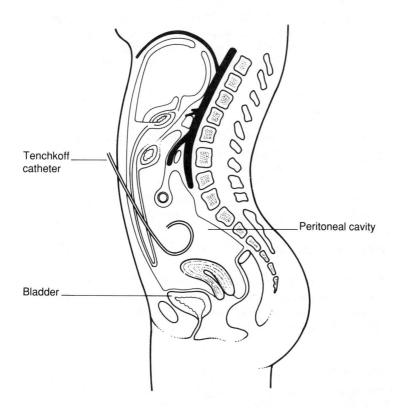

Tenchkoff catheter

Peritoneal cavity

Bladder

Figure 7.3 Peritoneal dialysis. The peritoneal cavity, showing the position of the Tenchkoff catheter.

Peritoneal dialysis

Dialysis is the removal of fluid and solutes across a semipermeable membrane. In the case of peritoneal dialysis this is the peritoneum, which has a large surface area and an excellent blood supply. The peritoneal cavity is filled with dialysate, which is a hypertonic solution to enable fluid removal and contains electrolytes and minerals such as sodium and calcium to avoid overdialysis causing low levels of these substances (Figure 7.3).

Indications

Peritoneal dialysis is suitable for the treatment of acute and chronic renal failure and to remove some poisons in all age groups. The equipment for peritoneal dialysis is simple and readily available. The technique is not difficult and, although there is no doubt that it is more successful in experienced hands, its simplicity lends itself to use by non-renal specialists, such as in intensive care. The most important aspect of care of a child on dialysis is a good understanding of fluid balance, which should be second nature to intensive care nurses.

For most ill children peritoneal dialysis is also the dialysis of choice for the following reasons:

1. There is no extra corporeal blood volume; therefore the method is suitable for very small and haemodynamically unstable children, who are notoriously difficult to haemodialyse.
2. Dialysis continues for 24 h/day, enabling slow gentle removal of fluid and electrolytes. Fluid can be removed at the same rate as fluid intake, keeping the circulation stable. Fluid removal can be more aggressive if necessary.
3. Interestingly, peritoneal dialysis is also often the choice of dialysis for children with end-stage renal failure awaiting transplantation who are allowed to choose their method of dialysis for themselves.
4. There is not a great deal of difference in cost between hospital haemodialysis and hospital peritoneal dialysis.

Peritoneal dialysis is not, however, suitable in all cases.

Contraindications

Contraindications to peritoneal dialysis include:

1. major abdominal surgery where the peritoneum has been opened;
2. severe scarring of the peritoneum, which can be caused by surgery or by repeated peritonitis;
3. abdominal burns;
4. abdominal crush injury;
5. severe clotting problems (it may be impossible to provide access to the peritoneum safely);
6. grossly catabolic state, e.g. following severe burns, when peritoneal dialysis may be inadequate;
7. poisoning, because peritoneal dialysis may not remove poisons effectively.

In these children haemodialysis would be the treatment of choice.

Insertion of peritoneal dialysis cannula

For acute use, the safest and easiest method of insertion of a peritoneal dialysis cannula is the Seldinger approach, using either a fairly rigid cannula or a very soft flexible Tenchkoff-type catheter. For chronic renal failure a cuffed Tenchkoff catheter is tunnelled subdermally. For acute use, an uncuffed catheter can be used without tunnelling. The rigid cannula is slightly easier to insert; the Tenchkoff catheter, although more difficult, gives excellent flows, does not block easily and is said by the children to be more comfortable. Both types of catheter can be inserted on the ward by a paediatrician or nephrologist without either a general anaesthetic or the aid of a surgeon. The procedure is as follows.

1. Reassure and comfort the child. Give sedation, for example pethidine compound 0.1 ml/kg intravenously over 20 min, followed by Diazemuls as required. Alternatively, intravenous ketamine 1–2 mg/kg (< 15 years) over 1 min administered by an anaesthetist.
2. Catheterize the bladder; if the bladder is not empty there is a danger of inserting the peritoneal dialysis catheter into it. The urethral catheter can be removed as soon as it has been established that the bladder is empty.
3. Clean the skin and drape with sterile towels. Inject the catheter insertion site with 1% lignocaine.
4. Insert the needle provided with the dialysis catheter set into the peritoneal cavity and fill it with dialysate, warmed to body temperature (to which 500 units of heparin has been added per litre of dialysate) until the abdomen feels slightly full and tense; this usually takes 30–60 ml of dialysate per kg body weight.
5. The Seldinger wire is passed down the cannula and the cannula removed; some dialysate usually leaks out at this point.
6. The catheter is passed over the guide wire; a blade may be needed to enlarge the hole. Once the catheter is in place the guide wire is removed.
7. Secure the catheter with a purse-string suture around the exit site and a dressing. Most catheter sets have some sort of device attached to secure the catheter; in an active child it may be helpful to protect the catheter with a gallipot.
8. Dialysis can now be started.

Dialysis circuit

The dialysis circuit should be set up and ready to use before the catheter is inserted so that dialysis can be started immediately. There are many peritoneal dialysis machines available on the market, but by no means all are suitable for the smallest babies. If dialysis is often undertaken, these are invaluable and save much nursing time. However, as most of these are available only in renal units, the following describes only manual peritoneal dialysis, which is most commonly used in intensive care. The principles are exactly the same whether manual or automatic dialysis is used.

Dialysis must be set up under aseptic conditions to prevent peritonitis; the warm glucose dialysate makes an excellent culture medium. As with intravenous feeding, the circuit should be broken as infrequently as possible and the connections soaked with iodine before disconnection. The circuit should be completely changed every 24–28 h.

Principles of peritoneal dialysis

A measured amount of warmed dialysate is infused into the peritoneal cavity, allowed to dwell so that urea, electrolytes, etc. can dialyse across the peritoneal membrane, drained out and measured; then the cycle starts again.

Temperature
The dialysate should be warmed to around body temperature; this is most conveniently achieved using a blood-warming coil and blood-warming bath. Cold dialysate is uncomfortable and can be painful; if continuously used, it will lower the child's body temperature. Obviously, hot dialysate could scald.

Volume
The usual volume of dialysate instilled in each cycle is 30 ml/kg body weight. (This is fairly conservative; some units use 50 ml/kg.) If the child has undergone abdominal surgery, the volume may be decreased for the child's comfort and to decrease the likelihood of a leak. Filling the peritoneal cavity with dialysate can splint the diaphragm and add to respiratory problems, making it necessary to use smaller cycles.

Cycle times
When dialysis is first started with a new catheter, cycling should be as rapid as possible. There should be no dwell time until the dialysate is no longer blood-stained, then cycles are usually set to enable two cycles per hour, depending on how quickly the desired volume will fill and drain.

A typical cycle is 5 min to fill, 15 min to dwell and 10 min to drain. The most common dwell time for acute dialysis is 10–15 min. The dwell time can be increased to decrease the rate of electrolyte and fluid loss.

Drugs

Some drugs can be added to the dialysate, using strict asepsis and changing the needle before injecting into the bag. Drugs may be added in the laminar flow room in the pharmacy department, where available, as this reduces the potential for infection.

Heparin
500 units/l dialysate is used until the dialysate is clear and no longer blood-stained, or if fibrin is seen in the drainage bag (stringy white fibres). With

a new peritoneal dialysis catheter it is safer to use heparin for the first 2–3 days than to stop it too soon, as fibrin easily collects around the catheter.

Potassium

Dialysis occurs across a concentration gradient; if that gradient is removed, dialysis cannot occur. If, for instance, 4 mmol potassium chloride is added to each litre of dialysate, the child's own potassium cannot dialyse below 4 mmol/l. However, the child's potassium level can still fall if potassium is lost through the gut or stored in cells. It is dangerous to add > 5 mmol potassium per litre to dialysate as it can cross the peritoneum and cause hyperkalaemia. If after 5 mmol/l has been added to dialysate the child is still hypokalaemic, intravenous potassium chloride can be given; if the serum potassium level rises too much, there will be a concentration gradient again and the excess will dialyse off.

Antibiotics

Antibiotics can be aded to the dialysate to treat peritonitis. Used dialysate should be checked at least daily that it is crystal clear. Cloudy dialysate should be sent for microscopy and culture. More than 50 white cells/l in the dialysate deserves treatment as peritonitis; treatment is usually started blindly until culture results are available.

Antibiotics most commonly used intraperitoneally are:

1. gentamicin 10 mg/l dialysate;
2. vancomycin 20 mg/l dialysate;
3. netilmicin 4 mg/l dialysate;
4. tobramycin 4 mg/l dialysate.

Antifungal drugs are also sometimes used, e.g. amphotericin, 5-flucytosine.

Dialysate

The amount of glucose in the dialysate controls the rate of fluid loss. The stronger the glucose solution, the higher the osmotic pull across the peritoneal membrane and the more quicky sodium and water will be removed.

Different manufacturers produce different strengths of dialysate. Some common strengths available are 1.36, 2.27, 3.86 and 6.36%. It is not necessary to stock all the strengths of dialysate as they can be mixed. Two strengths are adequate for most uses; 1.36% is essential, together with a stronger concentration (either 3.86 or 6.36%). If necessary, these two can then be mixed to provide a medium strength.

Unless a child is severely fluid overloaded it is sensible to start dialysing with 1.36% solution, as fluid loss in some children can be rapid even with this weak osmotic solution. The rate of fluid loss varies enormously from child to child, depending on the osmotic pressure of the circulation and the permeability of the peritoneum. Scarring following surgery, repeated use of strong dialysate and repeated episodes of peritonitis can all reduce peritoneal permeability. Infusions such as mannitol given intravenously can increase the osmolarity of the blood so there is little or no concentration gradient between the blood and dialysate; in this case, fluid loss will not occur unless the strength of the dialysate is increased. The 6.36% dialysate should not be used except in life-threatening situations such as pulmonary oedema. This is for several reasons: it can remove fluid very quickly causing hypovolaemia; prolonged use damages the peritoneum; and many children find it very painful.

In an acidotic child, dialysate based on sodium bicarbonate can be used to help correct acidosis.

Troubleshooting problems

Failure to fill or filling slowly.

1. First check the obvious: the fill bag must be above the patient: the clamps must be open; and nothing must be kinked.
2. Reposition the child, e.g. from lying flat to lying on one side.
3. Flush the catheter with 5 ml normal saline (push the syringe quickly to exert as much force as possible). *Remember to clean the connections with iodine before opening.* Try filling again.
4. Check that the child is not constipated; a full bowel can impede dialysate flow.
5. If the catheter is still not filling, it may be blocked with fibrin. Instill the catheter with 5000 units urokinase mixed with 10 ml normal saline and 500 units of heparin, leave for 1 h and try again.
6. If none of these work it is likely that the catheter tip is either in the wrong place or blocked by omentum, in which case the only solution is to replace the catheter. This is sometimes possible by passing a guide wire down the original catheter and replacing it via the guide wire.

In failure to drain or inadequate drainage, many of the steps to find the cause of the problem are similar to those taken to solve a drainage problem, but there are some differences.

1. Check that the line is not kinked, clamps are not on and the drainage bag is below the child.
2. Particularly when starting dialysis, drainage may be poor if the fill volume is too small. If the problem is inadequate drainage rather than failure to drain at all, it is worth filling again and trying to drain.
3. A hypovolaemic child may absorb the dialysate and will therefore not drain; this should correct itself as soon as the child is rehydrated.

4. Reposition the child.
5. Check the dressing for leakage. (If fluid is leaking out, measured drainage will be poor.)
6. Flush the catheter with 5 ml normal saline as for failure to fill.
7. Check that the child is not constipated.
8. Instill the catheter with heparin, urokinase and saline as for failure to fill.
9. If all else fails, replace the catheter.

Leakages

If dialysate is leaking around the exit site, the catheter can rarely be rescued; however, it is worth replacing the purse-string suture around the catheter. If dialysate still leaks out, the child will dialyse but infection is potentially a problem and fluid balance becomes difficult. The ideal solution if the child's condition allows, is to remove the catheter, suture the exit site, leave the child off dialysis until the following day to allow healing, and then resite the catheter on the opposite side, having minimized the risk of leaking from the old exit hole. Of course, the child's fluid and electrolyte state may not allow 12–24 h off dialysis, in which case the catheter must be replaced immediately.

Dialysate can also extravasate into the tissue around the exit site; this looks like a tissued intravenous site. Dialysis should be discontinued. Dialysate can also track down and cause vulval or scrotal swelling and dialysate hernias can appear.

Respiration

Dialysate splints the diaphragm, limiting movement with respiration, which can increase respiratory difficulties; in this case, the fill volume should be decreased.

A rare but important problem is a congenital hole in the diaphragm allowing dialysate to leak into the chest. If the child is lying flat this causes immediate respiratory distress, but the problem may not be obvious straight away if the child is sitting upright. The fluid can be seen clearly on chest radiography, and the only solution is to drain the dialysate and discontinue peritoneal dialysis.

Pain

Peritoneal dialysis is not usually painful, but if pain occurs it can be severe and require strong analgesia. It may be either local abdominal pain or referred shoulder pain.

Causes of pain can include peritonitis, displaced catheter or the use of a strong dialysate unmixed with a weaker solution.

Peritonitis

Peritonitis can cause severe abdominal or shoulder pain, pyrexia and cloudy dialysate. It can be mild or make a child severely ill very quickly. If peritonitis is suspected, dialysate should be sent for microscopy and culture. If there are more than 50 white cells/l in the dialysate or organisms are seen, the child should be treated with intraperitoneal antibiotics.

Treatment should continue for at least 5 days and certainly for 48 h after a clear dialysate specimen. If a child has repeated peritonitis with the same organism after it has been proved to be cleared, the catheter should be changed. Bacterial peritonitis usually resolves quickly once the correct antibiotic is administered. Fungal peritonitis is very serious and can quickly cause death. Usually the catheter has to be removed and the child converted to haemodialysis or haemofiltration.

Fluid balance

Any child on dialysis needs careful assessment and monitoring of fluid and electrolyte balance. A child undergoing peritoneal dialysis for acute renal failure needs at least daily blood tests for urea and electrolytes. Fluid balance should be assessed by monitoring pulse, respiration, blood pressure, and central and peripheral temperature differential; if the child's condition warrants it, central venous pressure monitoring is a useful addition.

If a child is very hypotensive, dialysis can be stopped until the acute problem is resolved and the child has been rehydrated. To minimize fluid loss, 1.36% dialysate should be used at first and the dwell time can be increased to 30 or 60 min.

Some symptoms of hypervolaemia can be alleviated by vasodilation; the only real solution is to remove fluid by dialysis. To maximize fluid loss as quickly as possible, the fill and drain times should be the shortest time needed to run the fluid in and out with a dwell time of 10–15 min. Strong dialysate should be used (6.36 or 3.86). Fluid loss can be dramatic with strong dialysate, so the child should be monitored carefully with BM Stix as glucose is absorbed from the dialysate. For less aggressive fluid loss, 1.36% dialysate can be mixed with the stronger solution.

Haemodialysis

Access

The most important aspect of haemodialysis involving the intensive care nurse is care of the vascular access. To haemodialyse a child there must be reliable access to the circulation to take and return blood at volumes of up to 200 ml/min in an older child. It is possible to take and return from a single access, e.g. a large central line, but dialysis is easier and more effective with a double access. Infection is a potential problem for all haemodialysis access, and in a seriously ill or immunosuppressed child can be life threatening. Access is therefore always treated with strict asepsis, used only for haemodialysis, and removed if there are signs of infection.

Flucloxacillin prophylaxis is a sensible precaution to minimize the risk of infection. As a child cannot be haemodialysed without vascular access, care of access is of paramount importance.

Double-lumen central-line access
This is designed for dialysis and inserted in the same way as a conventional central line. It has the following advantages:

1. quick and easy insertion;
2. availability for use as soon as radiography has checked the position;
3. effective adequate blood flows;
4. minimal scarring;
5. easy removal;

and the disadvantages that it is:

1. difficult to secure and often needs repositioning (catheters move, flows deteriorate and clots can form despite filling with a heparin lock);
2. liable to erode the major blood vessels or heart on insertion or subsequently causing tamponade;
3. uncomfortable.

Double-lumen soft-cuffed and tunnelled catheter (similar to Hickman)
This has the advantages that it:

1. is usable immediately after insertion and radiographic check;
2. is well secured, because the catheter is tunnelled;
3. gives excellent blood flows;
4. is comfortable for the child, although painful after operation;
5. is easy to remove.

The disadvantages are that it:

1. needs to be inserted in theatre under general anaesthesia by a surgeon;
2. can block despite a heparin lock.

Either type of central access, if blocked, can sometimes be rescued by infusing a mixture of urokinase 5000 units, heparin 500 units and normal saline 50 ml at a rate of 5 ml/h to each lumen (2–3 ml/h if fluid intake is a problem).

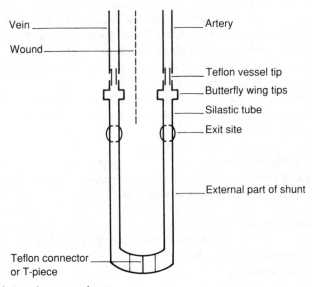

Vein
Wound
Artery
Teflon vessel tip
Butterfly wing tips
Silastic tube
Exit site
External part of shunt
Teflon connector
or T-piece

Figure 7.4 Arteriovenous shunt.

Arteriovenous shunt

The third type of vascular access used is the arteriovenous shunt (Figure 7.4). A silastic catheter tip is inserted into an artery and a vein in either an arm or leg. These are attached to two silastic tubes, which are then connected externally to complete the blood flow and disconnected for dialysis. A T-piece can be inserted to enable blood samples to be taken.

The advantages are that it:

1. provides excellent blood flow from a major artery;
2. can be used immediately;
3. can also be used for haemofiltration;
4. does away with the need for venepuncture (a big plus from the child's point of view);
5. is comfortable after the initial period, although very painful after operation;
6. allows cyanosis to be easily seen as arterial blood can be seen clearly.

The disadvantages are that:

1. if it is opened, bleeding is severe; clips must therefore be kept on the dressing, and it must be covered by a dressing so that the loops cannot be pulled;
2. it needs to be inserted by a surgeon;

3. it scars;
4. it can clot, needs to be warm and not kinked (care must be taken with dressing, tight clothes, etc.) and must be checked hourly for warmth, regular bright red colour and pulse.

A clotted shunt can often be declotted, especially if it has not been clotted for too long. This should only be attempted by experienced renal staff.

Principles of haemodialysis

Dialysis is the passing of solutes from a high to a low concentration across a semipermeable membrane, dependent on diffusion rates and selectivity by the membrane.

Haemodialysis is a very efficient intermittent form of renal replacement therapy. Because haemodialysis is intermittent, it is often difficult to provide adequate nutrition due to fluid restriction. Before the availability of volumetric dialysis machines, the control of fluid loss was variable and bed scales were required to determine the patient's weight. Access to the central circulation needs to be provided by either subclavian catheter or arteriovenous shunt. Unlike for continuous arteriovenous haemodiafiltration (CAVHD), specialist equipment and trained staff are necessary. This can be very time consuming because the trained dialysis nurse has to remain with the patient throughout the procedure.

Special considerations need to be applied when performing acute paediatric haemodialysis. The child's hepatitis B antigen status should be known before dialysis (Australian antigen test) and treated according to unit policy.

The extracorporeal guideline must be used to perform safe dialysis. No more than 8% of the child's total blood volume is removed; the priming volume of the dialyser and lines must not exceed this. If the child's extracorporeal blood volume is exceeded by the dialysis circuit or the child is anaemic, a blood prime of the dialyser and lines is necessary.

Children should have a dialyser that is not greater than their own body surface area. To calculate this the child's height in centimeters × weight in kilograms is plotted on a nomogram. For the first dialysis session, a dialyser that is two-thirds of the child's body surface area is used.

There are two types of dialysate available: acetate and bicarbonate. The use of bicarbonate dialysis is preferable as it is a natural buffer.

To prevent haemolysis, dehydration and disequilibration, the difference between the child's serum sodium concentration and that of the dialysate fluid should not be greater than ±10 mmol/l. If the child's blood urea level is >40 mmol/l, mannitol 20% is used. It is prescribed at 1 g/kg. Two-thirds of the total volume prescribed is infused over the first half of dialysis, the remainder during the second half.

Heparin may be given to prevent clotting of the dialysis circuit. It is prescribed at 10–30 units/kg if required. Sequential dialysis (in which dialysis and fluid removal occur separately) is used if the patient has excess fluid to lose. Peripheral and central temperatures are used as a guide to fluid removal. When the patient is peripherally warm and hypertensive, fluid removal can be commenced.

Paediatric dialysis is an involved procedure. It is very important to explain the procedure to the child and family according to their level of understanding. Dialysis can be a long procedure, and therefore suitable play equipment or a video should be provided to prevent boredom. During dialysis, observations are recorded as required and acted on accordingly. Routine observations include quarter hourly blood pressure, pulse, core–peripheral temperature differential and general appearance. Haemodialysis is now rarely used in intensive care since the advent of CAVHD, except in cases of hyperkalaemia or drug toxicity.

Continuous arteriovenous haemofiltration

Continuous arteriovenous haemofiltration (CAVH) is a simple manual filtration technique (Figure 7.5) controlled by the patient's cardiac output. It is a process by which whole blood is filtered and water molecules pull other molecules, e.g. sodium and potassium, with them. The filter consists of two compartments, the blood side and the filtrate side. These are separated by a semipermeable membrane.

Access can be provided for CAVH by wide-bore cannulation of an artery and vein, e.g. umbilical, femoral or arteriovenous shunt. If arterial access is difficult or contraindicated, venous access is used and continuous venovenous haemofiltration is performed. As there is then no driving force for the circuit, a pump is necessary. This method of haemofiltration is rarely used in paediatrics.

To ensure that CAVH is performed safely, no more than 8–10% of the child's blood volume must be used. This is calculated by:

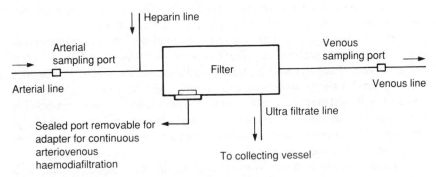

Figure 7.5 Continuous arteriovenous haemofiltration.

$$\frac{\text{weight in kg} \times 80 \times 10}{100}$$

e.g. for a neonate:

$$\frac{2 \times 80 \times 10}{100} = 16\,\text{ml}$$

Therefore the priming volume of the haemofilter and blood lines must not exceed 16 ml.

There are a variety of haemofilters available for neonatal and paediatric use. Each manufacturer provides instructions on how to prepare the filter for use. The basic objective is to prime the filter free of air and to rinse out the sterilizing agent. The filter is primed by gravity using 0.9% heparinized sodium chloride on the filtrate and the blood side. It is very important that only experienced members of staff undertake this procedure. Improper priming of a haemofilter can lead to air embolism.

The hepatitis status of the patient should be known before commencing haemofiltration and acted on according to unit policy. The patient should be as stable as possible with an adequate blood pressure to ensure that good flow is maintained through the filter. A normal albumin level of 30–40 g/l ensures that oncotic pressure can pull excess fluid into the circulatory system from the tissues. The difference between core and peripheral temperature should be $<2\,^{\circ}\text{C}$. The use of a space blanket is one way to help maintain this gap of $2\,^{\circ}\text{C}$ or less. Combining all these will ensure optimum fluid removal.

Before commencing CAVH, the filter should be rechecked to ensure that it is correctly primed and the filtrate line is closed. A sterile procedure is used, and the access is cleaned with betadine alcoholic solution and dried. Access is checked to ensure patency. Inadequate arterial flow will lead to clotting and poor filtration rate. The clamped arterial line is attached to the arterial end of the patient's access, and the venous line to the venous end. All connections are luer locking and should be checked for security. All clamps are removed and blood allowed to flow through the filter. At this stage, monitoring for hypotension and tachycardia is vital; CAVH may need to be discontinued if these are severe. Equipment should be ready to reinfuse blood from the circuit back to the patient.

Heparin (10–30 units/kg) is prescribed as necessary according to the results of the coagulation screen. Some children and neonates require no heparin. Coagulation screen should be checked at least daily to ensure that anticoagulation is adequate. The first bolus of heparin should be given according to prescription at the commencement of CAVH. The infusion of heparin helps to prevent coagulation of the haemofiltration circuit.

When a full circuit has been obtained, the lines are securely taped with no obstruction to blood flow. A space blanket/silver swaddler is used to keep the patient and filter warm. For safety, clamps should be at the bedside at all times in case of disconnection. All connections should be checked regularly for signs of disconnection.

Filtration may be commenced after this. The amount of filtrate removed depends on the pressure created by the distance between the haemofilter and the collection vessel (= negative pressure). By minimizing the distance between the haemofilter and the collection bag the filtrate will decrease and vice versa.

A gate clamp or volumetric pump may be used to help to regulate fluid removal. These are attached to the filtrate line. With a constant amount of fluid removal the life of the filter is extended because the patient's blood pressure will be more stable, therefore decreasing the risk of poor blood flow leading to sluggish flow through the filter. The amount to be removed per hour from the patient is determined by the doctor. The filtrate should be measured at least hourly. Depending on the fluid balance to be achieved, the filtrate is either replaced or treated as excess to obtain a negative fluid balance; a decrease in the amount of filtrate removed may indicate that the filter's ultra-filtrator capacity is failing and therefore should be replaced by a new system.

Haemofiltration is blood pressure dependent. Excessive depletion from the circulating system can cause hypotension, tachycardia, poor skin turgor, sunken fontanelle and an increase in the central peripheral temperature differential. With decreased blood flow due to hypotension, the filter is more prone to clotting. The filter should be observed for dark streaks along its length and at both sides.

If a filter clots, it is very important to preserve the patient's access. Obtaining and maintaining paediatric access can be problematic. If possible, the blood in the circuit should be reinfused; this should only be performed by experienced staff familiar with the procedure. If a shunt is used it should be connected immediately to maintain flow through the circuit. Other types of access should be treated according to type.

With the use of haemofiltration, practically unlimited nutrition can be given to the paediatric patient. This is extremely important as they can become catabolic. Good nutrition helps to maintain a low urea level and provides energy for growth and repair.

Haemofiltration is now becoming a standard feature in the intensive care unit. Renal nurses have been instructing intensive care staff to understand, care and maintain their patients on CAVH, the result being that the procedure has been performed well.

Continuous arteriovenous haemodiafiltration

Continuous arteriovenous haemodiafiltration (CAVHD) is fast becoming the

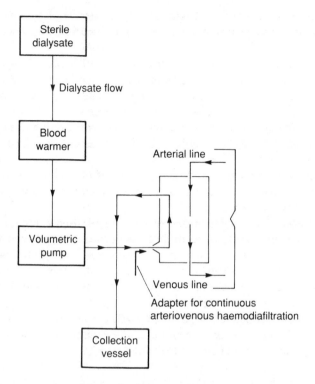

Figure 7.6 Continuous arteriovenous haemodiafiltration.

treatment of choice in intensive care units for patients requiring renal replacement therapy. It is especially useful for neonates, as the dead volume of present haemodialysis circuits is greater than their permissible extracorporeal blood volume. It is also ideal for patients who are haemodynamically unstable or where peritoneal dialysis is unsuitable. As for CAVH, the extracorporeal blood circuit should not exceed 8% of the patient's circulating volume.

CAVHD is a gentle process during which fluid removal and dialysis occur simultaneously by osmosis and diffusion. Using a conventional haemofilter adapted for CAVHD, sterile warmed dialysate is pumped across the filtrate side of the semipermeable membrane. A countercurrent flow is achieved by infusing the dialysate fluid through the filter in the opposite direction to blood flow through the filter (Figure 7.6).

The concentration of the dialysate provides the diffusional gradient required to achieve equilibration using a volumetric pump; between 500 ml and 1 litre of dialysate is pumped through the filter per hour, thus achieving adequate dialysis. The filtrate is measured hourly. The amount infused as dialysate is subtracted from the total filtrate obtained, which equals the excess fluid removed from the patient. As losses may be excessive, a volumetric pump may be connected to the filtrate line, thus controlling fluid loss at a prescribed rate.

Following the manufacturer's instructions, the haemofilter is primed as required for CAVH, using adapters provided to complete the circuit. The filter is attached to the patient's access using the same technique as for CAVH. Once a full circuit is established and the patient is stable, the filtrate line is unclamped and dialysis infusion is commenced. To prevent build-up of fluid in the filter and to avoid back-filtration, it is essential that the filtrate line remains unclamped throughout the process.

The general maintenance and management of CAVHD is as for CAVH with regards to patency of access and heparinization; the same guide lines for fluid removal also apply.

Blood urea and electrolyte measurements are required at regular intervals for dialysis requirements. As equilibration occurs, the dialysate flow may be reduced as necessary to maintain a satisfactory electrolyte balance.

Due to the continuous nature of this treatment the hypercatabolic state of the acutely ill patient can be controlled by the use of adequate nutrition, because fluid loss can be easily achieved.

The mechanical equipment used for CAVHD can be found in most intensive care units, and therefore does not significantly increase the cost of managing acutely ill patients with acute renal failure.

ACKNOWLEDGEMENTS

I thank Dr G. Haycock, L.J. Lee, V. Smith, E.C. Wright and Mrs T. Turtle.

FURTHER READING

Andreucci, V.E. (1984) *Acute Renal Failure*, Martinus Nijhoff, The Hague.
Assadi, F.K. (1988) Treatment of acute renal failure in an infant by continuous arteriovenous haemodialysis. *Paediatric Nephrology*, **2**, 320–2.
Behrman, R.E. and Vaughan, V.C. (1987) *Nelson Textbook of Paediatrics*, 13th edn, W.B. Saunders, London.
Coles, G.A. (1988) *Manual of Peritoneal Dialysis*, Kluwer Academic, London.
Drukker, W., Parsons, F.M. and Maher, J.F. (ed.) (1983) *Replacement of Renal Function by Dialysis*, 2nd edn, Martinus Nijhoff, The Hague.
George, J. (ed.) (1990) *Nursing Theories*, 3rd edn, Appleton and Lange, New Jersey.
Goodison, S.M. and Holmes, S. (1985) Acute renal failure: Aetiology and emergency treatment. *Nursing*, **42**, 1254–7.
Haas-Beckert, B. (1987) Removing the mysteries of parenteral nutrition. *Pediatric Nursing*, **13**(1), 37–41.

Holliday, M.A., Barratt, T.M. and Vernier, R.L (1987) *Paediatric Nephrology*, 2nd edn, Williams and Wilkins, Baltimore.

Hopkinson, R. and Davis, A. (1987) A guide to parenteral feeding. *Care of the critically ill*, **3**(3), 64–7.

Leaker, B. (1988) Acute renal failure. *Care of the Critically Ill*, **4**(3) 6–8.

Lieberman, K.V. (1987) Continuous arteriovenous haemofiltration in children. *Pediatric Nephrology*, **1**, 330–8.

Nursing 84 (1984) *Renal and Urologic Disorders*, Springhouse corporation, Pennsylvania.

Paganini, E.P. (1988) Slow continuous hemofiltration and slow continuous ultrafiltration. Transactions of the American Society for Artificial Internal Organs. *Nephrology Dialysis Transplantation*, **34**, 63–6.

Rigden, S.P. Start, K.M. and Rees, L. (1987) Nutritional management of infants and toddlers with chronic renal failure. *Nutrition and Health*, **5**(3/4), 163–74.

Roper, N., Logan, W.W. and Tiernay, A.J. (1980) *The Elements of Nursing*, Churchill Livingstone, London.

Van Geelen, J.A. Vincent, H.H. and Schalekamp, M.A. (1988) Continuous arteriovenous haemofiltration and haemodiafiltration in acute renal failure. *Nephrology Dialysis Transplantation*, **2**, 181–6.

Zobel, G., Ring, E. and Zobel, V. (1989) Continuous arteriovenous renal replacement systems for critically ill children. *Pediatric Nephrology*, **3**, 140–3.

Zobel, G., Ring, E., Trop, M. and Stein, J.I. (1986) Arterio-venous hemodiafiltration in children. *International Journal of Pediatric Nephrology*, **7**, 203–6.

8

Care of the child with polytrauma and thermal injury

Bernadette Carter and Dot Cooper

The aim of this chapter is to give an insight into the care and management of the child with polytrauma. It is impossible to be prescriptive when discussing the care of the child who is the victim of polytrauma, because the range of problems that the child may present with are very varied. Therefore the principles underlying the nursing management problems are highlighted and explored.

POLYTRAUMA: A SPECIAL CASE FOR INTENSIVE CARE

Statistics associated with the incidence, trends and types of trauma injuries admitted into intensive care are not available in the UK because paediatric trauma is not widely recognized as a separate specialty. However, in the UK in 1984 accidents were the most common cause of death in children aged 5–14 years (Zideman, 1986).

One of the major factors to consider in the child who is experiencing severe trauma is that the previously healthy child is usually suddenly and catastrophically ill. This means that there is no time for the child or the family to prepare for the experience, and the child's critical condition will pose a heavy immediate and ongoing strain on the physical and psychological resources of the intensive care unit.

Factors such as the time from injury to initial treatment and transfer to intensive care have also been shown to have a major effect on outcome and prognosis (Polley and Coran, 1986).

The main problems and needs of the child and the family are as follows and will be experienced either to a greater or lesser degree depending on the nature and severity of the trauma:

1. maintaining airway and breathing;
2. supporting comprised circulation;
3. relieving pain;
4. identifying and assessing injuries;
5. preventing further injury and deterioration;
6. facing the possibility, with the family, that the child may either die or have a considerably different quality of life as a result of the trauma;
7. helping the family to cope with the catastrophic situation.

THE CONCEPT OF TRAUMA

All nursing and medical care of the polytraumatized child is aimed at containing and reducing the effects of the trauma. The nature of the trauma, e.g. mechanical, thermal (heat and cold), electrical or radiant, must be considered as well as the degree and size of the trauma.

The degree or size of the trauma is dependent on, and can be affected by, many factors, including:

1. degree of tissue hypoxia;
2. degree of tissue damage;
3. location of the tissue damage;
4. amount (and type) of fluid lost;
5. severity and duration of pain;
6. time from injury to treatment centre.

Although the degree of trauma will depend on the previously discussed factors, the effects of the trauma on the child must be understood if the nurse is to understand the child's condition.

Trauma has both local and systematic effects which may be considered in the care and management of the child. The psychological effect is not dismissed but will be discussed later (Reynolds and Ramenofsky, 1988; Lanning, 1985).

The local effects may be inflammation or degeneration and necrosis. *Inflammation* is the specific reaction to vascular connective tissue caused by the trauma itself: heat, swelling, redness, pain, decrease and loss of function, and the release of chemical substances. *Degeneration and necrosis* of tissue occur as a local response to cellular damage (as well as in response to systemic hypoxia and poor perfusion). In the early stages degeneration may be reversible, but it may progress to necrosis.

The systemic effects may be circulatory or metabolic. The *circulatory* responses include adjustments to maintain blood pressure and perfusion by increasing heart rate, peripheral vasoconstriction and hormonal responses. The *metabolic* responses vary according to the intensity of the injury itself and the presence of possible complications, as well as other factors such as the age of the child, and nutritional and health status before the trauma.

In response to trauma there is an increase in the serum glucose level. Glucose is a ready source of energy, and increased concentration of glucose in the blood results in an increase in the serum osmolarity, which helps to attract fluid into the vascular spaces and to maintain the circulating blood volume.

Fat metabolism is also affected because fat becomes the major source of energy in the trauma patient. Polytrauma causes a massive protein catabolism, resulting in a negative nitrogen balance with a large amount of protein nitrogen being lost in the urine. Muscle, skeletal and general body tissue protein is catabolized after major trauma.

Changes in water and electrolyte balance also occur in response to trauma. Initially, the body tries to conserve water and sodium. In response to hypovolaemia, antidiuretic hormone and aldosterone secretions are increased and urinary output is decreased.

The management of polytrauma is not simply the care of each individual injury that the child has sustained; rather, it is the care of the cumulative and additive effects of all the injuries.

SHOCK SYNDROMES

Shock is a clinical syndrome characterized by a decreased cardiac output leading to a failure of the circulation to meet the metabolic demands of the tissues. This results in inadequate or inappropriate tissue perfusion and a general cellular hypoxia. (Rimar, 1988a; Mattson Porth, 1990; Muir, 1988). There are three major classifications of shock: hypovolaemic, cardiogenic and distributive. All may be involved in the child affected by severe trauma (Table 8.1). Hypovolaemic shock is the most common form of shock in the paediatric trauma patient.

Table 8.1 Major shock syndromes and possible causes

Syndrome	Possible causes
Hypovolaemic	Blood loss, visible and invisible
	Plasma loss
	Capillary leak syndrome
	Burns
	Hypoproteinaemia
	Water loss
	Glycosuria diuresis
	Diarrhoea and vomiting
	Diabetes insipidus
Cardiogenic	Drugs
	Metabolic imbalance
	Acidaemia
	Congenital heart lesions
Distributive	Anaphylaxis
	Sepsis
	Vasomotor paralysis
	Drugs

Shock is progressive and dynamic and is characterized by three major phases (Figure 8.1). The management and treatment of shock is aimed at preventing shock from progressing from compensated to uncompensated or irreversible shock. The importance of fast and effective initiation of treatment cannot be understated because it is impossible to measure or accurately predict the transition from uncompensated to irreversible shock (Rimar, 1988b). Many

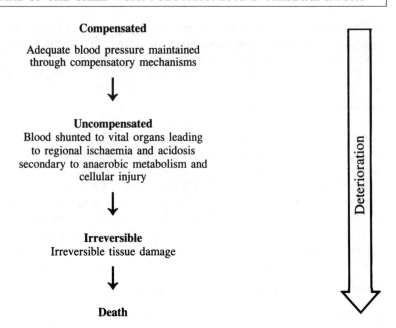

Figure 8.1 Dynamic phases of shock.

compensatory mechanisms are involved (Table 8.2) and the child's response to shock is greatly intensified compared with the adult's and can be almost too efficient.

Successful and effective management involves prioritizing the treatment that the child is to receive and being flexible and dynamic in the approach to treatment (Hurn and Connolly, 1983).

Hypovolaemic shock

Hypovolaemic shock results from the loss of fluid from the circulating blood volume which, if untreated or uncompensated, results in inadequate tissue perfusion. Blood, plasma and water losses or a combination of all of them can lead to hypovolaemic shock. In the polytrauma patient, visible and invisible haemorrhage are most likely to be the causes of shock.

Children in severe shock may appear to be coping quite well because they can maintain a normal systolic blood pressure even with a circulation blood volume deficit of 25–30%. Blood pressure in the child decreases only in profound shock (Coln, 1985).

The nurse should assess the child for tachycardia and decreased pulse pressure, poor peripheral perfusion, tachypnoea, decreased urinary output and a decreased level of consciousness, which more accurately indicate the

Table 8.2 Compensatory mechanisms in shock

Classification	Stimulated by	Involves	Results
Sympathetic	Decreased blood pressure	Baroreceptors	Increased heart rate Increased myocardial activity Constriction of peripheral arterioles and veins
	Decreased P_{aO_2} Increased P_{aCO_2} Increased $[H^+]$	Chemoreceptors	Increased alveolar ventilation Increased respiratory rate Increased depth of respiration
	Increased P_{aCO_2} Increased lactic acid Very much increased arterial blood pressure	CNS ischaemic reflex-extreme	Increased blood pressure Decreased carbon dioxide
Capillary fluid shift	Increased blood pressure Decreased capillary pressure	Movement of water from interstitial to vascular space	Increased blood pressure Increased carbon dioxide
Humoral or hormonal	Decreased P_{aO_2} Decreased P_{aCO_2}	Respiratory centre	Increased respiratory rate and depth Increased alveolar ventilation
	Sympathetic nervous system	Adrenaline, noradrenaline	Increased heart rate Increased CO_2 & blood pressure Increased arteriovascular constriction
	Decreased blood pressure	Renin–angiotensin	Vasoconstriction aldosterone secretion Na & H_2O retention Increased blood pressure & CO_2
	Increased blood pressure	Antidiuretic hormone	Vasoconstriction Increased blood pressure & CO_2

degree of shock, rather than relying on blood pressure as the major parameter.

The picture of the cool, pale child is characteristic of the child experiencing hypovolaemic shock, but this is not so for the child presenting with septic shock.

Septic shock

Septic shock is categorized as a form of distributive shock and because of its high associated mortality rate must be seriously considered and assessed by the nurse caring for the child with severe trauma. Septic shock is caused by the presence of microorganisms or their products in the blood, which can in turn lead to circulatory insufficiency and inadequate tissue perfusion (Littleton, 1988).

Septic shock in the severely traumatized child is an unwanted and all too often fatal complication. Septic shock is often associated with serious pathologic complications such as disseminated intravascular coagulation (DIC) and marked acute respiratory failure with pulmonary oedema.

Septic shock generally progresses through two haemodynamic phases, which are most easily recognized by assessing the child's skin temperature. The first phase is *hyperdynamic* or *warm* shock, in which the child feels warm; this occurs as a result of a marked reduction in peripheral vascular resistance, which is compensated for by a high cardiac output. The peripheral vaso-dilation results in the child feeling warm to the touch, can often mask an underlying picture of developing shock if the nurse is not aware that this must be taken into consideration. The second phase is *hypodynamic* or *cold* shock, which is more characteristic of the shocked patient. This stage occurs when the increased cardiac output is unable to maintain blood pressure and flow to the dilated peripheral vessels. At this point, the child appears cool and cyanosed and manifests the classic signs and symptoms of shock.

Cardiogenic shock

Cardiogenic shock occurs when, despite adequate ventricular preload, cardiac output is insufficient. In the polytrauma patient, cardiogenic shock is likely to develop as a result of sepsis, uraemic metabolic imbalance and the consequences of prolonged uncompensated shock of another origin.

DISSEMINATED INTRAVASCULAR COAGULATION

DIC is a complex syndrome, which is not completely understood. It is seen in critically ill patients and can be a major contributor to multiple organ failure. DIC is an acquired bleeding disorder that always develops secondary to another disease. These include infection, trauma, hypoxaemia, hypoperfusion, anaphylaxis, major surgery, liver damage and incompatible blood transfusions.

DIC is an accelerated, inappropriate and systematic activation of the clotting cascade, causing the simultaneous development of thrombi and haemorrhage (Caplin, 1984; Griffin, 1986). Normally the clotting cascade is a well balanced and finely tuned mechanism, only becoming activated in times of need, and deactivating itself once the initial trigger has been compensated for. However, in DIC this does not occur, once the cascade has been activated it becomes completely aberrant.

To appreciate the syndrome of DIC the normal coagulation pathways must be considered.

Haemostasis

Haemostasis is achieved through a balance between two mechanisms: prevention of the formation of unnecessary clots and fibrinolysis when coagulation is no longer required. In health, this balance is maintained and neither process is activated until a trigger is present (Machin, 1988; Gaspard, 1990).

The coagulation process can be triggered in two main ways:

1. by endothelial trauma: the intrinsic pathway;
2. by tissue trauma: the extrinsic pathway.

Either pathway, once triggered, can activate the final common pathway,

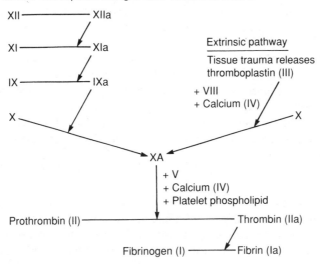

Figure 8.2 The blood coagulation cascade.

which results in clot formation, provided all coagulation factors are present in sufficient quantities (Figure 8.2). Problems arise if one or all of the necessary factors is unavailable; the cascade is interrupted and the development of the final clot is unachievable. In health this does not occur and clotting is achieved when and where required and acts as a protective and haemostatic mechanism. Once the body recognizes that the clot is no longer required, the process of *fibrinolysis* or dissolution of the clot commences. Plasminogen triggers the enzyme plasmin to break down the fibrin threads within the clot and the products of the clot are eventually removed in the circulation:

$$\text{plasminogen} \rightarrow \text{plamin} \rightarrow \text{clot dissolution}$$

Disorders of haemostasis can result from a variety of causes involving both genetic and acquired origins. DIC is a syndrome characterized by consumption of coagulation factors and inappropriate clotting.

Pathology

In DIC, thrombin formation holds the key to understanding the process of simultaneous clot formation and haemorrhage.

Clot formation

Free thrombin liberated into the circulation as a result of both the intrinsic and extrinsic cascade catalyses the activation of fibrinogen. The fibrinogen causes more fibrin to be produced and this travels in the circulation to the microcirculation, where it is finally desposited. Once within the microcirculation, the threads of fibrin form clots and cause decreased circulation and decreased flow of vital nutrients to cells and tissues. This can lead to tissue ischaemia, especially within the kidneys, lungs, brain, gastrointestinal tract, pancreas, adrenal glands and pituitary. These organs start to fail and are further compromised by platelet clumping, which is also activated by the formation of thrombin.

The clotting problem is further exacerbated by the release of phospholipids from damaged erythrocytes and platelets, which also act as clotting agents.

Haemorrhage

The rapid formation of harmful and unnecessry clots quickly uses up all the essential and readily available clotting factors so that clot formation can no longer occur anywhere in the body. The body no longer has any reserves with which to prevent possible terminal haemorrhage. This outcome is called consumption coagulopathy.

The activation of the fibrinolytic system may dissolve some of the fibrin clots and allow the release of fibrin degradation products. The FDPs interfere with fibrinogen and platelet aggregation, increase thrombin time and have an anticoagulant effect. In DIC, the normal balance between clot formation and lysis does not occur.

Trigger factors

It is a secondary disorder resulting from a primary disease that triggers the abnormal pattern of the clotting cascade: damage to either tissues involving blood vessels or the endothelial lining of blood vessels:

1. *Endothelial injury.* Collagen is exposed and the intrinsic coagulation cascade as well as the fibrinolytic system is triggered. Endothelial injury can result from shock, sepsis, anoxia, adult respiratory distress syndrome, transfusion reactions and amniotic fluid emboli.
2. *Tissue injury.* This results from diseases and disorders that allow the release of tissue thromboplastin into the circulation and thereby activates the extrinsic cascade. Tissue injury can be caused by shock, sepsis, tumours (especially those involving the brain and lungs), extensive surgery, burns and snakebites.

Diagnosis

Diagnosis of DIC is made by all or some of the above indications and is supported by laboratory results:

1. decreased platelet count;
2. decreased plasma fibrinogen;
3. prolonged prothrombin time;
4. prolonged partial thromboplastin time;
5. decreased haematocrit;
6. increased fibrin degradation products;
7. damaged or fragmented appearance to erythrocytes.

However, these values can be altered by other factors, such as multiple transfusions, which may dilute clotting factors and platelets.

MULTIPLE SYSTEM ORGAN FAILURE

Multiple system organ failure (MSOF) is the result of a major deficit in oxygen delivery to the tissues of the body. It is a sequential process associated with a high mortality rate. If it is to be treated effectively, prevention and early diagnosis of the triggering factors are essential.

MSOF occurs as a result of underlying pathogenic factors, the two major factors being existing organ dysfunction and sepsis (Marvin, 1988). Preventing these two factors from developing remains the primary goal in the management and care of the polytrauma patient. However, the nature of polytrauma itself predisposes to both factors presenting or developing. The incidence of MSOF is greatly increased if more than one organ system is failing and if sepsis is present. Other predisposing factors which may occur as a result of sepsis or organ dysfunction, include hypoperfusion and massive crystalloid and colloid therapy.

MSOF remains responsible for the death of children admitted with apparently reversible injuries but who subsequently develop sepsis. The complication further highlights the need for vigilance when assessing the polytraumatized child for signs of infection.

Pathogenesis

MSOF occurs when the normal response to hypoperfusion and sepsis is unable to meet the demands of the tissues and two major pathways are activated: a pathway designed to improve the supply of oxygen and energy to the cells, and a pathway designed to overcome the infective trigger.

Hypovolaemia, reduced cardiac output, hypoxaemia and sepsis, unless reversed, result in hypoperfusion and decreased oxygen delivery to the tissues and this triggers the process that leads to MSOF. Hypoperfusion triggers the release of adrenocorticotrophic hormone (ACTH), cortisol, adrenaline, noradrenaline and glucagon in a compensatory physiological attempt to improve oxygen and vital nutrient delivery to the tissues. The release of these factors has several consequences: first, constriction of non-vital and renal vascular beds, resulting in an increased blood flow to the heart and brain; secondly, elevation of serum blood sugar and reduction of glucose uptake in muscle and fat; and, finally, gluconeogenesis, which is triggered once glycogen stores are exhausted, so that muscle is broken down to release amino acids, which are transferred to the liver and used in the production of fuel and protein. This then results in increased protein catabolism, which creates excessive demands on the liver, which can in turn only inappropriately metabolize the amino acids.

Sepsis also triggers macrophage activity and activates the immune defence system. This activates the complement cascade, which results in endothelial injury and actively damages the tissue cells.

Eventually, the catabolic demands outweigh any possible response and the tissue cells have an insufficient supply of oxygen and an inappropriate or inadequate fuel supply. When this occurs, adenosine triphosphate (ATP) synthesis within the cells fails, and it is then impossible to restore the normal function of the affected cells, tissues and organs; end-stage MSOF results.

Treatment

Prevention, by removing the initiating and triggering causes, is the best means of dealing with MSOF. This can be achieved by ensuring that adequate oxygen is delivered to all tissues through achieving and maintaining adequate circulating volume, vascular integrity and cardiac output. Crystalloid and colloid solutions, pharmacological support in the form of inotrope–vasodilator and antibiotic administration are commonly used to treat the underlying causes of MSOF. Less commonly, corticosteroids may be used in conjunction with antibiotic therapy in an attempt to mediate the stress response that occurs as a result of trauma. Studies indicate that steroid therapy is most beneficial if used in the early stages of shock.

However, MSOF frequently proves to be impossible to treat effectively, and the goal of ensuring that adequate oxygen delivery to all tissues is unachievable. In this situation, management becomes increasingly problematic, with the demands of one failing organ system conflicting with the demands of another. The result is that intervention beneficial to one organ may compromise and endanger another. Antibiotic therapy essential in the treatment of sepsis may put an additional strain on the renal and hepatic systems. Fluid administered to maintaining circulating volume may escape through damaged vascular and cellular walls and contribute to pre-existing oedema, resulting in increased cerebral and pulmonary oedema. In this situation, treatment is almost always one step behind the failing systems and the patient rapidly deteriorates despite intensive and experienced intervention. As the process continues, additional systems fail and the possibility of recovery decreases; the patient eventually reaches end-stage MSOF and ultimately dies despite all the support and intervention provided.

THE NEED FOR AN INTENSIVIST

Preparation for the child includes informing the anaesthetist and other members of the medical and surgical teams likely to be required in the initial emergency assessment and management. At this point, it is imperative for an intensivist or child care coordinator to be named and recognized even if this is not a routine practice within the unit.

The polytraumatized child is likely to require the combined services of the nursing team, anaesthetists, physicians, neurosurgeons, general surgeons, orthopaedic, vascular and genitourinary surgeons, haematologist, radiologist, biochemist, pharmacist and physiotherapist. The complexity, speed and often unpredictability of the changing condition of the polytraumatized child require that input from these specialists should be at the highest level; that is, at consultant level. This ensures that the child is receiving care from the most experienced representatives from the speciality and that this experience is readily recognized by the other members of the trauma team. It has been suggested that optimal care can only be delivered in specialist trauma centres, but in the absence of these centres the paediatric intensive care unit must give the best possible care (Glass, 1985; Harris, 1987).

The aim of the trauma team must be to ensure that the separate specialists work together and are aware of all aspects of the child's condition. This is often highlighted in the case of fluid and drug therapy, where one specialist may decide to increase the fluid input while this contravenes the prescription of another specialist. If a suitably experienced coordinator is recognized, the clear lines of communication vital to the child's successful treatment may be established at an early stage. This not only improves the child's prognosis but can do much to reduce the stress that the nursing staff can feel if specialists countermand another's prescription without proper consultation.

To clarify some of the priorities of care and the interventions required to promote maximum recovery of the child, some aspects will be examined individually. This, however, may lead to a false scenario being described, because the medical and nursing problems that the child presents with will frequently occur together and require concurrent intervention and treatment; for example, a child who is unable to breathe spontaneously and is haemorrhaging will be receiving emergency treatment for both conditions at the same time. However, in all circumstances, the first priority must be secure an airway and establish respiratory support. Without adequate oxygenation of the tissues, other measures such as control of haemorrhage are pointless.

MANAGEMENT OF THE POLYTRAUMATIZED CHILD

The polytraumatized child will often present with many nursing management problems and needs, and these must be clearly established if nursing care is to be effective. Care of the child requires all the expertise and experience of the intensive care nurse, who must first identify the management problems and needs and then establish the aim of nursing intervention. Nursing care can then be planned, implemented and evaluated. This process is dynamic and ongoing. The care that the polytraumatized child receives is not simply the care and treatment of each individual injury, but care of all the injuries together. This requires that the nurse is capable of prioritizing care. The following management problems highlight possible injuries and some approaches to their effective management. Further details on specific care can be found in the appropriate chapters.

Problem 1: respiratory

Main aim: to establish and maintain airway, support respiration and prevent hypoxia.

Causes

Both airway and respiration can be compromised in the polytraumatized patient for many reasons, which are dependent on the type, site and degree of the injury. The type of treatment involved will therefore also be dependent on the injury.

Management problems and needs

Features commonly associated with trauma causing airway and respiratory problems include:

1. inability to self-maintain the airway due to decreased level of consciousness and/or maxillofacial/chest trauma;
2. hypoxia or anoxia due to local and systemic effects of trauma;
3. increased oxygen requirements due to increased metabolic rate after trauma and the urgent need to ensure that all tissues are adequately oxygenated;
4. presence of or potential for developing pneumothorax and haemothorax, and the presence of lung contusion.

Intervention and management

An immediate and ongoing consideration is to ensure that tissue perfusion is improved. Continuing untreated or undertreated hypoxia compounds the degree of trauma and injury. To try to increase the chance of perfusing all damaged areas, 100% oxygen is recommended; this should continue throughout all initial assessment procedures such as computer tomography and other radiographic procedures. The damaged tissues must be continually perfused if further damage and necrosis are to be minimized.

Maximal perfusion in the child with polytrauma usually requires *early elective* intervention with full intermittent positive pressure ventilation (IPPV). The child therefore requires intubation, which can be difficult in the child with polytrauma. Oral intubation is the fastest means of securing the airway (long term), but facial and oral injuries may make this impossible. Nasal intubation must be carefully considered because in basal skull fracture this could cause further damage by passing the endotracheal tube into brain tissue. A further factor that must be considered when intubating the child with polytrauma is cervical spinal fracture or injury. Until good-quality cervical spinal radiographs dismiss the possibility of trauma, it must be assumed that the spine is fractured, and some form of cervical support, such as a collar, must be used to immobilize the neck. This can cause difficulties by preventing the neck being extended to improve access for intubation.

The trauma may require a tracheostomy, and this must be cared for in the appropriate manner, again taking care not to manipulate the neck in an unsafe way. Elective paralysis may be considered appropriate, but before this the child should be observed for flail chest.

The child's colour may not be a good indicator of respiratory efficiency or inefficiency because, in severe hypovolaemia, when the haemoglobin level is <6 g/dl, even minimal respiratory effort may be sufficient to prevent the haemoglobin becoming desaturated, and it is desaturated haemoglobin that causes the skin to appear dusky.

Assessment of the child's respiratory condition remains a priority throughout their management, and regular frequent reassessment is necessary to ensure the early detection and prompt treatment of any deterioration, as well as accommodating improvements in condition.

It may be that the child's condition is so poor, owing to decreased level of consciousness, that emergency ventilatory intervention is required. In this case, the prognosis is deemed considerably poorer than in the child who receives early elective ventilatory support.

Nursing management

The nursing care aimed at overcoming respiratory problems centre on observation, monitoring and maintaining safe and effective ventilatory support.

Observation
The nurse must observe the child's chest for equality of chest movements, splinting, compliance with ventilation, colour and perfusion.

Monitoring
Respiratory monitoring in the critical situation involves the support of medical technology, which allows a greater variety of parameters to be assessed and measured. These may include blood gas analysis, preferably via arterial blood samples from an indwelling arterial line, transcutaneous oxygen or oxygen saturation monitoring using pulse oximetry. However, children in uncompensated shock or who are poorly perfused and peripherally shut down for some other reason are not good candidates for accurate asessment of oxygenation via either transcutaenous or pulse oximetry methods. Neither method is designed to cope with these situations.

Maintaining ventilation

Maintaining safe and effective ventilatory support will involve both effective humidification of and suction to the endotracheal tube/airway, which should ensure that the tube remains patent. Tracheal aspirate should be assessed in respect to amount, type and consistency, which can indicate underlying respiratory changes. Blood-stained secretions, beyond those which may result from a traumatic intubation, must be considered very seriously as they can be the first indication of a deterioration in the lungs. All routine care of the child requiring ventilation must be carried out.

Problem 2: cardiovascular

Main aim: to contain and prevent the damage caused by shock.

Causes

The management of the severely traumatized child, once the airway and breathing have been effectively dealt with, centres on the containment and prevention of shock.

Shock kills and, although children can initially compensate effectively, the efficiency of their compensatory mechanisms masks the severity of the condition. If shock is not quickly and effectively treated, the prognosis for the child inevitably deteriorates. To examine the interventions and treatments required by the shocked child, the shock syndrome must be understood.

To facilitate understanding of the support of the cardiovascular system two major areas of intervention must be examined:

1. fluid replacement therapy
2. pharmacological support.

Management problems and needs

Features commonly associated with trauma causing cardiovascular problems include:

1. uncompensated hypovolaemic shock due to internal and external haemorrhage caused by multiple injuries leading to hypotension, tachyardia and decreased cardiac output;
2. poor peripheral perfusion due to decreased blood pressure, and decreased capillary pressure due to hypovolaemia, sepsis and decreased cardiac output;
3. decreased urinary output due to decreased arterial blood pressure and renal injury.

Intervention and management

Hypovolaemic shock
Although the child may display the classic signs and symptoms of hypovolaemic shock the primary cause(s) of the hypovolaemic state must be determined if treatment is to be of long-term value. Polytrauma usually results in severe or even massive haemorrhage, which can be both internal and external, obvious or hidden, fast or insidious. All possible causes for haemorrhagic hypovolaemic shock should be considered.

The first aim of intervention is to prevent further loss. This is obviously easiest in external haemorrhage, where pressure can be applied either to the bleeding point or to the closest pressure point. Simple first-aid treatment is the first means of containing haemorrhage. Hidden loss, such as internal bleeding, may need to be treated by surgical intervention, but this requires that the child has been stabilized before theatre. Stabilization of the child usually results from a combination of fluid replacement and drug support.

Initial management Initially the child may receive an infusion of 0.9% saline before any colloid being prescribed. However, it is usual with deeply shocked children for plasma protein fraction to be prescribed. This helps to maintain the circulating blood volume, and the molecular weight of the plasma proteins helps to support blood pressure and prevent the loss of fluid from the circulation into the extravascular space (McClelland, 1990).

An immediate priority after gaining high-volume venous access is for blood samples to be sent to the laboratory for glucose, urea and electrolyte determination, full blood count, crossmatching, blood grouping and saving. It is important that the child in uncompensated hypovolaemic shock caused by haemorrhage receives blood products that will ensure or improve the carriage of oxygen to the tissues. It is also important, bearing in mind the likelihood that the child may need massive transfusions, that properly crossmatched blood is available, in sufficient quantity, as soon as possible. One problem that should be avoided, if possible, is the development of DIC as a result of poorly matched transfusions. However, giving unmatched group O positive blood may be required to save the child's life, and the potential of developing other problems must then be accepted (Hewitt and Machin, 1990).

Ongoing management Many difficulties lie within the realm of fluid replacement therapy and the child with polytrauma. First, a decision must be made as to the fluid and blood products to give and the potential problems associated with their infusion and transfusion. Secondly, the rate of administration of the chosen fluid must be considerable. Unless this is carefully monitored, there is the possibility of overtransfusion, with the child becoming hypervolaemic. This can produce equally undesirable effects, such as pulmonary and cerebral oedema (Baskett and Small, 1989).

Specialized blood products such as SAG.M blood may be chosen. Packed cells can be given when the child is normovolaemic but anaemic. A packed cell transfusion or reduced plasma transfusion that corrects anaemia can result in a vast improvement in the child's oxygen-carrying ability without the risk of overloading the child that whole blood carries.

Other blood products, such as fresh frozen plasma, are invaluable in helping to maintain blood pressure. It must be remembered that an important part of nursing management of fluid replacement therapy is the careful checking of the product with the prescription, following local policy guidelines (Ala, 1988).

Multivenous access To give adequate fluid replacement, more than one intravenous access site is often required and is generally considered safer. Relying on a single access site in the treatment of the child in uncompensated shock results in total dependence on that route: if the line fails for some reason, the child may quicky deteriorate, perhaps beyond the point where regaining access is possible. More than one access point also ensures that drug therapy can continue without having to interrupt infusion or transfusion. Drug and fluid incompatibilities also prove less of a problem if multiaccess is possible.

One major disadvantage of multiple venous access is that it creates more trauma and possible sites for infection in the already vulnerable patient, but this, at least initially, must be accepted as a necessary disadvantage.

Complications of blood replacement therapy The side-effects and complications that can result from massive transfusions of blood and blood products must always be considered and assessed, because they can fatally complicate the medical problems that the critically ill child is confronted with. These may include hyperkalaemia, microemboli, an elevation in temperature (which increases the already elevated metabolic rate) and anaphylactic reactions. Any of these side-effects occurring in an already debilitated, highly labile child can be fatal. It should be noted that the child who has received multiple transfusions becomes more at risk of developing complications because of the much increased number of antigens found in the circulating volume. It should also be remembered that blood which has been stored for more than 4 days is unlikely to contain any useful platelets; if a platelet insufficiency is diagnosed platelet concentrates should be given, and if clotting factors are required fresh frozen plasma is prescribed and transfused.

Other fluid support measures As the child becomes stabilized, fluid therapy will tend to move from the colloids to the crystalloids and simpler electrolyte solutions prescribed, such as dextrose saline mixes. Total parenteral nutrition is an important form of fluid therapy and nutrition, which is considered once the child is stable.

Careful monitoring is required to ensure that the child does not become overloaded or hypovolaemic as a reult of electrolyte solutions being lost into the interstitial fluid; this can happen where vascular integrity is poor.

Pharmacological support Drug support is frequently used in conjunction with fluid replacement therapy and plays a vital role in helping to maintain circulation and perfusion. The choice of drug therapy will often vary between units but will aim to increase cardiac contractility and cardiac output. Dopamine may be used.

Septic shock
The polytraumatized child is especially vulnerable to developing systemic sepsis that could lead to septic shock. Septic shock is associated with a high mortality rate and therefore it must be assessed for vigilantly and treated promptly. A major problem in diagnosing septic shock in the polytraumatized patient is that the symptoms can be masked and may not be obvious, especially in the early phase. The hyperdynamic, warm, pink phase may not be initially recognized as the first stage of septic shock, but may be thought to reflect a gradually improving condition following interventions for hypovolaemic shock, e.g.response to fluid and drug therapy.

The first aim of intervention is to establish and treat the underlying cause of sepsis. If practical, blood cultures are taken to allow the infecting agent to be identified so that the most appropriate antibiotic therapy can be instituted. However, blood cultures may be negative if antibiotic therapy commences before the sample is taken or if the sepsis is associated with extensive tissue necrosis.

Invariably, septic shock is diagnosed on clinical grounds in its early stages. Septic shock is characterized by pyrexia, tachypnoea, rigors, and occasionally by hypothermia and decreased urinary output. Blood samples demonstrate a 30–50% increase in circulating leucocytes, thrombocytopenia, hypoalbuminaemia, an increased blood urea nitrogen level and hypoglycaemia. The child would also present with respiratory alkalosis and metabolic acidosis.

Antibiotic therapy should be considered without delay, with the choice of antibiotic reflecting the possible cause of infection, which may result from both the intitial trauma and subsequent trauma caused by the use of invasive techniques for monitoring and fluid and drug support. Subsequently, therapy can be altered if the results indicate a specific infection.

Septic shock also requires intervention to maintain tissue perfusion through respiratory and gaseous support. Sepsis may result in a decreased cellular ability to extract oxygen, which means that septic patients often require a higher than normal P_{aO_2}. Intervention to maintain normal blood pressure and peripheral vascular resistance through pharmacological methods is of major importance in ensuring tissue oxygenation. Hypovolaemia resulting from capillary leak syndrome must also be considered and treated, although care must be taken not to overhydrate the child. Careful consideration should be made in respect of potentially disordered glucose metabolism.

Nursing management Nursing care is aimed at overcoming the circulatory problems that the child presents with, and centres on observation, monitoring and maintaining the circulating blood volume.

Observation The nurse must observe the child for changes in colour; the child in uncompensated shock (apart from the hyperdynamic phase of septic shock) will have mottled or grey peripheries, and generally appear very pale. The child's skin will appear dry, and skin turgor is poor with the mucous membranes also appearing dry. The child's eyes may appear sunken, and in babies the fontanelle may also be sunken.

The child who is not unconscious may appear to be either very quiet or restless, depending on the level of consciousness impairment.

Monitoring This may include physically assessing pulse pressure or monitoring the child's heart rate and rhythm via simple chest leads. Alternatively, increasingly sophisticated methods such as central venous pressure, arterial blood pressure and pulmonary artery monitoring may be employed. Temperature monitoring is also important.

Arterial blood pressure monitoring can be vital, because it can indicate changes in systemic blood pressure and stroke volume.

Central venous pressure (CVP) monitoring indicates right atrial pressure, which is indicative of the child's circulating blood volume and cardiac performance. When recording the CVP, several factors must be taken into consideration:

1. right ventricular function (the ability of the heart to accept and expel blood);
2. venous return (the volume of blood returning to the heart);
3. venous tone;
4. intrathoracic pressure (intermittent positive pressure ventilation (IPPV) and continuous positive airway pressure (CPAP) may cause inaccurate measurements).

CVP is reflective of various factors and must be interpreted in relation to known facts, otherwise the readings can be very misleading. Accurate CVP readings are of prime importance in assessing a child's volaemic state. One of the cardinal signs of hypovolaemia is a decrease in CVP; this occurs before any signs of a decrease in cardiac output such as pallor, sweating and reduced blood pressure. CVP is vital in estimating the success or otherwise of fluid replacement and drug therapy, but it is associated with many complications, which the nurse should be aware of, including local infection, septicaemia, infiltration, blockage, arrhythmias, air emboli, and nerve and vein damage.

Pulmonary artery monitoring is particularly useful in major trauma because it allows more definitive assessment of intravascular volume and the state of vasodilation than previously described methods. It is important in helping to determine whether the child is suffering from hypovolaemic or cardiogenic shock. Many complications can arise from this complex form of monitoring, and therefore these catheters are used only in selected cases and requires the child to be closely monitored.

Close and careful temperature monitoring allows assessment of the child's state of perfusion. The child's temperature should be continually measured via a rectal or oesophageal core temperature probe and a peripheral temperature probe. The hypovolaemic polytraumatized child who is peripherally shut down may demonstrate a temperature difference of 5°C or more. Care must be taken in positioning the probes so that they do not create areas of pressure, which may break down and add to skin trauma.

Fluid balance Ongoing care of fluid replacement therapy is based on the monitoring of the patient and on ensuring that fluids are infused and transfused as prescribed and that possible side-effects are considered and assessed.

Problem 3: neurological

Main aim: to promote continuing adequate perfusion of cerebral tissues and to maximally salvage compromised cerebral tissues.

Causes

Cerebral damage in the polytraumatized patient can result either from direct injury or as a result of hypoxia or anoxia leading to ischaemia and necrosis. Many factors associated with polytrauma, such as the site of the trauma and degree of resuscitation required, can influence the prognosis associated with the neurological aspects of the trauma.

Management problems and needs

Features commonly associated with trauma causing neurological problems include:

1. compromised circulation due to shock, leading to hypoxia;
2. cerebral haemorrhage resulting from bony injury;
3. cerebral oedema resulting from hypoxia and inflammatory responses;

4. postcardiac arrest;
5. fits of indeterminate cause.

Intervention and management

In attempting to prevent and contain neurological damage many interventions are necessary, some of which are specific to the particular trauma and some of which are more generally applicable. Aggressive treatment that is commenced promptly and continues is the key to eventual success.

Initially, IPPV can help to promote cerebral perfusion by ensuring that adequate oxygen is carried to the tissues and that carbon dioxide is carried away. Raised intracranial pressure (ICP) is a condition that must be assessed for and treated should it occur because it is a major cause of cerebral ischaemia and necrosis. It is therefore vital that arterial blood pressure (ABP) is treated to maintain it within normal limits and equally importantly that raised ICP is treated to reduce it to normal limits.

Hyperventilation, which 'washes out' carbon dioxide, leads to vasoconstriction of cerebral arterioles and a decrease in cerebral blood flow and volume, and therefore a decrease in ICP. A P_{CO_2} of about 3–4 kPa is aimed for; hyperventilation that causes the P_{CO_2} to drop below 2.5 kPa results in a grossly decreased cerebral blood flow and ischaemia.

Treatment of anaemia can improve oxygenation of cerebral tisues and can reduce potential damage.

More invasive intervention, such as surgery, may be required for skull fracture or cerebral bleeds. This may involve major neurosurgery or more simple burrhole surgery to allow escape of blood and relieve pressure.

Nursing management

Nursing management of the child with neurological involvement focuses on observation, positioning, minimal handling, and specific care of the child after surgery.

Observation and assessment
The vital signs that the nurse must monitor and record in respect to neurological care are extensive and to some degree dependent on the degree of sophistication of available equipment. However, all children with neurological trauma must have temperature, pulse, respiration, blood pressure, level of consciousness, pupil reactions, limb movements, and presence or absence of fits assessed and documented, because these can indicate improvement or deterioration in condition. Where possible, the nurse should monitor ICP, cerebral perfusion pressure (CPP) and cerebral function, which can more accurately reflect

the degree of trauma and efficacy of treatment. However, the nurse must be aware that drug therapy can alter some parameters, such as level of consciousness, pupil reactions and limb movements, without the child necessarily being as ill as the vital signs suggest. Drugs that commonly cause such side-effects include the opioids and paralysing agents.

If induced hypothermia is a prescribed part of the child's treatment, the nurse should also monitor this. A high degree of nursing skill is required to reduce and maintain a low core temperature successfully. This treatment can prove to be extremely upsetting to parents if the reasons are not adequately explained.

Positioning

Positioning can have both a therapeutic and a detrimental effect on ICP and CPP. Generally, the child will be nursed either flat or only slightly head-up because this causes the least harmful haemodynamic effects. However, in the polytraumatized patient, other injuries and considerations may make this difficult to achieve, and the best overall position for the child must then be chosen.

Minimal handling

The child with a poor CPP or at risk of deterioration in CPP should be allowed to rest without unnecessary disturbance wherever possible to help to reduce ICP, improve CPP and thereby improve outcome. However, this is easier to suggest than to practise because the polytraumatized child often requires frequent examination and handling.

Problem 4: breached skin integrity

Main aim: to contain and treat existing infection and minimize the potential for further infection.

Causes

Polytraumatized patients are almost unique in their susceptibility to infection. The nature of the trauma will have a marked effect, especially where the body's first line of defence against infection – the skin – has been breached. In these circumstances infection becomes a major potential problem. Also, the polytraumatized patient initially has a decreased immunological response.

Management problems and needs

Features commonly associated with the development of skin integrity problems and infection include:

1. contamination of the wound, caused by the initial traumatic incident;
2. immature immune response in the young patient;
3. compromised immune response due to the physiological response to trauma;
4. possible problems associated with reduced levels of T cells, which causes a decreased immune response, e.g. as a result of splenectomy;
5. infection resulting from the large number of invasive procedures;
6. decreased perfusion of damaged tissues, leading to delayed wound healing and increased risk for infection;
7. decreased nutritional status, resulting in delayed or absent wound healing.

Intervention and management

Tetanus prophylaxis
Prevention of infection is of major importance in the management of the polytraumatized patient. The child should be given tetanus toxoid cover, especially if the trauma resulted from a 'dirty' incident, or the adequacy of previous cover should be checked.

Antibiotic therapy
Early and effective broad-spectrum antibiotic therapy is essential to minimize the problem of infection. Broad-spectrum antibiotic therapy is given either to treat existing infection or prophylactically to decrease the risk of infection. This is particularly important because systemic infection has been shown to be the second most frequent cause of death in trauma patients surviving longer than 3 days (Littleton, 1988).

Antibiotic therapy itself poses problems to the patient. The route of choice is frequently intravenous, and this requires that the drugs are infused over a specific time in a specific dilution. This can lead to difficulties in respect to the child's overall fluid balance. In many situations the child's fluid requirements are given as colloids and only minimal volumes of crystalloids are able to be infused; this results in difficulties giving the appropriate antibiotic therapy. The possibility of major drug interactions must also be considered, especially as the number of drugs and fluids prescribed increases the likelihood of complex interactions.

Attention to damaged skin areas
Treatment of damaged skin can vary from basic cleansing and dressing with topical applications of lotions and other products to more radical management, which can include removal of damaged areas of skin and even amputation. The aim is to contain or remove a focus of infection that could become systemic.

Necrotic skin is a major potential focus for infection, and such areas should be debrided or surgically removed to reduce this risk. Effective cleansing of wounds may require anaesthetic cover to ensure that all debris is removed. Ongoing wound care, if not managed sympathetically, can be a source of both physical and psychological stress and distress to the child.

Nutritional support

Nutritional support plays a vital role in aiding recovery and preventing unnecessary delays in wound healing. Hypermetabolism is one of the initial responses to trauma, and as soon as the child is stabilized either enteral or parenteral nutrition must be considered. The child should not be allowed to suffer from a nutritional deficit for longer than is absolutely indicated by their condition.

Delayed wound healing, MSOF and sepsis are potential complications from inadequate nutrition. The nature of the injuries sustained will largely dictate the type and timing of nutritional intervention. If possible, the enteral route is chosen because this is most similar to normal nutrition. However, many injuries, including facial, oesophageal, abdominal and pulmonary, can preclude the use of enteral nutrition and total parenteral nutrition is then required.

Prevention of stress ulcers

The polytraumatized patient is at risk from developing stress ulcers and this risk can be reduced by administering antacids such as magnesium trisilicate mixture to reduce the acidity of the gastric fluids. This therapy is usually given as required and titrated to gastric pH. Other drug therapy involves administering anticholinergic agents and histamine antagonists, which reduce the secretion of gastric fluids.

Nursing management

The nursing care aimed at overcoming the problems related to infection and breached skin integrity centre on observation and monitoring, prevention of infection and promotion of wound healing.

Observation and monitoring

The nurse has many varied responsibilities in respect to observing the polytraumatized child for problems associated with breached skin integrity.

Vital signs Initial observations of the child's vital signs must be made. Core and peripheral temperature should be monitored as these can be good early indicators of sepsis and septic shock. Peripheral temperature may be difficult to record if the child's extremities have been badly injured. It should be remembered that the septic child may present as either hypothermic or hyperthermic.

Heart rate and rhythm, respiratory rate and arterial blood pressure must also be recorded to assess for sepsis, ischaemia and necrosis.

Skin integrity Visual observation of the child should not be forgotten; this is a very important means of assessing the extent and possible deterioration of external soft tissue trauma. The nurse should assess wounds, ecchymoses and sites of invasive lines as well as general skin integrity for potential purpura and petechiae.

Compartmental syndrome The nurse should also be aware that the child displaying signs of neurovascular compromise, muscular tension and unrelievable pain may be developing compartmental syndrome. These symptoms may result from the build-up of pressure from blood or oedematous tissue within a fascial compartment. Compartmental syndrome is a major potential problem for the child with a large degree of soft tissue trauma, especially if a pneumatic antishock garment has been used. If pressure is allowed to build up irreversibly, nerve damage may result and fasciotomy will be necessary to relieve the symptoms (Proehl, 1988).

Fat embolism This is another potential problem in the child with extensive soft tissue trauma. The nurse should monitor the child for tachypnoea, tachycadia and decreased level of consciousness, all of which may indicate that the child has suffered fat embolism. These signs and symptoms generally appear 24–28 h after the injury. The child may eventually display petechiae, haematuria and retinal changes. If any of these signs are present, the nurse should be alerted to the possibility of fat emboli.

Myoglobinuria If the polytraumatized child has suffered a crush injury or compartmental syndrome, myoglobinuria may present and the nurse should be aware of the signs and symptoms. These include a decreased urinary output and elevated relative density, and occur when the circulation to the traumatized tissue has been restored. Damaged muscle releases myoglobin once circulation to the area is re-established and this is then released into the general circulation. The myoglobin may precipitate in the renal tubules and lead to myoglobinuric renal failure. This is classically characterized by black urine.

Prevention of infection and promotion of wound healing
Prevention of infection in the child with breached skin integrity is a vital part of the nurse's role and the golden rule that prevention is better than cure should always be remembered. Wound healing must have a high priority as soon as possible, and can be promoted by satisfactory care of the wound, promotion of mobility, careful positioning and maintaining adequate nutritional input. Wound care protocols can be of real value in caring for the trauma patient,

who can present with a variety of differing wounds, including traumatic deep tissue injury, abrasion, laceration and surgical wounds. Passive and active movements improve circulation, oxygenation and perfusion of traumatized tissue and aid recovery. Careful positioning can ensure that damaged tissues are not further traumatized by excess pressure, and the use of special pressure-relieving aids such as sheepskins, beanbags and waterbeds are also of value in a patient who is 'difficult' to manage.

Problem 5: renal

Main aim: to maintain adequate renal function and reduce factors that may compromise function.

Causes

Depressed or potentially compromised renal function may result from direct injury, inadequate renal perfusion or unreasonable demands on renal function. A major goal in treatment is to preserve renal function and prevent the necessity for more complex interventions such as dialysis. However, if dialsyis is required, the already vulnerable and critically sick child has to face additional risks associated with such treatment.

Management problems and needs

Features commonly associated with trauma causing renal problems include:

1. compromised renal perfusion, due to decreased arterial blood pressure as a result of shock, which may cause tubular necrosis;
2. renal failure as a result of massive blood transfusion;
3. direct trauma to the renal tract;
4. nephrotoxic effects resulting from complex drug regimens.

Intervention and management

A major aim in the management of potential or existing renal problems lies in maintaining adequate renal perfusion. Without satisfactory perfusion, renal failure and its resulting complications ensue. Shock should be prevented or treated by treating the primary cause and by giving supportive therapy in the form of fluids and drugs.

The child with no obvious indication of renal trauma should also be carefully and systematically assessed for the possibility of renal trauma. Urinary assessment should be performed and radiography and other investigations may be required to eliminate or diagnose renal trauma.

In view of the probability that the child will require multiple blood transfusions, extreme care should be taken in crossmatching blood to reduce the possibility of an adverse transfusion reaction.

Careful consideration should also be taken in the administration of prescribed drugs, which may have nephrotoxic effects. Management of complex drug regimens can be problematic in the child with renal trauma.

Surgical intervention may also be required to treat the damaged renal system, and other supportive therapy may also be required.

Nursing management

The nursing management of the child with renal injury focuses on observation, positioning and special requirements indicated by the more intensive aspects of intervention.

Observation

Vital signs should be recorded as indicated by the child's condition and should include all routine shock observations that indicate possible problems associated with decreased renal perfusion pressures.

Urinary assessment is a vital means of recording renal function and, unless contraindicated by the presence of haematuria, the child should be catheterized to allow accurate hourly diuresis measurements to be made. Diuresis should be assessed against the child's expected urinary output, response to fluid regimens and challenges, and drug therapy.

The child's abdominal girth should also be assessed; an increase can be indicative of internal bleeding or swelling. This is only a crude indication, but often proves to be useful if used in conjunction with other information. Abdominal bruising indicates the possiblity of underlying injury.

The nurse should also record all intake, including drug therapy, and all output to allow a fluid balance estimation to be made. Separate subtotals of the different intakes and losses facilitates record keeping. The nurse should also observe for signs of fluid retention, which can occur even where the child is apparently hypovolaemic. If cell membranes are compromised, intravascular and interstitial fluid can leak into the cells, causing oedema and further compromising the circulating volume. The child should be observed for signs of periorbital and peripheral oedema as an indication of fluid retention.

Careful positioning

Care must be taken in positioning the child with possible renal trauma or after renal surgery to ensure that the renal bed drains effectively so that further compression of renal tissue is not possible.

Special consideration must be made in respect to the turning, positioning and pressure area care of a child who is oedematous or who has other injuries.

Intensive supportive management

The nursing care of the child who requires more intensive renal support will often need specialist nursing skills and interventions such as ultra-filtration.

Problem 6: gastrointestinal

Main aim: to preserve long-term gastrointestinal function and to reduce the risks of infection associated with gastrointestinal trauma.

Causes

Direct trauma to any part of the gastrointestinal tract can result in specific functional problems. The care and intervention required will depend on the site and extent of the injury. Gastrointestinal function may also be compromised as a result of drug therapy (which may cause paralytic ileus or severely reduce bowel motility), reduced perfusion of the bowel and gastric tract, surgery and other interventions.

Management problems and needs

Features commonly associated with polytrauma resulting in gastrointestinal problems include:

1. decreased vascular supply to the bowel as a result of shock, which may eventually result in ischaemia and necrosis;
2. direct trauma to specific areas, such as duodenal rupture and oesophageal trauma;
3. paralytic ileus as a result of administration of paralytic, anaesthetic or sedative agents;
4. disordered bowel function due to sepsis.

Intervention and management

An essential goal in the treatment of the child with bowel trauma is to treat the primary disorder and to effectively rest the bowel. Unless contraindicated by trauma to the nasopharynx and upper regions of the gastric tract, a large-bore nasogastric tube should be passed to allow drainage of the stomach contents. This is especially important if the child ate or drank shortly before the trauma occurred.

If specific intervention such as gastric or bowel surgery is required, care of the appropriate drainage tubes, bags and wounds is necessary. The polytraumatized patient with bowel involvement will often require a short-term stoma because of either direct trauma to the bowel or local ischaemia as a result of poor perfusion. This must be cared for and assessed by observing colour, size, perfusion, and type and amount of losses.

Polytrauma often involves laceration to the liver and the spleen, which requires surgical repair. If possible, the spleen is not removed and lacerations are sutured, because the spleen plays an important role in maintaining an effective immune response which is vital in the child's recovery from polytrauma (Polley and Coran, 1986).

Appropriate antibiotic therapy will be precribed if the gastrointestinal tract is involved because it is vitally important that the bowel does not become a focus of infection, which could trigger septicaemia and MSOF. If the gastrointestinal tract is compromised, normal nutrition will not be possible and a suitable alternative method such as parenteral feeding should be instituted.

Nursing management

The nursing care aimed at overcoming gastrointestinal problems in the polytraumatized child centre on assessment of fluid balance, prevention of infection and wound care, and maintenance of satisfactory nutrition.

Assessment of fluid and electrolyte balance
Trauma and compromised gastrointestinal function can have a major effect on both fluid and electrolyte balance, particularly if the child has had a stoma fashioned or has chronic paralytic ileus. It is likely that the child will lose large quantities of electrolyte-rich fluid from the stoma and wound drainage tubes and via the gastric tube. These losses must all be recorded to allow appropriate replacement therapy to be administered to prevent electrolyte and fluid imbalances. The child should also be assessed for signs of hypovolaemia or hypervolaemia. This is particularly important if the child has either splenic or hepatic involvement, as haemorrhage is a possible complication.

Prevention of infection and care of wounds
While the child is not receiving oral fluids, great care should be taken in repect to oral hygiene; antifungal gels and solutions may be prescribed to decrease the possibility of oral *Candida albicans* infection. This is especially important if the child is receiving comprehensive antibiotic therapy.

If the child has had a stoma fashioned, the nurse must pay particular attention to the colour, perfusion and size of the stoma. The unstable child will be more at risk of perfusion problems to the newly formed stoma and this must be taken into consideration.

The nurse must also take particular care of all surgical wounds associated with gastrointestinal trauma to reduce the risk of infection.

Maintenance of satisfactory nutrition

Until normal nutrition is resumed, alternative nutritional options may be used and the nurse must be aware of the complications associated with them. One of the responsibilities of the nurse is to assess serum blood sugar at regular intervals to ensure that the child is not becoming either hypoglycaemic or hyperglycaemic. This is especially important in the polytraumatized patient, where the physiological stress response can cause a labile serum blood glucose level during the first few days of treatment.

Problem 7: pain

Main aim: to provide a pain-free recovery and to reduce the psychological and physiological trauma associated with the experience of pain.

Causes

Pain has physiological, physical, psychological and spiritual components, and all of these must be addressed if the child is not to be distressed by the experience of injury and the intensive care of those injuries. The child has the right to be free of pain and to have their pain acknowledged and treated effectively even when other aspects of care and intervention would seem to have higher priority.

Management problems and needs

Features commonly associated with pain resulting from polytrauma include:

1. the underlying pathology of the trauma itself, which can cause the physiological component of pain;
2. the nursing and medical care, which can compound the pain experience;
3. the memory of the original trauma, anxiety about recovery, separation from family and many other factors, which can contribute to the psychological component of pain.

Intervention and management

Management of the underlying causes is an essential means of treating pain and this may include treating sepsis, immobilizing fractures, and reducing and relieving oedema. Administration of appropriate analgesic and sedative regimens can relieve pain and reduce anxiety. Drugs with amnesic properties may also be of benefit during the first few very traumatic days.

Nursing management

Nursing management aimed at relieving the child's pain will require careful planning and assessment, and involvement of the child and the family.

Appropriate intervention

Initially this will involve the judicious use of continuous intravenous opioid or analgesic infusions. Alternative routes must also be considered. Topical creams such as EMLA cream should be used whenever possible to reduce the pain and trauma associated with the insertion and reinsertion of arterial and venous lines. At all times the child should be assessed as a unique individual with changing needs and problems that will require sympathetic, effective and varied nursing interventions.

Problem 8: potential disseminated intravascular coagulation

Main aim: to re-establish haemostasis and to contain potential tissue damage caused by inappropriate clotting and bleeding.

Causes

DIC is a complication that frequently occurs in the polytraumatized patient. It can be a mild condition that responds to treatment, but more often it is a very damaging or even fatal complication.

In some respects, DIC can be said to be an iatrogenic disorder. Increasingly sophisticated care for patients with a wide range of problems means that more are surviving to be at risk of the secondary problem of DIC.

Management problems and needs

Features commonly associated with the secondary development of DIC in the polytrauma patient include:

1. massive tissue injury;
2. a period of uncompensated shock;
3. septicaemia;
4. blood transfusions;
5. a combination of the above factors.

Intervention and management

Early recognition, detection and treatment of DIC is of prime importance; all patients should be carefully observed for the very early signs of onset of the syndrome, and prompt action should be taken.

Treatment of underlying disorder

The treatment of DIC remains controversial, with many often apparently opposing methods being advocated. However, all approaches begin with the premise that the underlying condition that triggered the aberrant clotting picture must be treated if the DIC is to be managed effectively. This initial treatment depends on the underlying cause. For example, antibiotics may be prescribed intravenously to treat infection, and hypovolaemic shock will be treated with fluid replacement.

Supportive measures

Supportive measures that do not directly attempt to control the clotting but aim to improve the patient's condition and thereby prevent an increase in the number of trigger factors play an important role. These may include oxygen therapy to improve tissue perfusion, and specific fluid replacement with monitoring of the child's haemodynamic status. These measures are generally obvious and non-controversial; however, the specific measures discussed below can cause difficulty and dissent (Machin, 1988).

Blood product replacement This is also complicated and controversial and requires close coordination and cooperation between the medical and haematology staff and the Blood Bank.

Blood product administration is used to:

1. replace red cell loss due to haemorrhage;
2. prevent or treat existing shock;
3. replace depleted coagulation factors.

The response to the problems presented by DIC must be immediate and ongoing to be effective. Commonly used blood products include the following.

Fresh frozen plasma acts as a plasma expander (and is therefore useful in treating the shock component of DIC) and also contains all the coagulation factors and two major indicators antithrombin III and protein C.

Platelet concentrates are used to boost the number of circulating platelets and to improve the clotting capacity of the blood.

Cryoprecipitate is of major importance in the treatment of DIC because it is rich in factor VIII, which is rapidly utilized in the clotting process. Cryoprecipitate also contains fibrinogen and fibronectin.

Packed red cells and *red cell concentrates* are used to maintain or improve the haemotocrit levels so that tissue perfusion is optimized. Owing to the difficulty in transfusing red cell concentrates with a mean packed cell volume of 70–75%, many red cell concentrates are diluted by electrolyte and/or colloid solutions to produce a haematocrit of 60%. These solutions include ADSOL and SAG.M blood. SAG.M blood is the most frequently used blood product.

Human plasma protein fraction is used to maintain circulating blood volume, cardiac output and thereby tissue perfusion, although it does not contain any products that are of value in treating the aberrant clotting cascade.

Antithrombin III is a relatively recent addition to the specific treatment of DIC and has been shown to be successful especially in the treatment of severe cases.

As the child is frequently reviewed and assessed the further often very heavy requirements for specialist blood products can place a strain on local availability of a particular product.

Although it is necessary to intervene with the use of blood product replacement therapy, this can exacerbate the problem because transfusions can fuel the vicious cycle of clotting and bleeding, promoting clotting and fibrin deposition. The child must be carefully assessed to ensure that this is not occurring.

Heparin The decision to use heparin remains controversial. It is used to try to stop the cycle of clotting and haemorrhage. The literature describes both benefits and disadvantages of using heparin. The arguments against are that giving heparin to patients is a great risk, especially to patients with open wounds or intracranial haemorrhages and during the postoperative period. Heparin may interact with other drugs and this may make finding the correct dose problematic.

Heparin is administered via a slow continuous infusion. It is suggested that it is used only in severe cases where the initial treatments have been inadequate and provided replacement therapy is continued. If heparin is used, protamine sulphate should be available to reverse the effects if necessary.

Prostacyclin Prostacyclin can also be used where the main trigger factor is thought to be platelet activation. It also has beneficial effects in supporting pulmonary and renal function.

Plasmaphaeresis or exchange transfusion This is also controversial, although some benefits have been seen to result from the use of plasmaphaeresis or exchange transfusion. The theory behind this therapy is that by removing plasma loaded with toxic bacterial components and abnormal proteolytic activity and replacing it with fresh frozen plasma the original trigger to DIC is removed and the secondary disease process halted. This is still not a routine practice in older children and adults although exchange transfusion in babies has proved to be of value.

Hyperbaric oxygen treatment This can be used in conjunction with other forms of treatment. The aim is to increase perfusion to the ischaemic or poorly perfused areas of tissue by providing a steeper oxygen concentration gradient, and thereby to decrease the risk of severe ischaemia, and gangrene and amputation. The patient must be transferred to a hyperbaric chamber, and there may be problems in continuing other forms of treatment during the patient's stay in the chamber. The logistics involved in this procedure make it a difficult proposition.

Nursing management

The nursing care of the child with DIC centres on the observation and assessment of the progress of the syndrome and the efficacy of the treatment in minimizing organ damage and soft tissue injury.

Observation and assessment

In assessing the child who may develop DIC, the nurse must be aware that the onset can be either insidious with a gradually deteriorating blood picture (subclinical manifestation) or acute with massive haemorrhages occurring concurrently with multiple thrombi forming. The following areas should be considered.

1. At-risk patients must be considered especially carefully.
2. DIC causes decreased tissue perfusion and potential ischaemia, and therefore the patient should be observed for subtle changes in level of consciousness.
3. Haemorrhage is the most obvious and common manifestation of DIC and can be the first sign. Prolonged bleeding times from needle-stab sites may indicate the need for further investigation.
   (a) Frank haemorrhage includes bleeding and oozing from wound sites, gums and traumatized areas, haematuria, malaena, petechiae, purpura, ecchymoses and mottled or blue extremities.
   (b) Occult bleeding may occur in the gastrointestinal tract, skin, etc., and may primarily be indicated by headache or other non-specific symptoms. Assessment can be achieved by measuring abdominal girth, and skin, haemodynamic and neurological status.
   (c) Acrocyanosis is characterized by sharply defined irregularly shaped cyanotic patches, which may be the result of fibrin deposition in the microcirculation and are diagnostic of DIC (and of Raynaud's syndrome). These areas can become gangrenous and may require radical intervention, including amputation of affected limbs, and/or deep tissue removal, which will need months of skin grafting.
   (d) Thromboemboli are often concurrently deposited in many organs of the body.

Monitoring

Continuous and close haemodynamic monitoring appropriate to the child's condition is essential to allow the early detection of potential shock and organ failure resulting from inappropriate thrombus formation and haemorrhage. Peripheral pulses should be palpated regularly to ensure that there is adequate capillary filling. If the peripheral pulses become unpalpable despite intervention, they can be checked using Doppler ultrasonography.

The child should also be monitored for signs of invisible haemorrhage by monitoring temperature, neurological status, renal output and gastrointestinal function, including bowel sounds and abdominal girth.

Maintaining optimum skin integrity

This is a major consideration of both immediate and ongoing importance. The child who has suffered soft tissue damage as a result of the initial trauma and who develops DIC is at extreme risk of developing major skin lesions that will affect both short-term and long-term outcomes.

The nurse must protect the child from unnecessary trauma resulting from needle punctures. This can be achieved by the judicious use of an arterial line for obtaining blood samples, optimum care of existing venous lines to reduce the need for them to be resited, and minimization of the number of blood samples that cannot be taken from the arterial line.

If possible, low-adhesive tapes and electrodes should be used to minimize skin trauma when the tape is removed. Equally, splinting and bandaging techniques should be optimized.

The intramuscular route for medication should be avoided because this causes further potential trauma and can result in erratic absorption of the drug.

The appropriate use of pressure-relieving aids such as bean pillows, 'burns' beds, waterbeds, gentle handling, and careful turning and positioning help to reduce further trauma and provide improved conditions for wound healing. Scrupulous examination of the skin and the early initiation of appropriate treatment of affected areas is essential if the degree of damage is to be contained.

Oral hygiene practices may require adaptation if the child has fragile buccal mucosa. Extra care will also be required when performing tracheal and pharyngeal suction in an attempt to reduce the possibility of trauma.

THERMALLY INJURED CHILDREN

Children experiencing thermal injuries make up a sizeable proportion of attenders in accident and emergency departments across the UK. The analysis of the Home Accident Surveillance system data (Department of Trade and Industry, 1985) concerning the incidence of non-fatal thermal injuries in 1983 provided data on 2604 children according to age group, sex and whether the injury was a burn or scald. A further 798 children received fatal injuries. McFarlane (1979) pointed out that most fatalities could be attributed to carbon monoxide poisoning. He concluded that although 34.4% of deaths in children between 1968 and 1974 were from fires, only 5.3% of these were directly due to thermal injury.

The 14 centres specializing in the treatment of serious thermal injuries in children could be a source of valuable data on mortality, morbidity ratios and the effectiveness of nursing and medical intervention, but as yet no standardized method or form of data collection has been agreed. Certain trends are apparent; for example, Pearce (1989) in a study carried out in the Paediatric Accident and Emergency Department at the Queen's Medical Centre, Nottingham concluded that children under 5 years of age were more at risk from thermal injury. Over 70% of such accidents occur in the 1–2 year age group, with boys more likely to be injured than girls except in the 5–9 age group, where more girls sustain scalds (Table 8.3).

Table 8.3 Distribution of burns and scalds by age group and sex, 1983

	Age (years)			
	0–4	*5–9*	*10–14*	*Total*
Burns				
Male	446	60	90	596
Female	291	46	74	411
Unknown	2	1	1	4
Scalds				
Male	687	107	95	889
Female	493	115	86	694
Unknown	7	2	1	10
Total	1926	331	347	2604

Children differ from adults in that they have a larger body surface area in relation to their weight and are more at risk from dehydration because of different intracellular and extracellular fluid ratios, and their efficient reaction to shock may mask a severe reduction in circulating blood volume. A partial thickness injury involving over 10% of the total surface area in the infant or more than 15% in the 4-year-old is potentially life-threatening. In any large area of population there is a need for a specialist unit, and children with thermal injuries above the quoted percentages should not be nursed in paediatric surgical wards and never in adult areas (recommendation of the Working Party of the Accident Prevention Trust, 1985). The care of these children should be 'undertaken in specialist units and special attention paid in the training of all health professionals – medical, nursing and auxiliary staff working in this field'.

Serious thermal injury can tax the skills and ingenuity of the nursing team in coordinating, communicating and liaising with other members of the multidisciplinary team to ensure that the family are sustained and supported, the rights of the child protected and the quality of care maintained. The availability and utilization of psychological and social support for parents and families of thermally injured children is recommended. To sustain the child throughout the life-threatening, life-maintaining and rehabilitation phases of illness, the particular knowledge, skills and attitudes of the paediatric nurse are required. At all times the parents and the child and siblings, if applicable, need to be closely involved in the aspects of the caring role with which they feel comfortable and to be consulted when decisions regarding changes in management and treatment are being made.

A knowledge of child development is vital, as most injuries occur during the transitional stage when the child is passing from passivity to autonomy. Erikson (1964) suggested that life is not only a sequence of developmental transitions but of accidental crises as well. The under fives are particularly vulnerable because of their natural inquisitiveness, their need to explore and experiment, and their lack of appreciation of danger. A child will display proximity-seeking behaviour when separated from parents, in pain, tired or perceives threat: all aspects present in the traumatized child (Bowlby, 1983). It should be no surprise that children between 1 and 3 years of age are at greatest risk of permanent emotional problems related to hospitalization. A child may interpret present suffering as a punishment for imaginary naughtiness, and their level of cognitive development and immature linguistic skills causes extreme difficulty when explaining that painful procedures are helping to make them better. Immobilization is also stressful for a child who is normally 'always on the go'. The recognition that this child has a tendency towards magical thinking will result in reassurance and understanding if the toddler shows fear of the machinery and alarms, perceiving them as monsters who eat children (Reynolds and Ramenofsky, 1988).

Reference to normal anatomy and physiology aids understanding of the effects of thermal injury on cells, tissues, the process of inflammation, wound healing, and the subsequent susceptibility to infection. The child who has inhaled heat or smoke requires the highest standard of nursing observation, as ventilatory support may prove necessary. Correct alignment of limbs, positioning of joints and the extension of the neck, if involved, will help to minimize contracture formation. The involvement of many members of the multidisciplinary team, each using their special skills, cannot be over-emphasized in the holistic approach to the seriously burned or scalded child.

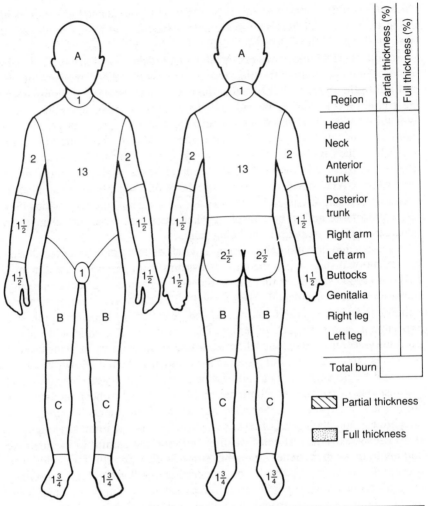

Percentage of body surface affected					
Area	Age				
	0	1	5	10	15
A: half of head	$9\frac{1}{2}$	$8\frac{1}{2}$	$6\frac{1}{2}$	$5\frac{1}{2}$	$4\frac{1}{2}$
B: half of one thigh	$2\frac{3}{4}$	$3\frac{1}{4}$	4	$4\frac{1}{2}$	$4\frac{1}{2}$
C: half of one leg	$2\frac{1}{2}$	$2\frac{1}{2}$	$2\frac{3}{4}$	3	$3\frac{1}{4}$

Figure 8.3 The Lung and Browder chart for estimation of severity of thermal injury.

The first-aid measure of flushing thermal injuries with cold water at the time of the injury reduces further tissue damage. On admission, an estimation of the extent of the injuries is made and converted to a percentage (Figure 8.3). An assessment criterion is used to estimate the depth of the thermal injury. Table 8.4 suggests a clear demarcation between the levels, but in reality the boundaries may be blurred. Areas of superficial damage are not included in the estimation. The percentage is then used in calculating the fluid replacement necessary to counteract burns shock.

Table 8.4 Degrees of burn

Depth of burn	Appearance	Circulation	Sensation	Healing
Superficial Germinal layer is unaffected	Erythematous Red and swollen	Blanches on pressure Reddens when pressure is released	Painful	3–7 days
Partial thickness All the epidermis and part of the dermis are involved	Pink or red Blisters and areas of wet exudate present	Blanches on pressure Reddens when pressure is released Capillaries dilated	Extremely painful	10–14 days May require grafting
Full thickness Both the epidermis and dermis are destroyed Underlying tissues may be involved Epithelial element lost	Dry brown or white Surface may appear leathery Thrombosed blood vessels present	Looks dead No change when pressure is released	Painless as nerve endings are destroyed At edges of wounds sensitivity to pain is present	By granulation Grafts needed to promote healing and prevent septicaemia

Burns shock

An important factor to remember when considering thermal injury is that the fluid compartment ratios alter as the child grows and develops, and these have a marked effect on the way the child reacts to burns trauma and treatment (Table 8.5) (Lung and Browder, 1944).

Table 8.5 Fluid compartment volumes and ratios

	Plasma ml/kg	litres	Interstitial fluid ml/kg	litres	Extra-cellular fluid (litres)	Intracellular fluid ml/kg	litres	Total (litres)	Solid: fluid ratios
Adult (65.5 kg)	42	2.750	200	13.000	15,850	400	28.000	42.050	40 : 60
Baby (4.5 kg, 3 months)	42	0.180	420	1.575	1.755	350	1.710	3.465	20 : 80
Child (18 kg, 5 years)	42	0.756	200	3.600	4.356	400	7.200	11.556	35 : 65

Babies exchange half their extracelluar volume daily, the adult only one-sixth. Compensatory mechanisms ensure that homeostasis is maintained. Fluid shifts across the various fluid compartments under the control of the hypothalamus by the action of blood pressure and capillary dynamics, plasma proteins, electrolytes and hormonal influences.

Severe thermal injuries upset homeostasis by disturbing the equilibrium of the internal environment. If plasma, metabolic water requirements and electrolytes are not replaced, the child's survival is threatened.

Treatment

The priorities are to establish a patent airway, evaluate vital signs and coordinate prompt treatment of life-threatening problems. Oxygen therapy, endotracheal intubation and ventilator therapy may be necessary.

All children with thermal injuries involving 10–30% of their body surface area are transfused for at least 36 h. If the thermal injury involves more than 30% of the surface area, this period is extended to 48–72 h.

Human plasma protein fraction is the intravenous solution of choice to commence resuscitation. Plasma replacement is calculated using the following formula:

$$\frac{\text{weight in kilograms} \times \% \text{ area of burn}}{2}$$

The answer in millilitres is the amount to be transfused in each period:

Period	1	2	3	4	5	6	etc.
Hours after burning	4	8	12	18	24	36	

Metabolic water requirements are required as follows:

100 ml/kg for first 10 kg body weight
50 ml/kg for next 10 kg body weight
20 ml/kg for remaining kg body weight

The total is then given for a 24 h period in equally divided amounts.

For an 18 kg child with 20% full and partial thickness burns, the plasma requirements are therefore:

$$\frac{18 \times 20}{2} = 180 \text{ ml in the first 4 h period}$$

Rate of infusion = 45 ml plasma over the first hour

and the metabolic water loss rate is:

100 ml/kg for the first 10 kg body weight = 1000 ml

50 ml/kg for next 8 kg body weight = 400 ml
Total   1400 ml

This total is divided by 24 h, which equals 58 ml h. Therefore a total of 103 ml would be transfused in the first hour.

At the end of each period the child's response to therapy is reassessed and is related to the following important aspects; urine output, haematocrit readings, insensible fluid loss, loss from burned areas, central venous pressure, ability to take oral fluids, vital signs, peripheral perfusion and altered level of consciousness. These are all of importance when evaluating response to emergency measures.

Changes in physiology due to thermal injury

Following thermal injury, metabolic requirements increase. To keep up with demand protein is broken down, fat is mobilized and the amount of circulating triglycerides is reduced (Rosequist et al., 1985). For every 1°C increase in temperature, the basal metabolic rate is raised by 10%. The action of angiotensin results in the retention of sodium and water, leading to oedema, which is worsened by the leakage of serum albumin from leaking capillaries. Raised amounts of albumin in the extracellular space increases tissue osmotic pressure, and water is attracted out of the systemic circulation so that blood pressure drops as cardiac output falls and hypovolaemic shock worsens.

Heat loss due to the disturbance of the thermoregulatory function of the skin and the evaporation of fluid leaking from the injured areas requires the child to be nursed in a constant temperature of 24–28°C and a humidity of 30% to offset these changes. Tissue breakdown leads to the release of nitrogen, phosphorus, potassium, calcium, zinc, magnesium, sulphur and creatinine, which are excreted in the urine.

Hypokalaemia is corrected at the end of the shock phase, by which time a considerable amount of potassium has been lost in the urine. Haemolysis in the area affected by thermal injury and a shortened life-span of red blood cells results in anaemia, which may become severe. Haemoconcentration due to hypovolaemia gives false high levels of circulating haemoglobin if a haematocrit reading is not taken for comparison. As the haemolytic effects also act on the transfused blood, a transfusion may be deferred for a few days.

The development of metabolic acidosis 12–14 h after injury results from the acid release from damaged tissues and inadequate tissue perfusion. As a reduced urine output is associated with falling arterial pH, prompt correction of acid–base deficits is important.

The following formula is used to restore acid–base balance:

MEq (milliequivalent) of bicarbonate required = base deficit × body weight (kg) × 0.3
(when 8.4% sodium bicarbonate is used 1 MEq = 1 ml).

After 24 h, further catabolism leads to loss of muscle and subsequent loss of weight. Hormonal activity increases, leading to an increase in catecholamine (adrenalin and noradrenaline) production resulting in an increased oxygen uptake, heart rate and breakdown of glycogen to mobilize glucose for energy. Glucagon, glucocorticoids and growth hormone release are stimulated and glycosuria may be present as the balance of insulin and catecholamine antagonism is disrupted (Kemble and Lamb, 1987). Nitrogen released from protein breakdown appears in the urine and faeces, followed by a reduction in muscle bulk and lowered resistance to infection as immuno-globulin production is affected by the lower availability of protein for utilization.

Problems and needs of the burns-injured child

The main problems and needs of the thermally injured child and the family depend on the extent and depth of the injuries and the child's reaction to trauma:

1. asphyxiation, anoxia, and hypoxia due to inhalation of smoke or steam fumes may result in the need for ventilator support and/or tracheostomy; these signs may be delayed, so vigilant review of progress is essential;

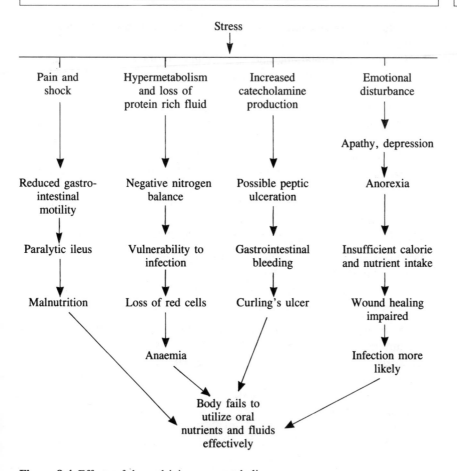

Figure 8.4 Effects of thermal injury on metabolism.

2. hypovolaemia due to fluid, protein and electrolyte loss from the burned areas;
3. pain, fear and the sudden admission to hospital, and the possibility of neurogenic shock and later long-term morbidity;
4. circulatory collapse due to loss of fluid and the effects of shock; possible constriction of blood vessels exerted by circumferential burns;
5. renal impairment due to low blood pressure, renin release and reduced filtration efficiency of the kidneys; oliguria and anuria are possible sequelae; blood protein, glucose and ketones are present on ward testing of the urine.
6. susceptibility to infection due to destruction of part of the body's natural defence against the invasion of potentially pathogenic organisms; plasma

protein depletion and loss in the exudate result in lowered immunity to infection;

7. difficulty in maintaining nutritional balance following trauma, the loss of nutrients via burned areas and a marked decrease in red blood cells (Figure 8.4);

8. Psychological trauma related to altered body image, disfigurement, deformity and contracture; management is aimed at minimizing this potentially severe problem by involving those skilled in counselling, recognizing adverse signs and knowing when to intervene;

9. long-term emotional and social disruption due to trauma, hospitalization and appearance;

10. potential problems of paralytic ileus, gastrointestinal ulceration (Curling's ulcer) and marked weight loss;

11. guilt, grieving and possible rejection affect family dynamics.

All of these areas must be considered by the nurse caring for the child and his or her family to ensure that optimum care is delivered.

The management of the thermally injured child is complex. Effective management can be facilitated by the use of the 'Imperative To Act' mnenomic

Immediate assessment by named nurse in collaboration with other multidisciplinary team members;
Maintenance of environment; internal external;
Pain and fear reduction;
Extent of thermal injury calculated;
Rehabilitation started;
Analgesia reviewed, amended, and evaluated;
Transfusion regime carefully tailored to meet needs;
Intake and output accurately monitored hourly;
Vital signs recorded – abnormalities responded to quickly;
Emotional status monitored;

Therapy ongoing; – including physiotherapy and play;
Outcome – multidisciplinary approach;

Application of pressure garments;
Counselling of child and family;
Teaching.

Dietary management

The objective is to avoid weight loss of more than 10–20%. A high-protein high-calorie diet is drawn up by the dietitian in consultation with the child, parents and the primary nurse to ensure that the child accepts and enjoys the diet.

The dietary intake needs to include amino acids for wound healing and for the synthesis of proteins and collagen, carbohydrate for energy and for normal white cell function to aid resistance to infection, and 10% fat to prevent fatty acid deficiencies, as these are essential components of cell membranes. Elements such as iron for oxygen transport, zinc for wound healing and copper and magnesium for collagen production should also be included. Minerals and trace elements ensure the normal function of cells as well as acting as cofactors in enzyme reactions. Vitamin A level is reduced following severe trauma and is related to increased catecholamine release, which is implicated in the stress-induced peptic ulceration known as Curling's ulcer. Vitamin K helps to prevent haematoma formation, which provides an ideal medium for bacterial growth. Vitamin C binds cells together and so is a vital factor for the new epithelial cohesion of burned areas during the healing process and is also a component of collagen. Thiamine and nicotinamide are used in carbohydrate metabolism and oxidative processes, and riboflavine in amino acid metabolism (Kemble and Lamb, 1987).

Principles of feeding the severely thermally injured child

Feeding should be instituted once resuscitation measures have proved effective, oedema no longer threatens the airway and absorption is confirmed. The use of 'bendy' straws, attractively coloured fluids (for example, blackcurrant drinks, banana milkshakes and Hycal) in frequent small amounts initially may help to alleviate anorexia. The identification of favourite foods and drinks allows a diet high in protein and calories to be drawn up and increases the possibility that it will be acceptable to the child. The intake is planned to reverse negative nitrogen balance, promote healing and maintain acceptable growth patterns. Diet should be varied, easily digestible and attractively served. Mineral and vitamin supplements should be prescribed in the most acceptable form and given by the parents or primary nurse to encourage the child to take them. If the diet is refused, a substitute of Complan or a milk-based drink should be offered. The avoidance of too hot, too cold or spicy food will minimize the complication of gastrointestinal ulceration.

Vomiting, diarrhoea or constipation should be reported immediately, the diet evaluated to pinpoint the cause, and changes made. All intake needs to be accurately recorded and if refusal or adverse gastrointestinal signs persist a regimen of total parenteral feeding may be indicated as a short-term measure to prevent further weight loss and to restore nitrogen balance. Insufficient intake during the day because of the child's lack of appetite, and where there are no adverse gastrointestinal signs, may be offset by giving intragastric drip feeds overnight. The use of a volumetric device ensures that the calculated amount is run in continuously according to the child's needs. This has the advantage of not disturbing sleep and rest as well as maintaining fluid and calorie requirements, and will minimize the danger of making mealtimes stressful during the day.

Evaluation of the success or failure of the dietary regimen is estimated according to the weight curve plotted regularly on a percentile chart. The catabolic state persists and weight gain may not occur until more than 10 days after the trauma, but weight loss should be declining during the latter part of this period.

Skin grafting

Accurate assessment of the depth of the burn is often difficult at the time of admission. However, early excision of dead tissue and skin grafting is the norm for full-thickness skin loss if fatal bacterial invasion is to be avoided. Other areas may be grafted after separation of the slough occurs, which may take place up to 3 weeks after the injury.

Types of graft

Homografts
Skin is taken from donors or from cadavers. The advantage of such grafts is that they can be used for the seriously burned child whose life is threatened. Adequate cover is possible and the grafts can be applied without an anaesthetic being required. The drawback is that they are viable for an average of 3 weeks only and will be rejected.

Autografts
Skin is taken from the patient and has the advantage that it will not be rejected unless infection is present. Alternate strips of autografts and homografts may be used to cover large areas of skin loss and this method has proved effective as lateral migration of epithelial cells from the autograft bridge the exposed tissue left when the homograft has been rejected. Autografts are used in the hands, face and around joints, ensuring that these functional areas heal quickly. The disadvantage is that the areas from where skin is taken cause pain and discomfort and are unsightly initially, but can be recropped if further grafts are needed later.

Xenografts
Freeze-dried porcine skin is used when autografts or homografts are unavailable. These act only as dressings and have to be replaced, but appear to reduce fluid loss from burned areas.

Advances in the care of the thermally injured patient were previously related to control of burn shock and prevention of secondary infection by the introduction of effective topical antibacterial therapies (Burke, 1990). A more recent advance offers the hope of skin cover without using large areas of the patient's undamaged skin. If further research solves the specific problems of smoke inhalation and MSOF the next decade should improve the outlook even more for the seriously thermally injured child.

Cultured autologous epithelium

This technique affords permanent cover for partial and full-thickness injuries and was described by Hancock (1989) as an advance where 'science fiction seemed to be meeting reality'. Epithelia cells are taken from a small full-thickness skin biopsy and carefully excised from the dermal layer. Groups of cells are then grown in a tissue culture medium in a flask. Seeding to other flasks allows growth of thin sheets of epithelium so that if the initial cover from the first flask is unsuccessful the procedure can be repeated. An enzyme is used to lift the sheet of cells from their bed on a layer of feeder irradiated fibroplasts, and the epithelial culture is clipped to vaseline gauze. The gauze and small surgical staples used to secure the graft can be lifted off in 7–10 days.

Graft failure

Haematoma formation and insufficient fixation are non-infective causes of graft failure. Bacteria that prevent a graft from 'taking' include *Streptococcus pyogenes*, which prevents the formation of connecting capillaries between the underlying tissues and the graft. *Pseudomonas aeruginosa*, *Klebsiella* spore-bearers and *Proteus* spore-bearers may also cause partial graft failure. Once the sensitivity is known, a course of the appropriate antibiotic is commenced.

REFERENCES AND FURTHER READING

Ala, F.A. (1988) Red cell components – plasma proteins and albumin: current transfusion cocktails. *Care of the Critically Ill*, **4** (4), 14, 16–19, 22.

Asensioua, J.A. *et al.* (1988) Trauma: a systematic approach to management. *American Family Physician* **3**, September, 97–112.

Baskett, P. and Small, D. (1989) Blood substitutes: a review *ITCM* November, 283–4, 286.

Bowlby, J. (1983) *Attachment and Loss*, 2nd edn, Basic Books, New York.

Burke, J.F. (1990) From desperation to skin regeneration; progress in burn treatment. *Journal of Trauma*, December, S40.

Caplin, M. (1984) Disseminated intravascular coagulation: a multisystem approach. *Dimensions of Critical Care Nursing*, **3** (2), 76–83.

Coln, D. (1985) Pediatric trauma medical aspects. *AORN Journal* **42** (3), 338–42.

Department of Trade and Industry (1989) *Home and Leisure Accident Research, Eleventh Annual Report.* Home Accident Surveillance System, Oxford University Press.

Erikson, E.H. (1964) *Childhood and Society*, W.W. Norton, New York.

Fifield, G.C. (1984) Multiple trauma in children. Initial management, key to improved survival. *Postgraduate Medicine* **75**, 111–23.

Gaspard, K.J. (1990) Alterations in blood coagulation and hemastasis, in *Pathophysiology Concepts of Altered Health States*, 3rd edn, (ed. C. Mattson Porth), J.B. Lippincott, Philadelphia.

Glass, B.L. (1985) Pediatric trauma units nursing's input into development. *AORN Journal*, **42** (3), 353–6.

Griffin, J.P. (1986) Be prepared for the bleeding patient. *Nursing 86*, **16** (6), 34–42.

Hancock, K. (1989) Cultured keratinocytes and keratinocyte grafts. *British Medical Journal*, **229**, 1179.

Harris, B.H. (1987) Recommendations for pediatric trauma care in hospitals. *Emergency Care Quarterly*, **3** (1), 65–72.

Hazinski, M.F. (1984) *Nursing Care of the Critically Ill Child*, C.V. Mosby, St Louis.

Hewitt, P.E. and Machin, S.J. (1990) Massive blood transfusion. *British Medical Journal*, **300**, 107–9.

Hurn, P. and Connolly, C. (1983) The polytrauma patient management problems and nursing management. *Focus on Critical Care*, **10** (6), 15–20.

Kemble, J.V.H. and Lamb, B.E. (1987) *Practical Burns Management*, Hodder and Stoughton, Sevenoaks, Chapter 3.

Lanning, J. 61985) Pediatric trauma emotional aspects. *AORN Journal*, **42** (3), 345–51.

Littleton, M.T. (1988) Pathophysiology and assessment of sepsis and septic shock. *Critical Care Nursing Quarterly*, **11** (1), 30–47.

Lung, C.C. and Browder, N.C. (1944) Estimation of areas of burns. *Surgery, Gynaecology and Obstetrics*, **79**, 352–8.

Lyonel, S.H. (1981) Critical care of the child with multitrauma. *Nursing Clinics of North America*, **16**, 658.

Machin, S.J. (1989) Coagulopathy and its control. *Care of the Critically Ill*, **5** (2), 49–51.

MacFarlane, A. (1979) Child deaths from accidents: place of accident. *OPCS, Population trends, No. 15*, Spring, 10–15.

Marvin, J.A. (1988) Nutritional support of the critically injured patient. *Critical Care Nursing Quarterly*, **11** (2), 21–34.

Mattson Porth, C. (ed.) (1990) *Pathophysiology Concepts of Altered Health States*, 3rd edn, J.B. Lippincott, Philadelphia.

McClelland, D.B.L. (1990) Human albumin solutions. *British Medical Journal*, **30**, 35–7.

Muir, B.L. (1988) *Pathophysiology An Introduction to the Mechanisms of Disease*, 2nd edn, Wiley, New York.

Polley, T.Z. and Coran, A.G. (1986) Special problems in management of pediatric trauma. *Critical Care Clinics*, **2** (4), 775–89.

Proehl, J.H. (1988) Compartment syndrome. *Journal of Emergency Nursing*, **14** (5), 283–92.

Ramenofsky, M.L. *et al.* (1984) Maximum survival in pediatric trauma: the ideal system. *Journal of Trauma*, **24**, 818–23.

Recommendations of Working Party of Accident Prevention Trust (1985) Bedford Square Press/NCVO, pp 53–4.

Reynolds, E.A. and Ramenofsky, M.L. (1988) The emotional impact of trauma on toddlers. *Maternal Child Nursing* **13**, 106–9.

Rimar, J. (1988a) Recognizing shock syndromes in infants and children. *Maternal Child Nursing*, **13**, 32–37.

Rimar, J. (1988b) Shock in infants and young children: assessment and treatment. *Maternal Child Nursing*, **13**, 98–105.

Rosequist, C. *et al.* (1985) The nutrition factor. *American Journal of Nursing*, January, 45.

Ross, D.M. and Ross, S.A. (1988) Assessment of paediatric pain: an overview. *Issues in Comprehensive Pediatric Nursing*, **11**, 73–91.

Spence, M.T. *et al.* (1988) Trauma audit – the use of TRISS. *Health Trends*, **20**, 94–7.

Zideman, D. (1986) Paediatric resuscitation. *Care of the Critically Ill*, **2** (4), 137–8, 140.

Bernadette Carter

Pain is a critical ethical issue because of its capacity to dehumanise the human person and complicated by the fact that it is a subjective, qualititative experience being treated in a objective, quantitative empirical minded health care environment. (Lisson, 1987)

Pain is important. It is important not only to the child experiencing the pain but also to the nurse caring for the child. Pain is a complex concept that remains difficult to define, but it is clearly both a physical and a subjective response to some form of noxious stimuli (Melzack and Wall, 1988). In intensive care, the noxious stimuli, such as inflammation, trauma and surgery, may seem obvious, but other stimuli such as isolation, fear and anxiety may not be considered as factors that can affect the child's perception of pain.

It is both the physical response and the subjectivity of the pain experience that makes pain assessment and its effective management of vital importance to the nurse caring for the child who is critically ill. Initially, the nurse may be most concerned with dealing with the adverse physiological effects that result from pain, but the nurse should also be aware of the equally damaging and often long-term effects that poorly managed pain may have on the child's psychosocial development (Quinton and Rutter, 1976).

CHILDREN'S PERCEPTION OF PAIN

The younger child

Children's understanding of pain is dependent to a great degree on their age. Young children see pain as being an immediate frightening punishment, whereas older children have reached a level of reasoning where they understand that pain has a cause which can be treated. The young child will often feel that pain can magically be taken away by 'kissing it better'. This age group have little understanding of the link between medicine and the pain disappearing some time later, and will often find it difficult to locate the pain exactly when asked. It is not unusual for a young child to tell the nurse that they have a 'headache in their tummy'.

The older child

The older child is able to relate the disappearance of pain with the administered treatment. As the child's understanding of pain matures, they have a greater perception of the psychological aspects of pain and may associate bad pain with death and dying. Children will also go to extraordinary lengths to show that they are 'brave'.

Regardless of the age group, all children experiencing pain require reassurance and comfort. Effective pain management is important, as it can help to strengthen the relationship between the child and the nurse by creating trust. Equally, the child soon learns to distrust the nurse who promises to 'make it all better' and fails to do so.

PAIN ASSESSMENT

In assessing a child for pain, the nurse must be aware that both the child's admission to hospital, especially to the intensive care unit, and the pain itself may cause the child to regress and display pain signs that would normally be associated with an earlier developmental stage. This is a natural reaction to pain, and children should feel safe enough to express themselves in this way. Lack of behavioural expression does not preclude the child's experience of pain (Jay *et al.*, 1983).

What must be made clear is that children have the right to be involved in the assessment of their pain. This is fundamental to good practice and can be implemented if the nursing staff are truly committed to providing high-quality pain management.

Not all children in intensive care units are fully paralysed, sedated, passive recipients of care, and the nurse may be able to involve the child in his or her own pain management. A child's reaction to pain may not fit in with what the nurse expects, and this may lead the nurse to underestimate the degree of pain that the child is experiencing. Great skill and patience must be used if paediatric pain assessment is to be accurate (Davitz and Davitz, 1975). Equal care must be shown in the evaluation of the effectiveness of the treatment.

Pain assessment is greatly enhanced if appropriate pain-assessment tools are used. Many tools are available (Eland 1981, 1985; Hester, 1979; Molsberry, 1979; Beyer and Aradine, 1987, Wong and Baker, 1988). Careful consideration must be made before choosing one. It is insufficient to have one standard pain assessment tool on the unit; a range should be available, and the child should whenever possible be consulted in the choice of the most suitable tool for assessing their pain. The young child may feel happiest using the Wong and Baker faces scale (Wong and Whaley, 1986), whereas the older child may prefer to use a linear scale. The Eland colour scale is also a widely accepted and useful means of assessing children's pain (Eland 1981, 1985). The nurse should also be adept at using an initial pain assessment sheet so that all of the child's pain can be documented. All too often, nurses imagine that they are correctly assessing a child's pain but are ignoring the pain that the child may be experiencing from venous access sites and machinery. Invasive procedures are particularly stressful to children requiring intensive care (Tichy *et al.*, 1988).

However, the very sick child or the child who is paralysed and/or sedated may be unable to cooperate in the assessment of their pain and in these circumstances the nurse should rely on an alternative expert: the child's parents. Next to the child, the parents are most likely to be able to give an accurate assessment of the child's pain because they have previous experience of how the child reacts to pain and what behaviour and signs to look for. By working together with the parents, the nurse should attempt to make an accurate assessment through the means of non-verbal and physiological clues.

In the absence of formal documentation, the nurse's perception of the type, intensity, location, aggravating and relieving factors associated with the child's pain should be recorded. The efficacy of any intervention, both nursing and medically based, should be documented with information useful to the other nurses caring for the child. This information may include the exact dosage of the drug given in the case of a prescription that allows some leeway, and whether or not the dose kept the child comfortable and able to rest between prescribed doses. This can easily be done using a flowchart (McCaffery and Beebe, 1989).

Paediatric pain management within the intensive care unit should not simply be the safe administration of prescribed analgesic; rather, a holistic view should be taken. As new and more sophisticated pharmacological methods of pain relief are introduced, relying on technical gadgetry, other skills must not be forgotten or dismissed as being of little importance.

Indicators of paediatric pain

Fully ventilated, electively paralysed children can experience pain. Paralysing agents such as tubocurare and pancuronium bromide have *no analgesic properties*; they merely prevent movement. The ventilated paralysed child is often the most difficult to assess for pain, but it is possible for the nurse to assess the child for pain and evaluate the effectiveness of the treatment given. Usually, the child's vital signs change, with the heart rate and blood pressure increasing. The child may appear pale and sweaty and feel cool to the touch. Blood gases may be affected, with a decrease in P_{O_2} and an increase in P_{CO_2}. The child may display signs similar to those of shock, and often pain is diagnosed when other causes for these changes have been excluded.

Children who are not paralysed, but are able to communicate, benefit from being involved in their pain assessment. Some children may be too sick or, for some other reason, not able to communicate easily with the nurse, but may display some of the more obvious signs of pain, such as restlessness, distress, crying, altered position and guarding of the painful area, as well as alterations in the physiological parameters (Table 9.1).

It must be stressed that parents almost always see pain relief as being of prime importance and can become very distressed at the thought that their child may be experiencing pain. This distress may be exacerbated by the thought that the child is unable to indicate this in a normal manner. The parents should be involved wherever possible in helping to assess their child for pain; their knowledge of their own child can be a most important part of pain assessment.

Table 9.1 Indicators of paediatric pain

Physiological	Behavioural
Increased heart rate	Restless or irritable
Increased blood pressure	Crying or screaming
Altered blood gases	Altered position, e.g. fetal
Increased P_{CO_2}	
Decreased P_{O_2}	
Cool, pale, sweaty skin	Anxious or distressed
	Sleeping or unnaturally alert
	Guarding

Back to basics

Skilled therapeutic nursing care is of prime importance and must continue within the unit. Comfort, reassurance and positioning are important ways of relieving pain and may be all that is required in mild pain. The skilled use of sheepskins, rolls, soft bedding, beanbags and careful handling can help to reduce the degree of pain experienced by the child. Protecting the child from unnecessary noise, light, disturbance and handling can reduce the number of stressors that can influence pain.

Reassurance, comfort, honesty and good preparation for unpleasant procedures can all be used to reduce the psychological component of the pain experience for the child, especially when aimed at the unique and specific needs of each child (Whaley and Wong, 1989).

Distraction and imagery are also useful methods of relieving pain and can be used very successfully by nurses who have no formal training in alternative pain management techniques (Kuttner, 1988; Ross and Ross, 1984; McGrath and de Veber, 1986). Children can be distracted with suitable toys, games, television, video and music, and the child's fertile imagination can be used to encourage the child to imagine something that is personally reassuring and friendly. Children requiring intensive care can be encouraged to play, even if it is somewhat limited play. This can be of great value in helping them to come to terms with what is happening to them and relieving their anxieties, fears and pain.

PHARMACOLOGICAL METHODS OF PAIN RELIEF

There are many different methods by which safe and effective pain management can be achieved. These depend not only on what might be the most appropriate to the child but also are largely dependent on the actual resources, in respect to both specialist skills and technology, of the area in which the child is nursed.

It is important to have a basic understanding of pain physiology, which in turn ensures an understanding of how the treatment that has been prescribed works, to be able to care fully for the child. The most widely recognized pain mechanism is the gate-control theory (Melzack and Wall, 1988). There are three possible sites at which the pain can be blocked.

1. First, at the level of the nociceptors. This prevents the initial stimulation of the pain impulse and therefore pain is not experienced. Damaged tissue releases algogens (pain-producing substances), which in turn cause the nerve endings to fire and to become more sensitive to stimulation by other algogens. Mild analgesics, such as paracetamol, intervene at this level by preventing the manufacture of some algogens, which reduces the possibility of pain impulses being transmitted.

2. Secondly, by affecting transmission of input at the level of the spinal cord. Transmission of nerve impulses requires the normal flow of ions across nerve membranes. If this is either partially or completely disrupted or blocked, the excitability of the nerve fibres is altered. Unmyelinated nerve fibres, such as the C fibres involved in pain impulse transmission, are the most easily affected by pharmacological intervention in this way. The effect of the drug used is dependent on the strength of the solution; weak solutions have only a partial effect and stronger solutions may completely block transmission of pain impulses.

3. Thirdly, central nervous system blockers can be used in pain management. The opiates exert their effect on the higher centres. Morphine is an example from this group; it works by binding to specific receptors in the outer region of the dorsal horn of the spinal cord and in other regions of the central nervous system. Morphine prevents the impulses that reach the dorsal horn of the spinal cord from being transmitted onwards. It also increases the activity of the descending inhibitory pathway.

METHODS OF ADMINISTERING PAIN RELIEF

Oral

This can be continued if the treatment is appropriate, provided several factors are taken into consideration, such as the cough and swallow reflexes, gastric emptying and the absorption of the drug.

Topical

This includes drugs such as EMLA cream (Eutectic Mixture of Local Anaesthetics). This continues to be of prime importance in the paediatric intensive care unit. The nursing and medical staff must still consider using EMLA cream to anaesthetize the skin before venepuncture. The cream must be applied half an hour before the procedure to ensure maximum effectiveness. It is pointless applying the cream and then allowing the procedure to take place too soon. This simply means that the cream does not work and the child mistrusts the nurse and the 'magic' of the cream. Frequent, repeated venepuncture can often be the child's main source of uncontrolled little-considered pain in intensive care.

Rectal

This route can be used when other methods are deemed inappropriate. However, it is a deeply personal invasive procedure for the child and if it is necessary to administer analgesia such as paracetamol or volteral suppositories via this route the child's feelings must be considered and their dignity maintained. The rectal route can be used when the oral route is not thought to be safe, and when only a mild analgesic is required.

Intramuscular

This route is used to give stronger analgesia and although it can be an effective route it has many disadvantages. If it is to be the only route for pain relief children, even if they are experiencing severe pain, will often not admit to being in pain because they are generally more frightened of the needle used for giving the injection. Young children under the age of about 7 years, despite being told that the injection will 'make the pain go away', will not be able to link the sharp, 'ritual' pain of the injection with the magical disappearance of the pain 20–30 min later. If the intramuscular route is to be used, preparation, comforting and reassurance of the child assumes critical importance. Disadvantages apart from the psychological effects it can have on the child include the unpredictability of drug absorption into the blood stream in some situations. Poor peripheral perfusion can have a marked effect on the rate of absorption of the analgesia, which means that a drug given to relieve pain can have a sudden and marked effect several hours after administration with the child suddenly becoming drowsy and possibly hypotensive for no apparent reason.

Intravenous

This is now the commonest route for administering analgesia within the intensive care unit. Although it requires special and constant observation of the child and special nursing skills, it is generally seen to be the kindest and most effective route. Drugs can be given in two different ways: by intermittent slow boluses or by continuous infusion.

Intermittent slow boluses have an advantage in that no special technology is required; if analgesia is administered at regular intervals this can be a very effective method. There is the possibility, however, of the child experiencing pain towards the end of the interval. There can be delays between doses, and nurses are notoriously bad at giving pain relief frequently enough to keep the patient pain free, especially if it is prescribed 'as necessary'.

Continuous infusion is very effective because a continuous amount of the drug is present in the circulating blood. Small bolus doses of the drug can also be used in conjunction with a continuous infusion to control breakthrough pain episodes, as well as to give extra cover to the child during unpleasant procedures. Problems arise with intravenous analgesics when vascular access is difficult and when the infusion 'tissues'. In this situation the child is temporarily deprived of analgesia, the circulating analgesia is used up and the child can quickly experience severe pain. Re-establishment of the intravenous line is very important and a bolus dose of the drug is usually required on recommencing the infusion. Drugs and infusion fluid incompatibilities must always be considered when giving analgesia via the intravenous route, and bolus doses of other drugs should not be given via the analgesia line. If this happens, an unprescribed bolus of the analgesia should be given followed by a period of time without the analgesia infusing once the other drug has been administered.

A new area that must not be overlooked is that of patient-controlled analgesia, which is successfully being used in the effective management of even very young children, who have control over their own medication by the use of a special giving device. Failsafe features ensure that it is impossible for the children to overdose themselves. The number of times that a child 'requests' a dose as well as the number of times that a dose has been delivered is recorded and can be examined by the nurse. This method of administering analgesia reduces the waiting time between a child requiring analgesia and having it given that is associated with the more traditional methods of administration. Research has also shown that children usually require less analgesia if they have control over it in this manner.

Epidural

This route for analgesia is now becoming increasingly popular, and it has many advantages over the intravenous route. Analgesia and anaesthesia via this route can be used in some cases to relieve postoperative pain or provide intraoperative cover to children unable to tolerate a general anaesthetic.

The drugs commonly used in this procedure are used either solely for their analgesic properties, such as diamorphine, or for their combined analgesic and anaesthetic properties, such as bupivacaine and lignocaine. Drugs can be given either as single intermittent or as continuous doses, and the effect is dependent on the type and the strength of the drug used. Epidural analgesia requires the support of skilled committed anaesthesiology staff in placing the catheter, administering the treatment and selecting children who would benefit from the treatment. Specialized nursing care, including minimizing the risk of infection, observing the child for possible side-effects and preventing the formation of pressure sores by frequently changing the child's position, is required when the epidural route is used. Adequate preparation of the child is essential because some children may become very distressed about the lack of sensation they experience as a result of anaesthesia.

NEONATAL PAIN: A SPECIAL CASE?

After many years of people expressing misguided notions about the issue of neonatal pain, most people now believe that *neonates do feel pain*. However, there is some question about whether or not they are capable of experiencing subjective distress as a result of a pain episode (Booker, 1987). Increasing evidence now supports the view that the neonatal cerebral cortex is functioning to a degree where subjective distress seems likely. Many deleterious side-effects of neonatal pain have been highlighted (Owens and Todt, 1984; Williamson and Williamson, 1983; Beaver, 1987; Brown, 1987; Anand *et al.*, 1985; Grunau and Craig, 1987; Johnston and Strada, 1986; Emde *et al.*, 1971). These make the treatment of pain and the reduction of side-effects of prime importance (Table 9.2).

Table 9.2 Neonatal indicators of pain

Physiological	*Behavioural/psychological*
Increased heart rate	Decreased level of activity[†]
Increased blood pressure	Decreased level of alertness[†]
Decreased transcutaneous oxygen levels	Altered facial expression, angular squarish mouth and closed eyes
Decreased oxygen saturation levels	Altered sleep patterns: prolonged periods of non-rapid eye movement and inactive sleep
Increased serum glucose levels	
Increased glycerol levels*	
Increased adrenaline levels*	
Increased noradrenaline levels*	

* Physiological stress response
[†]Behavioural stress response

One of the problems in pain relief in the neonate, especially the preterm baby, is the lack of choice and availability of appropriate drugs. Technical difficulties in administration, possibilities of serious side-effects and the inability of the neonate's immature liver and kidneys to break down and eliminate the drugs all ensure that it has been generally easier to decide not to give analgesia. However, new drugs and techniques of administration are now being developed and this is resulting in a new and exciting approach to the treatment of neonatal pain.

A resistance to the use of opioids due to the perceived high association between opioid administration and serious side-effects such as respiratory depression, carbon dioxide retention and hypotension, as well as the possibility of addiction, does persist, but the judicious use of continuous opioid infusion such as morphine and fentanyl have been shown to enhance the general physical condition of the neonate (Koren *et al.*, 1985). It has been shown that such infusions have improved the outcome of procedures.

Neonatal epidural analgesia or anaesthesia is another method by which effective and safe pain relief can be achieved, although it is generally confined to specialist areas with highly skilled practitioners in control.

CONCLUSIONS

For effective pain management in the intensive care unit, the nurse should always be aware of the possibility of the child experiencing pain. Pain signals should never be ignored or dismissed as being of lower priority than other signals that are 'routinely' acted on. Pain, once assessed, should be seen as an ongoing priority, and pain management should be seen as a combination of nursing and pharmacological therapy. The nurse should be aware of the different pain relief options available and should ensure that the most appropriate route and type is used. Pain assessment should occur regularly and appropriate action be taken if analgesia is ineffective.

The child has the right to be pain free, and nurses should be aware that because they are in close continual contact with the child they are in the ideal position to ensure that this right is upheld.

REFERENCES AND FURTHER READING

Anand, K.J.S., Brown, M.J., Causon, R.C. *et al.* (1985) Can the human neonate mount an endocrine response and metabolic response to surgery? *Journal of Pediatric Surgery*, **20**, 41–8.

Beaver, P.K. (1987) Premature infants' response to touch and pain; can nurses make a difference? *Neonatal Network*, **5** (13), 13–17.

Beyer, J.E. and Aradine, C.R. (1987) Patterns of pediatric pain intensity: A methodological investigation of a self-report scale. *Clinical Journal of Pain*, **3** 130–41.

Beyer, J.E. and Aradine, C.R. (1988) Convergent and discriminant validity of a self-report measure of pain intensity for children. *Child Health Care*, **16**, Spring, 274–82.

Beyer, J.E. and Byers, M.L. (1985) Knowledge of pediatric pain: the state of the art. *Children's Health Care*, **13** (4), 150–9.

Brooker, P.D. (1987) Post operative analgesia for neonates. *Anaesthesia*, **42**, 343–5.

Brown, L. (1987) Physiological responses to cutaneous pain in neonates. *Neonatal Network*, **6** (3), 18–22.

Davitz, L. and Davitz, J. (1975) How nurses view patient suffering. *Registered Nurse*, **38**, 69–74.

Eland, J.M. (1981) Minimizing pain associated with prekindergarten intramuscular injections. *Issues in Comp Pediatric Nursing*, **5**, 361–72.

Eland, J.M. (1985) The child who is hurting. *Seminars in Oncology Nursing*, **1**, 116–22.

Emde, R. N. and Koenig, K.L. (1969) Neonatal smiling, frowning and rapid eye movement states. II. Sleep study cycle. *Journal of the American Academy of Child Psychiatry*, **8**, 637–56.

Emde, R. N., Harmon, R.J., Metcalf, D.J. *et al.* (1971) Stress and induced neonatal sleep. *Psychosomatic Medicine*, **33**, 491–7.

Grunau, R.V. and Craig, K.D. (1987) Pain expression in neonates: facial action and cry. *Pain*, March 28, (3), 395–410.

Hester, N.O. (1979) The preoperational child's reaction to immunizations. *Nursing Research*, **28**, 250–4.

Johnston, C.C. and Strada, M.E. (1986) Acute pain response in infants: a multidimensional description. *Pain*, **24**, 373–82.

Jay, S.M., Ozotius, M., Elliott, C.H., *et al.*, (1983) Assessment of children's distress during painful medical procedures. *Health Psychology*, **2**, 133–47.

Koren, G., Butt, W., Chin Yanga, H., *et al.* (1985) Post operative morphine infusion in newborn infants: assessment of disposition characteristics and safety. *Journal of Pediatrics*, **107** (6), 963–7.

Kuttner, L. (1988) Favorite stories: a hypnotic pain-reduction technique for children in acute pain. *American Journal of Clinical Hypnosis*, **30**, 289–95.

Lisson, E.L. (1987) Ethical issues related to pain control. *Nursing Clinics of North America*, **22** (3), 649–59.

McCaffery, M. and Beebe, A. (1989) *Pain: Clinical Manual for Nursing Practice*, C.V. Mosby, St Louis.

McGrath, P.A. and de Veber, L.L. (1986) The management of acute pain evoked by medical procedures in children with cancer. *Journal of Pain Symptom Management*, **1**, 145–50.

Melzack, R. and Wall, P.D. (1988) *The Challenge of Pain*, Penguin, Harmondsworth.

Molsberry, D. (1979) *Young Children's Subjective Quantifications of Pain following Surgery*. Unpublished master's thesis, University of Iowa.

Owens, M.E. and Todt, E.H. (1984) Pain in infancy: conceptual and methodological issues. *Pain*, **20**, 77–86.

Quinton, D. and Rutter, M. (1976) Early hospitalization and later disturbances of behaviour. *Developmental Medicine and Child Neurology*, **18**, 447–59.

Ross, D.M. and Ross, S.A. (1984) Childhood pain: the school aged child's viewpoint. *Pain*, **20**, 179–91.

Tichy, A.M. *et al.* (1988) Stressors in paediatric intensive care units. *Paediatric Nursing*, **14**, 40–2.

Whaley, L.F. and Wong, D.L. (1989) *Essentials of Pediatric Nursing*, 3rd edn, C.V. Mosby, St Louis.

Williamson, P.S. and Williamson, M.L. (1983) Physiological stress reduction by a local anaesthetic during neobera circumcision. *Pediatrics*, **71** (1), 36–40.

Wong, D. and Baker, C.M. (1988) Facing pain: how much does a child hurt? *Pediatric Nursing*, January–February.

Wong, D.L. and Whaley, L.F. (1986) *Clinical Handbook of Pediatric Nursing*, 2nd edn, C.V. Mosby, St Louis.

10	# Care of the dying child

Jackie Browne and Pip Waddington

I know all about any display of emotion by you being unprofessional but it can help parents, it really can ...

... If your child is going to die it becomes vitally important that the child dies as a person, as an individual, not as yet another patient, another statistic. (Davies, 1977)

Recent surveys on stress in intensive care units show that, even though equipment is becoming complex and a greater demand is placed on the technical skills of nurses, it is death and caring for the dying patient and their family that causes nurses most stress (Lochoff, 1977). In most instances in nursing, there is a procedure to follow which allows some control. However, there is no standardized procedure for care of the dying and death; nor can there be, as every death should be treated as unique, death still tends to be ignored or regarded as failure.

This chapter aims to provide a more positive approach to death and dying in intensive care. Nurses cannot cure all their patients, but they are in the unique position of being able to help and support the child and the family through one of the worse tragedies they can face (Ballard, 1980, personal communication, cited in Hazinski, 1984).

Recently, much has been written about bereavement, and more specifically the death of a child. However, most of the literature looks at the child who is dying of cancer, and little is written about the child who dies in the intensive care unit. To avoid overlap with other works about the terminally ill child, this chapter concentrates on the child who is critically ill and ventilated, or who dies suddenly and unexpectedly in intensive care. What follows has been derived from talking to many bereaved parents and from personal experiences, although it should be stressed that there is no 'ideal' way of approaching death in intensive care.

WHEN DEATH IS EXPECTED

Whenever a child is admitted to intensive care the parents are immediately under stress. Obviously their main fear is whether their child will survive or not (Miles, 1979), but they are also anxious about the environment and the change in their parental role. When their worse fear is confirmed and they are told that their child is unlikely to survive, they may begin to experience 'anticipatory or preparatory grief' (Lindermann, 1944). It is often difficult for them to express their grief in an unfamiliar and machine-dominated environment (Lipsky, 1979). Anticipatory grief is similar to the stages of grief identified by Kubler-Ross (1973):

1. initial shock and denial;
2. feelings of anger, rage and envy;
3. bargaining or an attempt to postpone the inevitable;
4. depression, in which previous anger is replaced with sadness and a sense of great loss;
5. eventual acceptance involving a decrease in previous agitation and a sense of developing quiet expectation.

As well as these, parents may experience *guilt* and feelings of *failure* and *loss of control*. They may feel that they should have realized that something was wrong earlier and taken action sooner, or that they didn't spend enough time with their child. They may feel guilty for punishing the child for something they did earlier. They may feel that they have failed as parents, being unable to ensure their child reaches adulthood and powerless to effect what was their basic role as a parent. As the care for the child is taken over by hospital staff, they may feel that they are losing their responsibility.

These stages and emotions do not always follow a set pattern and will overlap and interrelate. Parents may experience more than one reaction at any time, or miss some completely. It is important that nurses are aware of and recognize the stages of grief parents can go through so that they can provide appropriate support.

Parental involvement

An important way to help parents is to encourage them to give as much time as they can and become as involved in the care of their child as they feel able to; but nurses should not make them feel guilty if they cannot provide this care. Often parents are embarrassed as they feel that they are being watched continually. They are also nervous because of all the equipment, tubes and wires; even changing a nappy becomes difficult. Encouraging them to carry out basic care and, if they feel confident enough, some of the more technical care, will help them to feel able to fulfil their parental role and gain self-confidence. They will also feel less of a failure if they know they have cared for their child to the best of their ability. In the words of one parent: 'Don't just pity us and feel sorry for parents – use them as a key to their child's treatment . . . Help them to give what they have so they can be positive, so that they can be left with triumph and not just a feeling that they have failed as parents' (Davies, 1979).

Nursing support

It is very easy for nurses to take over the total care of the child. This can non-verbally communicate the impression that the parents are incompetent (Gyulay, 1978). If parents feel unable to perform physical care, they can still talk to, touch and cuddle their child, read stories and play tapes.

It is important that the child is made as comfortable as possible, maintaining their dignity and being surrounded by familiar things, toys, their own bedclothes and photographs. If a child is ventilated and sedated it is important that the nurses carry on talking to them, and telling them their names and what they are going to do, in a way they will be able to understand. The child may be able to hear long after they are unable to respond, but if they are approached and procedures carried out without warning their stress and anxiety levels may rise (Reichle, 1975). By acting as role models, nurses give parents permission to talk to their child without feeling silly or offering false hope. It may reassure the parents that their physical presence is helpful even if the child appears unaware (Gardner and Stewart, 1978).

If the child is able to communicate but is unable to talk, it is important that everyone knows how they communicate, e.g. by nodding the head, squeezing the fingers or closing their eyes, and that they are given plenty of time to communicate their needs. If children can talk, it is important that they are able to communicate their fears and worries about their illness and dying. Questions should be answered openly and honestly and at the child's pace. Some children prefer to talk to staff rather than their parents as they don't want to upset their parents by talking about dying. Parents are often afraid of telling their child, but very often the child will already know, so it is much better to have everything out in the open. This does not mean that all conversation needs to be doom and gloom.

Parents should be encouraged to see to their own physical needs, sleeping and eating. They are often afraid to leave the child in case something happens while they are away. It is often helpful if a nurse stays with the child while parents have a break.

Parents will have many fears about the child's illness and death itself, especially if the child is unable to communicate. Is their child in pain? Do they know what is happening? Will there be a lot of blood when their child dies, or choking? How will they know when the child dies? One way to relieve this anxiety is open, honest communication. An answer that is kind but dishonest will eventually lead to a loss of faith in the nurse.

Poor communication, such as being told different things by different people, use of jargon, not being told the results of tests and treatment, and not being told the names and titles of staff (Miles and Carter, 1982) are all sources of stress to parents.

To avoid confusion, the minimum number of doctors should talk to the family about the course of the illness. Parents will detect and magnify any slight difference in optimism or pessimism; even using different words such as septicaemia or bacteraemia can confuse them, leading to doubts about their child's care (Friedman *et al.*, 1963).

Fewer nurses caring for the child minimizes the amount of adapting the child and family have to do, and allows the nurse to be familiar with every aspect of the child's care (Lyth, 1982).

It is very easy for intensive care nurses to hide behind equipment and observations, avoiding relationships and conversation. The impression of 'availability' is very important (Lugton, 1988). Sitting down with the family, with a cup of tea if appropriate, talking about everyday matters can be very reassuring to the parents. Often this leads to them talking about their fears. It is important to talk to the child, getting to know him or her as a person and not just a shell, and invite the parents to bring in photographs of the child; this all helps to show that the nurses care, and also makes it much easier to nurse the child as an individual and not a 'head injury' or 'meningitic'.

Parents, while they are sitting by their child's bed, will watch the staff and how they relate to each other and to the children; their confidence may be shaken if they observe what they think is inappropriate levity or inadequate emotional involvement. Even though the unit may be very busy, it is important that if the nurse says they will do something or come back in five minutes that they keep their promise, as this reliability is very reassuring. Some parents may concentrate on what seems to be a minor problem, such as a dirty sheet, but this allows them some control, something they can change (Parfit, 1975).

Parents often try to find out as much as they can about their child's illness and treatment; a coping mechanism known as intellectualization. This can often be seen as threatening by the nursing staff, leading to parents being labelled as 'difficult' or 'overprotective', but it is important that it is recognized as their way of coping. Sometimes, although the parents know the technical words, they may not understand their real meaning, so it is important that nurses ensure that parents do comprehend what they have been told.

APPROACHING DEATH

Sometimes it is difficult for parents to see a deterioration in their child's condition. The clinical deterioration may not be matched by physical appearance, so it is hard for parents to accept that although they may look the same as yesterday, they are now so poorly they are likely to die.

When treatment is withdrawn, often following intensive consultation with the parents or even at the parents' request, it may still be difficult for the parents to adjust from 'high-power' nursing to 'tender loving care' nursing.

When it is known that the child is not going to survive (as, for example, when the diagnosis of brain death is made) and no further treatment is available, parents should be aware that they still have a certain amount of choice in how that death takes place. Sudden death may still occur and parents should be warned of this. However, often there is some forewarning, especially if death occurs under controlled circumstances, such as discontinuation of ventilation following the diagnosis of brain death.

Parents have rarely been in this situation before, so are unsure what is expected of them. They are usually guided by the nursing staff, so all the choices should be available to them. Obviously each unit, parent, child and death, is different, but parents may be able to decide where they want the death to take place; in a side room, in a quiet area of the unit, or in their usual bedspace. They can help to decide what equipment remains in place, whether they remain with their child, and whether they hold them or lie on the bed with them. They may even decide to take their child home.

The parents may wish to have their child baptised or have other religious requirements carried out, according to their faith. On many intensive care units a chaplain visits regularly and is introduced to all the families. Whatever their religion, the family should be aware that someone from their own faith is available to talk to them.

As the child nears death some parents gain great comfort in seeing routine care continuing and all the equipment functioning. Others may become angry that their child is disturbed for a routine observation. Therefore a plan of care should be worked out with the parents. Often what nurses do for the parents' sake can turn out to be more harmful than beneficial. For instance, before the removal of unnecessary equipment, it is important to check with the parents or they may see this as 'clearing away' before their child has died.

When the child's condition deteriorates so that death is imminent, the family should be given as much privacy as they want. They may want all their family and friends to visit to say goodbye, or they may wish to be on their own. Some parents gain comfort from a favourite nurse being present or within earshot. They may wish to hold their child or lie on the bed with them or hold their hand. Some parents are unable to face the death; they should not be forced to be present but many parents who were not present when their child died later regretted their decision, feeling that they let their child down.

The death itself may be very peaceful or frightening for the parents, and they need to be warned. The child may leak body fluids and appear to panic as they fight for breath. Pain relief may be prescribed by the doctor so that the parents can be reassured that the child is not suffering. Sometimes, when brain death has been diagnosed, some movement may still occur owing to spinal reflexes, and parents need to be warned of this. When the child has died, the parents may display any number of emotions; they may scream, appear numb, or push the child away or cry. Whatever their reaction, they should be supported and reassured.

The doctor who comes to certify the child's death should preferably be one who knows the child and the family, rather than a stranger. The request for an autopsy may be made at this point if appropriate, or can be left until later, depending on the parents' emotional state.

It is important to remember that, even when a death is expected, when it actually occurs it can be devastating for everyone involved, especially the parents.

SUDDEN DEATH

Several studies have shown that sudden death is much more difficult to grieve than an anticipated death (Harvard Bereavement Study and Harvard Omega Project Study). There is not time to prepare and no time to say goodbye.

Despite recent trends for parents to stay during resuscitative procedures, there are times when parents may choose not to be present or when it may be inappropriate. In the case of accidents or sudden collapse, the parents may not even be at the hospital. These situations are often more difficult as the parents will not have had time to form a relationship with the staff.

It is now recognized that if the parents have to wait outside the unit it is helpful to have someone to stay with the parents to act as go-between. This person may be a nurse, an auxiliary nurse, a social worker, a clergyman or anybody appropriate for that family, and may or may not have some counselling skills (Epperson, 1977; Green, 1976). This person can help to prepare the parents for the death of their child, if appropriate, by becoming increasingly pessimistic with their information. There is no need for detailed medical reports, just short explanations without jargon, reassuring them that everything possible is being done.

This may be a good time to obtain a history which may help to take their mind off what is happening behind the closed doors. Because of the stress and shock, parents may find it difficult to answer even simple questions. They need to be reassured that this is quite normal. Because of the nature of some of the questions, parents may feel they are being blamed for the accident or illness, especially as they often feel guilty anyway. It is therefore important that the reasoning behind the questions is explained and that they are asked sensitively.

It can be very difficult to sit with parents, who may display any number of emotions and behaviour, such as anger (which may be directed at the go-between), shock, guilt, disbelief and immense grief. Nurses should not judge parents by their reactions; everyone will react differently and nurses should not add to their problems by showing disapproval. There may be many silences, but the presence of the go-between will be much appreciated, if not at the time then later. It is tempting to go along with the parents' denial of the seriousness of their child's condition, but it is essential to be honest and begin to prepare them for the death of their child.

If possible the parents should have a quiet area, away from curious looks. They will need access to a telephone and may wish to smoke. Drink and food should also be provided, although they may well be refused. Often the admission or incident takes place at unexpected times; the parents may be unsuitably clothed and they may have no money, so practical help as well as emotional support is needed. Other children need to be taken care of; they may be with the parents and may benefit from being entertained by the play therapist, or arrangements for collecting from school may need to be made.

Press interest is intense in the case of an accident or untoward incident, so the parents need protection from a barrage of questions. Ideally, no information should be given out without the parents' permission; depending on hospital policy, it is best to issue one statement rather than speaking to everyone individually. Relatives and friends also want to know what is happening, and parents should be asked whether they wish to talk to them or have a message delivered.

Everything possible should be done to avoid one parent being on their own. The police may have to be contacted if tracing parents proves difficult. Divorced or separated parents may have difficulty in talking to each other. It is important to ensure that the information is given to all parties involved; otherwise, it may become distorted. There may be hostility and blame, so staff should reinforce the fact that the child is omnipotent and the parents should overcome their problems and pull together.

Minutes will seem like hours to waiting families. They may be wondering if they are being told the truth or whether the staff are competent. The doors will appear forbidding, and as noises carry they will think every noise pertains to them. If possible the parents should be given the chance to see their child, even if for a few seconds. It may be the last chance they have of seeing their child alive, and seeing all the equipment helps them to realize how sick their child is and that all is being done to save the child's life.

Families from ethnic communities or foreign countries, and deaf parents or those with communication problems, may have difficulty understanding what is happening. An interpreter should be contacted. It is essential that during such a crisis the information is understood by everyone.

As well as the go-between, a doctor and a nurse should meet the parents and tell them what is happening at frequent intervals. When a child dies, the parents should be told the news together, if possible, in private by the same doctor and nurse. The explanation should be short and carefully worded, avoiding ambiguous phrases such as 'passed on' or 'slipped away' which could be misconstrued. Parents often find it difficult to ask questions as they are too numb or shocked; they may be afraid it will make them appear stupid or cause them to break down. Things may need to be repeated many times before the parents are able to take them in. Most parents gain comfort from seeing that the staff are saddened by the ordeal; others may be angry that staff are upset when 'they didn't even know him'. If relevant, the need for the coroner to be involved may have to be mentioned at this point. Most parents are very upset that their child has to have an autopsy, 'to be cut up' after all they have been through.

Parents should be given some time to themselves, ensuring that they know staff are available to answer any questions they may have or help in any way they can. They should be allowed to see their child as soon as possible. The resuscitation equipment should be cleared away and the child should be covered and wearing pants or a nappy if possible. The parents should not be forced to see their child, but it does help them to accept the reality of death and begin grieving. Holding or touching their child allows parents to say good-bye and feel that they are accepted as loving and caring parents by the staff.

CARE OF THE CHILD AND FAMILY IMMEDIATELY AFTER DEATH

When the child has died, the parents should be given every opportunity to stay with their child for as long as they wish, touching and holding them as much as they want to. They may want other relatives to see the child before they leave.

Before seeing their child they should be warned of the child's appearance and how this may change as time goes on. Some children feel cold to the touch immediately; others may remain warm for a while, and parents may be upset by this, as they often expect them to feel cold immediately. Some children may just look as if they are asleep, which may make it hard for parents to accept that they really are dead. Others look grotesque or scared, which is obviously very distressing for the parents. The child's skin often goes very pale, almost translucent or waxy – especially the lips, which may lose all their colour. The skin then gradually becomes mottled, usually from the back to the front and they can appear very cyanosed.

The child should be positioned to look as natural as possible, preferably flat, before rigidity makes repositioning difficult. Where possible the child's eyes and mouth should be closed, as staring eyes or a gaping mouth can be very upsetting. Children who have donated organs should have their wounds covered, although some parents may wish to see the scars. Some children look very peaceful, but the nurse should not be tempted to say so unless they really do. Some children appear to have a slight smile, which can be very reassuring for the family.

It is very important to maintain the dignity of the child, even in death. They should be given privacy, without everyone coming in and out.

Some parents may want to wash their child themselves and should be given the choice, as it is the last time they can perform care for their child. Others may want to do it with help, watch while the nurse washes the child, or go away and come back when the child has been washed and dressed. If parents are helping, they should be warned that as the child is moved air escaping from their lungs may produce a 'groan'; this can be very frightening for the parents. The leakage of body fluids can also be very distressing and may leave a lasting impression on the parents.

Most children are now dressed in clothes rather than a shroud. If appropriate, the parents should be given the choice of dressing them in day or night clothes. They may have a particular garment they wish them to wear.

A child's death has to be referred to the coroner in certain cases, such as sudden death or death following an accident or within 24 h of admission to hospital. Different authorities vary as to which tubes have to be left in position; however, to have permission to remove all the tubes around the face can mean a lot to the parents. Other tubes can be made to look as unobtrusive as possible. If the child has had a long-term tracheostomy, it is best to check with the parents whether they wish it to be removed or not.

The parents may wish to take a lock of their child's hair or have a photograph taken. When the child goes to the mortuary, their favourite toy may accompany them; this can be very reassuring for the parents and they can choose what accompanies their child.

The child's body should be labelled according to hospital policy. Some parents may not wish to leave the unit until their child has gone to the mortuary; others may wish to go with their child to the mortuary doors, or to leave while their child is still on the unit.

The mortuary trolley is usually ugly and obvious; it is helpful to try to disguise it with bright sheets, but it can still be very upsetting for parents when they see it. Babies can be carried in the nurse's arms, well wrapped up, or in a Moses basket; young children may be carried or placed in a pram, but older children usually have to go in the trolley. If possible, a nurse should accompany the child to the mortuary.

LEAVING THE INTENSIVE CARE UNIT

Leaving the unit after the death of a child can be very difficult for the parents and the staff. The parents may feel abandoned as they leave the security of the unit for the unknown, and staff that they are letting the parents down. The unit is the parents' last link with their child, and the staff have become part of the 'family', so the parents may not want to let go.

At home, the child's belongings are often just as they left them and are a very painful reminder to the parents of their loss. They may go to stay with relatives or friends, or if the child dies in the evening or at night they may prefer to stay at the hospital overnight and return home in the daylight.

Most units have a bereavement booklet to give to parents when they leave. This should reinforce information which has already been given verbally to parents. The booklet should explain the need for a coroner's case or autopsy, how to obtain the death certificate, when and where to go to register the death (including a map showing the registrar's office) and how to get help with funeral costs and information about arranging the funeral. Local support groups should be listed and the unit's telephone number given. Also, some information about how the parents and other children are likely to feel and act over the next few days or weeks. It should be stressed that there is always someone available on the unit to listen or help.

If death occurs over the weekend, a long time may pass without the parents seeing their dead child, so if possible they should be able to visit their child in the chapel of rest. This helps them to accept the reality of their child's death and allows them to begin to grieve in earnest.

Where possible, the death certificate should be given to the parents before they leave the hospital, so they do not have the trauma of returning to the hospital to collect it. When an autopsy has been requested or when the death is a coroner's case, it is usually carried out as soon as possible and the parents need to know how to collect the death certificate. Some units may have a bereavement office.

Some parents may gain comfort from visiting the hospital chapel, where they may enter their child's name in the Book of Remembrance. Some units may have their own book where parents may write their own poem, script or verse and mount a photo.

The general practitioner and health visitor should be contacted as soon as possible so that someone visits the family at home to help to ease their feeling of abandonment, offering help and advice and support. Some areas may have a bereavement counsellor who visits the family at home.

The child's belongings should be given to the parents, if appropriate, just before they leave the unit. If the child has been involved in an accident and the clothes were torn or bloodied it should be tactfully suggested to the parents that they were ruined in the accident. However, some parents are adamant that they want everything connected to their child, especially as it may be the last thing their child touched.

Some parents may decide it is too painful to keep their child's toys and belongings. However, it is a good idea to keep the belongings for a while because they sometimes change their mind, then regret they didn't keep them, especially their child's favourite toy.

It is usual for the child's consultant to see the parents 6–8 weeks after the child's death. This enables the parents to ask any questions they have thought of and to discuss the autopsy results. A nurse is often present at this meeting. The appointment should be sent to the parents near the time, although they should be informed about the meeting before leaving the unit.

When parents leave the unit, at least one member of staff should go to the door with them to say goodbye. Staff should ensure that the parents have transport home and that if they are going to drive they are fit to do so.

Often the parents inform the unit of when and where the funeral is to take place. It is up to individuals whether they attend the funeral or not. Some people find it too distressing; however, some find it helps them to work through their grief. Some staff worry that their presence may make the family relive their ordeal, but it is usually much appreciated and helps the parents to realize how much the staff cared.

The parents often like to keep in touch with the unit, especially with staff they formed a close relationship with. They may begin to raise funds for the unit, which helps them to work through their grief. They often return to the unit at least once because they need to see where their child died again. This can be difficult, as the staff often don't know what to say, especially if they are new and never nursed the child. Staff are often afraid to mention the child's name in case it causes the parents to cry, but it is often the desperate need to talk about their child to someone who knew them and the events that led to their death that drives them to come back to the unit.

When talking to parents it is often advisable to avoid platitudes such as 'it was for the best', 'you'll forget in time' (often they don't want to get over it or forget); these can cause the parents a lot of distress, although the person only means well. Instead it is best to express sorrow and show care and concern.

Some staff feel that their relationship with the family is such that they wish to visit them at home; again, this a personal choice and can be very beneficial to all concerned.

Parents may be alarmed by the length of time their grieving is taking. They should be reassured that this is quite normal. Where possible, parents should be put in touch with others who have had a child who died, as they can give a lot of help, support and advice because they have more insight into how the newly bereaved family are feeling than anyone else.

SIBLINGS

Parents often turn to the nurses for advice on how to cope with their other children. Parents often try to protect their children from the true situation (Lieberman, 1979). They perhaps feel that the children would be unable to cope with the truth (Cain *et al.*, 1963) or that because of the parents' own grief they would be unable to provide the children with the support they would need. However, if their parents are not honest, children soon sense that something is wrong and is being kept from them. This may mean that they try to find the answers to their own questions, and begin to fantasize over what has happened and whose fault it is (Rosen and Cohen, 1981). The sibling's age, experience and relationship with the dead child and their parents' reaction to death all have a bearing on their reaction to the death (Vernon, 1970). Children under 5 years old often see death as a reversible, non-permanent state similar to life, and may upset their parents by repeatedly asking when their dead sibling is returning. Children aged between 5 and 9 years often personify death as 'the bogeyman' or 'a skeleton', who takes you away, seeing death as a punishment. Children over 9 years are beginning to see death as a permanent state and inevitable (Anthony, 1940; Nagy, 1959; Bluebond-Langer, 1978; Scripen *et al*;, 1975). All children will vary in their view of death depending on whether death has been discussed within the family in the past.

Children may show grief differently from adults; their grieving is often missed as parents are grieving themselves. Young children may outwardly appear unconcerned, and carry on playing and laughing. Parents are understandably upset and concerned by the apparent lack of emotion; they should be reassured that this is quite normal. Some children may regress in behaviour, displaying temper tantrums, attention-seeking behaviour and withdrawal. Older children have a wide range of emotions and are unsure how to react. If adults are able to share their own feelings, it allows the children to talk about their own emotions. If the parents are unable to face the reality of death, the child may well distrust them and grow up fearing hospitals and death. If parents try too hard to be brave and hide their emotions and grief, the child may well believe that their parents don't care and wouldn't care if they themselves died.

Older children experience guilt and anger. They may blame themselves for the illness or death (Cain *et al.*, 1963). Arguments where the sibling 'wished' the other dead are often believed to have caused the sibling's death, so the child will need reassurance that this was not the case. They may feel guilty for being the survivor, or be angry at their parents for not paying them enough attention or for the disruption in their life, or feel anger at the sibling for causing the parents pain.

Children can be helped by being allowed to participate in the affairs of the family during the crisis, by being involved in decisions, given choices and allowed to help. They may be given the choice of visiting the sick child or not. If they decide to visit, they should be prepared for how their sibling will look and whether they can move or talk. The equipment should be explained in a way that they can understand, at a pace at which they want to know. This is a good time for the nursing staff to form a relationship with the siblings and talk to them about their feelings. The child should be given the chance to say goodbye to their brother or sister. They may wish to draw a picture or take a present for them when they visit. Some families gain comfort from being together at the time of death; others may feel it is too traumatic. Whether the child sees the dead sibling or not is another difficult decision, but again reality is often kinder than fantasy. 'I thought when you died your skin peeled off', one child said.

Care should be taken when explaining death to children. 'Went on a trip' may make children fear journeys. 'Went to sleep' may made the child fear bedtime, and 'died because they were sick' may make them fear illness and hospitals.

Following death of a sibling, children can feel very insecure and have a fear of losing someone else close to them. When a sibling is dying or has died, parents can be advised that although inclusion of other children may be painful exclusion may be worse (Gyulay, 1978).

GRANDPARENTS, OTHER RELATIVES, BABYSITTERS, FRIENDS

There are often many people who care for the child who may be forgotten when the child is dying. There may be a favourite uncle or childminder who need to show that they care. These 'forgotten others' are often a great source of comfort and help to the parents of the dying child. They may look after the other children, the house or the pets, or just be there for the parents when they need to talk or cry, so they need to be supported as well.

Grandparents play a major role in many families and it is important that their grief is not overlooked, especially as their grief is twofold, grieving for their grandchild and their own child's loss. They often find it more difficult than the parents to accept that their grandchild is dying (Friedman *et al.*, 1963). Therefore nurses need to help the parents prepare them for the death; this can be stressful to the parents, as they may feel they are betraying their child.

OTHER PARENTS IN THE INTENSIVE CARE UNIT

Fellow parents are usually a great source of comfort to one another; they gain a tremendous amount from comparing their children: name, age, illness, treatment and prognosis. Their sense of isolation is eased by realizing that there are others in a similar situation.

While on the unit they may see children deteriorating and dying and, although this may help to prepare them for the death of their own child, it is obviously very distressing. Parents are very aware of what is happening on the unit and are quick to sense when the atmosphere changes. When a child dies on the unit it is better to tell other parents the truth and give them time to discuss how they feel. Obviously, the other parents may become very depressed and they are often unsure what to say to the bereaved family, although they wish to express their sorrow. They may feel a mixture of relief that their child is still alive and then guilt because the other child has died.

THE EFFECT OF DEATH ON NURSING STAFF

Nursing the dying child involves an investment of time, energy and technical skills. Meeting their needs and those of their family can be most challenging and emotionally draining, but at the same time rewarding, aspect of nursing children. When dying people are cared for in as near ideal conditions as possible, it can bring great satisfaction for the staff, compensating for the emotional stress. However, if constant anxieties and frustrations arise in providing for the needs of patients and their families, burnout becomes a distinct possibility (Robbins, 1989).

Burnout can be described as an extension of stress; the person experiences a depletion of energy through feeling overwhelmed by other people's problems (Iveson-Iveson, 1983). The nurse who is beginning to burn out has various stress symptoms plus a compulsion to overwork, no interests outside work, guilt about personal 'inadequacy', compulsion to succeed, feelings of being trapped and powerless, and an unwillingness to delegate. Although some degree of stress is inevitable where death is a frequent visitor, much can be done by the individual nurse, the unit staff and managers to recognize stress and avoid burnout.

The role of the nurse caring for the dying child will vary; some nurses find it easier to give more of themselves, and others feel safer hiding behind the machinery. 'One can hide behind a uniform, a title or medical terminology only so long before facing the reality of the human situation' (Gyulay, 1978). Some nurses feel a sense of failure if the child they are caring for dies; others find a challenge in making the child's remaining time comfortable.

Nurses have their own grieving process, although the stages may not correspond to those the family are going through. These emotions are normal and enable nurses to be caring, but they need to be handled and channelled properly so that they don't become destructive.

Traditionally, 'good' nurses did not become 'involved' with their patients; however, as soon as a nurse begins to look after a patient she becomes involved. They find out little things about the child, their likes and dislikes, their personality; even if the child is unconscious, the family builds up a picture for them. Family-centred care and primary nursing reinforce this emotional bond between the nurse and the patient, making the patient's death more difficult for the nurse but also allowing them to provide genuine sympathetic care and support.

Nurses are often led to believe that they should not show emotions. Some nurses prefer not to show their emotions and wait until they are alone or at home; however, those who do wish to cry and find themselves 'bottling up' will find this transmuted into stress. Many parents have said how it helped them to see that the nurse cared. One parent said: 'Your eyes, your hands and your personal gestures say so much ... Obviously I am not advocating the wholesale opening of floodgates, but your pain, your grief, your personal involvement, your humanity and your understanding are immeasurably reassuring. Don't shut us out behind your professional front' (Davies, 1979). Tears can be helpful, but not to the extent that the family end up consoling the nurse! If grief begins to overwhelm, it is best for the nurse to withdraw for a while, to regain control and allow a return to a supportive role again.

Showing emotion is not a sign of weakness, neither is appearing emotionless a sign of coldheartedness. Our colleagues' responses should be recognized and understood and not judged as 'right' or 'wrong'; colleagues should also be given time and support. A nurse who has looked after a dying child and supported their family should be given time after the family leaves the unit before taking on the care of another patient. This should enable her to vent her feelings and regain control without expecting her to switch her emotions immediately to a new patient.

When a nurse is caring for a dying child and their family day after day, it can occasionally become too stressful, but the nurse may feel that to ask for a change of patient would be seen as a sign of weakness. Sensitive senior staff should be aware of this and offer chances to look after different patients before the nurse needs to ask.

Intensive support may be needed for new staff and students, especially if they have never nursed a dying child before. They may be upset by what they interpret as callous or offhand behaviour by more senior staff. Joking and laughing may appear grossly misplaced. It should be explained that this is often just defensive denial and tension release; it is often said 'if we weren't laughing, we'd be crying' (Jacobson, 1978).

Nurses often need to 'get things off their chest', either formally or informally. Talking to a friend or colleague can be helpful, as long as the talker is also prepared to listen; otherwise, the person may become stressed. A nurse can feel isolated by stressful events, and it is reassuring to find that others are feeling the same. However, 'letting off steam' at non-medical partners or friends can cause a strained relationship, as they often do not understand the work involved on intensive care (Hay and Oken, 1972).

Regular staff meetings are helpful as they allow projections of points of view, increasing everyone's sense of value and preventing feelings of frustration or isolation. Ethical dilemmas can be discussed, priorities organized, and particular events such as reactions to a cardiac arrest, talked through. Differences of opinion can be worked out at these meetings, thus sparing the families seeing staff disagree. Sometimes more formal counselling sessions are necessary or chosen, either within a group session or on a one-to-one basis. However, nurses are often wary of the stigma often associated with appearing to need professional help. Whatever sessions the unit decides on, they should begin and end promptly and last a reasonable length of time. All grades of staff should be represented, and the atmosphere relaxed.

The Health Education Authority report 'Stress in the Public Sector' (1988) says of nurses that 'they need to support both patients and relatives through such times yet receive little support or training themselves to handle these traumatic events'. Staff should be encouraged to attend study days and courses in counselling, bereavement and any other relevant training programmes. This is reflected in the UKCC Scope of Professional Practice, section 9 (1992). By increasing their knowledge of the process of dying and the grieving process, nurses will gain confidence and this will in turn gain the family's confidence and that of colleagues.

The death of a child is often more difficult for nurses to cope with than that of an adult because of the child's unrealized potential. This apparent unfairness can make nurses feel angry; some form of relaxation or physical activity can help them to work through this anger and so relieve some of the tension. Nurses should be able to recognize their own stress: 'Accept your limitations! Everyone has some . . . Accept your emotions! Everyone has those too . . . Accept that feeling stressed is ok, a sign of sanity! Learn what your individual stress symptoms are, and when you get them and seek the cause' (Swaffield, 1988).

Managers can relieve staff stress by having an 'open door' for staff with problems or suggestions, maintaining regular contact and giving praise when appropriate. Additionally, ensuring that staff have regular breaks and a fair off duty allocation, selecting staff suited to the intensive care atmosphere and encouraging quality care can be helpful.

'The nurse should formulate a professional philosophy so that her success as an ICU nurse depends on the ability to give good nursing care and emotional support to the patient and family rather than on the survival of patients.' (Newlin and Wellisch, 1978).

ESTABLISHING BRAIN STEM DEATH

'The irreversible cessation of brain stem function implies the death of the brain as a whole. It does not necessarily imply the death of every cell in the brain.' (Pallis, 1983). To establish brain stem death, certain criteria must be met. Each intensive care unit should have a written protocol or tests, which must be followed. These tests are designed to prove that there is no brain stem function and should be carried out by doctors of suitable standing. The UK Code of Practice recommends that one be a consultant and the other a consultant or senior registrar. One set of tests should be carried out by a doctor who has nothing to do with the patient's case or care, and therefore has an unbiased opinion. Both sets of test should be performed separately and independently. The time between the two sets of brain stem tests is up to the doctors, but should be done with sympathetic timing and agreement with the patient's family, ensuring that they understand the full implications of the tests. Nursing and medical staff should be aware of the emotional difficulty that some families encounter in accepting the death of their child, especially when their heart is still beating and they are 'breathing' by means of the ventilator.

Brain stem function can only be tested when:

1. there are no circulating sedatives or neuromuscular blocking drugs (no drugs that will impair brain stem function). This should be checked with staff and on the treatment card. Use of a peripheral nerve stimulator will detect residual neuromuscular blockers. If renal or hepatic impairment is suspected, brain stem tests should be deferred for 24 h. Antibiotic treatment should be continued.
2. the patient is not hypothermic. (The core temperature should be above 35°C.) A space blanket or warming blanket may have to be used.
3. there is no metabolic or endocrine disorder that may contribute to the coma persisting. Serum electrolytes, acid–base balance and glucose measurements should all be within normal limits.

The following tests that the doctors carry out during each assessement should be documented. These tests refer to brain stem reflexes.

1. Pupils should be fixed in diameter and unresponsive to light.

2. No eye movement or nystagmus should be seen to occur when ice-cold water is slowly syringed into each ear. (Each ear drum should be clearly visualized before this test is performed to ensure that there is a clear passage for the water to reach the ear drum.) This is called the caloric test.
3. There should be no corneal reflex. This can be tested by gently touching the cornea with a wisp of cotton wool.
4. No eye movement should occur when the head is rotated to either side. This is often called the 'doll's eye' test.
5. There should be no spontaneous or reflex movement within the cranial nerve distribution.
6. There should be no gag reflex or reflex to a suction catheter passed into the trachea (no coughing during endotracheal suction).

The last test that doctors are required to perform is the apnoea test. Before this test is performed, the arterial blood gas should be analysed to ensure that the P_{CO_2} is above 5.3 kPa (to stimulate respiration when ventilation is diconnected). If the P_{CO_2} is below this, ventilation should be reduced until subsequent tests show a value of 5.3 kPa or above.

The patient should be preoxygenated for a least 10 min with 100% oxygen. During the test, 100% oxygen should be delivered to the patient at 6 l/min by passing a catheter into the trachea via the endotracheal tube. These measures should prevent hypoxia during the test.

When ready, the doctor will disconnect the patient from the ventilator for a timed 5 min and observe whether there is any spontaneous respiratory effort. The chest should be uncovered and clearly visible. If no spontaneous breathing is observed, this is a sign of lack of brain stem function. The ventilator should be reconnected following the apnoea test.

When the second set of tests confirms brain stem death, this is the official time of the child's death, and the doctors should inform the parents without delay that their child has died. Parents should be given time to come to terms with the situation, and then given the opportunity to discuss how they wish the child's death to be handled.

ORGAN DONATION

Approaching parents

Individual circumstances will dictate who is best qualified to approach the relatives. It may be the clinician in charge of the patient or the nurse who has been looking after the child and has formed a trusting relationship with the parents. It requires sensitivity and a positive belief in the successful outcome of transplantation, and is something an unmotivated member of staff should never be pressurized into doing. In the majority of cases, the best time to discuss the matter will be after the first set of brain stem death tests have been carried out. These discussions may need repetition to ensure that the parents fully understand. There is no need by law for parents to confirm their lack of objection in writing, but any record of enquiries made and the outcome should be recorded in the child's medical notes.

If an autopsy is necessary, it is advisable to mention this to the parents before a request for organ donation is made; this information should not be used to apply pressure to the family who has said no. If parents have consented to organ donation, it should be explained that it is not possible for them to be present when ventilation is discontinued in the operating theatre. Therefore, the parent and family should be encouraged to say their goodbyes earlier. They should be aware that they can see their child again after donation. This could be later on in the intensive care unit, but timing is difficult as operating time is unpredictable. It may be better to suggest that parents go home, and if they wish to see the child again arrange a time when they can all be present.

The role of the transplant coordinator

Each Health Authority employs a transplant coordinator. Their role includes education, organization or the donor referral system, and informing and supporting the families and staff involved. Early recognition of potential organ donors and subsequent referral will ensure the optimum use of donor organs.

Suitability for organ donation

For successful organ transplantation to take place, various selection criteria need to be met in order to find a suitable donor. The potential donor should meet with the brain stem death criteria. The child should be maintained on a ventilator and the correct fluid balance and cardiovascular support given. Blood will be taken for tissue typing, and chest radiography, electrocardiography and measurements of the chest will be necessary.

There should be no evidence of:

1. major untreated system infection;
2. malignancy (except primary brain tumour);
3. chronic severe hypertension;
4. positive Australia antigen and/or human immunodeficiency virus (HIV) antibodies.

There should be consent from relatives and the coroner's approval. Victims of non-accidental injury are not usually considered suitable for organ donation.

Age, function and finding a suitable recipient play a part in the use of organs that the family has consented to be retrieved.

The *kidney* donor should be aged over 2 years, have no history of renal disease and have adequate renal function. An inotrope infusion may be necessary in combination with intravenous therapy to main good perfusion of the kidneys.

The *liver* donor should be aged over 3 months, have no history of liver disease, drug abuse or alcoholism, and have adequate liver function.

The *heart* donor should be aged over 3 months with no history of cardiac defect or disease. This patient should be stable without excessive inotropic support.

The *heart/lung* donor should be aged over 6 months. There should be no history of cardiac defect or disease or of pulmonary dysfunction. The donor should not be a heavy smoker. There should be good arterial blood gases and good lung compliance. This patient should not have been ventilated for a lengthy period.

The *pancreas* donor should be aged over 14 years and have no history of diabetes. If the liver is also being retrieved, this donor must not have had a splenectomy.

The *corneal* donor may be any age. There should be no corneal scarring and no rare infectious eye disease; therefore, eye care is extremely important.

The donors of *heart valves* should be aged over 6 months. The heart valves can be retrieved up to 72 h after death and therefore in patients where brain stem death cannot be diagnosed this is an ideal organ to be retrieved to help the donor's family achieve their wishes.

In any case of organ donation the consenting family are entitled to state which organs they wish to be retrieved for donation. Wight (1987) says, 'Undoubtedly a death with a difference when organ donation takes place'.

RELIGION

Many families find great comfort and support from their own religious groups. It is important that nurses are aware of the special needs of everyone in a multicultural society on the death of a child. Great anxiety and upset can be caused for the grieving family if a nurse is unaware of their religious customs. The following are guidelines (in alphabetical order) of some religious customs that nurses should respect, where possible, when a death occurs. Due to circumstances some customs may have to be waived.

1. *Church of England*: Some families of critically ill children may wish to have their child christened; therefore, the option and opportunity to do so should be offered.
2. *Hinduism*: Hindu families may ask to take a child home to die as this is of religious significance. If this is not possible, after death

the family may wish to wash the body themselves and dress the child in new clothes.

3. *Judaism*: The rabbi may join the family at the bedside to recite prayers. After death, the body is normally washed and then bandaged and wrapped in a white sheet without further interference. It is thought disrespectful to leave a body unattended, but of course this is not always possible in hospital.

4. *Islam*: Special prayers are said for the dying in Arabic (irrespective of nationality or culture). The family may ask for the child to lie facing Mecca. After death, the family may wish to wash the child's body themselves, as the body should not be touched by non-Muslims.

5. *Roman Catholic*: Families may ask for the Roman Catholic chaplain to come and give the sacraments of the sick. When the priest peforms the last offices, the family may ask for the child's hands to be placed in an attitude of prayer, holding a flower, crucifix or rosary.

6. *Sikhism*: The Sikh family may wish to read passages from their holy book at the bedside. There are no particular last offices.

These days there are no religious objections to organ donation, so any family may be approached for consent when circumstances dictate.

REFERENCES

Anthony, S. (1940) *The Child's Discovery of Death*, Harcourt, New York.

Bluebond-Langer, M. (1978) *The Private Worlds of Dying Children*. Princeton University Press, Guilford.

Cain, A.C., Fast, I. and Erikson, M.E. (1964) Children's disturbed reactions to death of a sibling. *American Journal of Orthopsychiatry*, **34**, 741–52.

Compassionate Friends. *Helping Bereaved Parents* (leaflet).

Davies, J. (1979) Death of a child. *World Medicine*, 17 November, 23–6.

Epperson, M. (1977) Families in sudden crisis. *Social Work Health Care, 2*, 265.

Friedman, S. B., Chodoff, D.B. and Mason, J.W. (1963) Behavioural observations of parents anticipating the death of a child. *Pediatrics*, **32**, 610.

Gardner, D. and Stewart, N. (1978) Staff involvement with families of patients in critical care units. *Heart Lung*, **7**, 105.

Green, M. (1976) The family and the critical host. *Report of the Sixth Round Table*, Ross Laboratories, 5706, 53.

Green, J. (1989) Death with Dignity series. *Nursing Times*, Islam, 1 February, 56–7; Hinduism, 8, February, 50–1: Sikhism, 15 February, 56–7; Judaism, 22 February, **85** (5, 6, 7, 8) 64–5.

Gyulay, J.E. (1975) The forgotten grievers. *American Journal of Nursing, 75*, 1476.

Gyulay, J.E. (1987) *The Dying Child*. McGraw-Hill, New York.

Hay, D. and Oken, D. (1972) The psychological stresses of intensive care nursing. *Psychosomatic Medicine, 34*, 109.

Hazinski, M.F. (1984) *Nursing Care of the Critically Ill Child,* C.V. Mosby, St Louis.

Health Education Authority (1988) *Stress in the Public Sector.* Health Education Authority, London.

Iveson-Iveson, J. (1983) Banishing the burnout syndrome. *Nursing Mirror,* 4 May, **156**, 43.

Jacobson, S. (1978) Stressful situations for neonatal intensive care unit nurses. *American Journal of Maternal Child Nursing,* **3**, 1.

Kubler-Ross, E. (1973) *On Death and Dying.* Tavistock, London.

Laurent, C. (1989) A death with a difference. *Nursing Times,* 18 January, **85**, 16–17.

Lieberman, F. (1979) *Social work with Children.* Human Sciences Press, New York.

Lindermann, E. (1944) Symptomatology and management of acute grief. *American Journal of Psychiatry,* 101–41.

Lipsky, K. (1979) *A Practical Guide to Paediatric Intensive Care,* (eds Levin, Morris, Moore), CV Mosby, St Louis.

Lochoff, (1977) *Intensive Care Environment.* Direction for Nursing. Noble.

Lugton, J. (1988) *Communicating with Dying People and their Relatives.* Austen Cornish/Sainsbury Foundation, London.

Lyth, I.M. (1982) *The Psychological Welfare of Children Making Long Stays in Hospital: an Experience in the Art of the Possible.* (Occasional paper No. 3) Tavistock, London.

Miles, M.S. (1979) Impact of the intensive care unit on parents. *Issues in Comprehensive Paediatric Nursing,* **3**, 72–90.

Miles, M.S. and Carter, M.C. (1982) Sources of parental stress in paediatric intensive care units. *Journal of the Association for the Care of Children's Health,* **11**, 65–9.

Nagy, M. (1959) The child's view of death, in *The Meaning of Death,* (ed. H. Fenfel), McGraw-Hill, New York.

Newlin, W. and Wellisch, D.K. (1978) The oncology nurse: life on an emotional roller coaster. *Cancer Nurse,* **1**, 447.

Pallis, C. (1983) *ABC of Brain Death.* Devonshire Press, London.

Parfit, J. (1975) Parents and relatives. *Nursing Times,* **71**, 1512.

Reichle, A.W. (1975) Psychological stress in intensive care. *Nursing Digest,* 3 December.

Robbins, J. (1989) *Caring for the Dying Patient and Family.* Harper and Row, London.

Rosen, H. and Cohen, H. (1981) Children's reactions to sibling loss. *Clinical Social Work Journal,* **9** (3), 211–19.

Scripen, G. *et al.* (1975) *Comprehensive Paediatric Nursing.* CV Mosby, St Louis.

Swaffield, L. (1988) Burnout. *Nursing Standard,* 9 January, **2**, 24–5.

UKCC (1992) *The Scope of Professional Practice.* London 6, 9.2 and 9.3.

Vernon, G.M. (1970) *Sociology of Death.* Ronald Press, New York.

Wight, C. (1987) Concerns of the family. *Nursing Times,* (April–June), **83**, 53.

Working Party of the Health Department of Great Britain and Northern Ireland (1983) *Cadevric Organs for Transplantation: A code of Practice Including the Diagnosis of Brain Death,* DHSS, London.

The ongoing care of the child

Christine Oldfield

The care of the child and their family in the intensive care unit is not simply crisis intervention; it also involves the care required throughout the admission and during the preparations for discharge. Often the child and the family spend only a relatively short period of time in the intensive care environment before being transferred to a lower dependency area before discharge home. However, there is a small but significant number of children who require prolonged high-dependency or intensive care. These children and their families have special needs and pose particular challenges for the nurses caring for them. Obviously some children's families require the unique support of the nursing staff through bereavement, and some children who survive their illness and admission may leave the intensive care unit tragically different. The child's family in both these circumstances require special support, counselling and consideration (Farrell, 1989). However, this chapter explores the principles underpinning both the transfer of children from intensive care and the strategies that can be used in caring for children requiring prolonged admission to an intensive care unit.

It should be remembered that no two transfers are the same and each child requiring chronic care is unique. The admission of a child into an intensive care unit is one of the most stressful times in the life of a parent. Nurses working in this environment care for both the mental and physical well-being of the child. They also care for the child's parents and recognize the mental stress and anguish that can stay with them for many years.

Tender loving care, in the form of comfort, reassurance and support, is of prime importance throughout the child's stay in the intensive care unit and especially during the period leading up to and during the transfer of the child. After the admission of the child, the nurse starts to build a good relationship with the parents, and this will often include preparing them for the eventual discharge. It is possible in some circumstances to predict roughly the time that will be spent in the intensive care unit and at what stage the child will be transferred either back to his own hospital or to another ward. It is also important to explain to the parents that, as the child improves, it may be necessary to transfer him or her at short notice to make room for another sick child.

TRANSFER OF THE CHILD TO ANOTHER HOSPITAL

Transfer of the sick child to another hospital can be a daunting task, and must be undertaken with meticulous care if the safety and comfort of the child are to be achieved. Discussion with the parents is paramount before any arrangements are made. The nurse in charge of the patient needs to sit with the parents and talk about any problems or worries they have about the transfer. A trusting relationship will normally have built up during the child's stay on the unit. The move to another hospital can be perceived by both the parents and the child as being very stressful, and often parents are extremely anxious about leaving a trusted and 'secure' environment for one that is unknown by them They will need to know that the nurses at the new hospital will be equally skilled in this specialized area. Time must be given to allow parents to talk about their worries and reassurance must be given. If possible the opportunity should be given for the parents to travel with their child in the ambulance. However, this is often impossible because of the lack of available space; it is often necessary for the nurse, doctor and/or anaesthetist to accompany the child as well as the numerous pieces of equipment needed.

The parents may prefer to make their own arrangement and should be advised not to drive if they feel very stressed. The help of the social worker may be welcomed if problems occur. Often a close friend or relative can be contacted who would be willing to drive them. If they decide to drive themselves, they must be warned not to try to follow the ambulance as this could be dangerous. A simple road map can be useful if they are not familiar with the locality.

After the arrangements have been made by the medical staff for the child to be accepted at another hospital, the nurse in charge of caring for the child must ring the accepting ward to discuss the child's condition, special medical and nursing needs, special equipment needed, and details about the family. A suitable time for the transfer can then be arranged. This ensures that the nurses receiving the child are fully informed. Arrangements are then made with the ambulance control centre and the appropriate details, which may include the age and condition of the child, are given. They must be made aware of the equipment needed to monitor the child en route and the number of persons accompanying the child. A check must be made that there will be oxygen and suction in the ambulance. A police escort, if necessary, will be arranged by the ambulance personnel.

Medical and nursing notes will be taken if this is the policy of the hospital. If possible a copy of the nursing care plan should accompany the child. If this is not policy, letters are written by the doctor and the nurse in charge of the patient. The accompanying nurse must be fully aware of all aspects of the child's care so that the parents feel that continuity of care has been achieved.

An incubator is used to transfer a baby. An older child may require blankets or a space blanket, depending on the weather and the patient's condition.

No two patients are alike, but if a patient is ventilated it is usually safer and more comfortable for the child if sedation is given immediately before transfer. Endotracheal tubes, intravenous lines, catheters and drainage tubes must be well secured. Intravenous lines which are not absolutely necessary can be heparinized. A resuscitation box, which has been scrupulously checked, must be taken, containing appropriate reintubation equipment, i.e. an endotracheal tube of the correct size cut to the required length, Magill introducing forceps, a largyngoscope with an appropriate sized blade, sterile lubricating jelly and scissors, suction catheters, syringes and needles. Emergency drugs must be included. All necessary spare batteries should also be taken.

Appropriate drugs may be drawn up in advance and labelled in consultation with the doctor accompanying the child. Portable syringe pumps are useful for several reasons: to keep lines open, to continue maintenance fluids and to give sedation as required. An electrocardiograph monitor, oxygen saturation monitor, oxygen cylinder and portable suction machine should all be prepared and checked as necessary.

Often the ambulance will arrive early, or circumstances will have delayed the preparation of the child. It is crucial, however, that the nurse responsible for the transfer is not hurried. Positive checks must be made with the ambulance crew that all connections on the suction machine and the oxygen cylinder are compatible with those in the ambulance. The nurse must ensure that everything is ready before leaving. It must also be remembered that the fastest journey is not necessarily the safest, and that the ambulance crew should be made aware of the need for a gentle, safe journey. The receiving ward should be informed when the ambulance leaves so that they can estimate the child's arrival time.

TRANSFER OF THE CHILD TO ANOTHER WARD WITHIN THE HOSPITAL

During the time spent in intensive care, which in some cases can be many weeks or even months, a close relationship builds up with the child and the parents and they can become very dependent on both staff and equipment. The transfer to another ward can be traumatic, but with thought and preparation this can be eased to some degree. Time for talking to parents must be found to allay fears. This can be done casually at the bedside while nursing the child, or more formally during a time set aside perhaps with the medical staff. Time is needed for the weaning process. This means that monitors and equipment can be removed gradually and appropriately. The parents can be encouraged to become more involved in the amount of care they give to the child so that they become increasingly confident. Confidence in their own ability to care for the child is important for parents who are contemplating the thought of their child being transferred to a ward where the staff are strangers and the routine is very different from the intensive care environment. Arrangements can be made with the new ward for the parents to visit and chat to the staff. Sometimes staff will visit the unit to introduce themselves to the child, but on many occasions the ward and the staff are well known to the family and the discharge may present fewer problems.

If the child needs to be transferred while still requiring a relatively high degree of dependency, owing to a shortage of intensive care beds, parents will need more reassurance. The parents will have built up trust and confidence in the staff during the time spent on the unit and they will need to know that the staff on the receiving ward are equally competent. The nurse transferring the child can help by spending a little time on the ward with them; even a few minutes can make all the difference. They should know that they can call into the unit at any time for a chat. Most parents will be aware that there may be times when staff are busy with an emergency and will be unable to talk to them, but knowing that they can return later when the unit has returned to normal will be reassuring.

CARE OF A CHILD REQUIRING PROLONGED OR CHRONIC CARE

When a child needs to be ventilated for a long period and is conscious and mentally alert, much ingenuity and effort has to be made to entertain and occupy them to prevent them becoming withdrawn and apathetic. Help from other disciplines can be sought, e.g. school teachers and nursery nurses. The majority of children in the toddler age group become accustomed to their ventilator tubes, infusion lines and monitoring equipment and need not be restrained. However, being naturally inquisitive, they will want to explore them. As long as somebody is with them at the bedside to supervise their exploration, they should be allowed to do this.

In most cases, children will not try to dislodge equipment once it has become familiar. However, there is always the 'little one' who will not, under any circumstances, tolerate them and will insist on trying to dislodge them at any opportunity. These children will need to be carefully, thoughtfully and appropriately restrained for their own protection. The younger child, once trusted not to disconnect any vital equipment, and when appropriately supervised, need not be kept in a cot. Play is a vital part of development; toys may be brought from home and it is especially important that a favourite toy stays with the child. A teddy can have a tracheostomy with connections and small pieces of tubing, bandages and electrodes so that teddy shares the experience of hospital. Blowing soap bubbles, which all children love to do, can be an excellent way of encouraging them to do deep breathing during physiotherapy. A nursery nurse is of great value in this age group. Parents will feel more able to spend time at home if they so wish when they see their child playing happily.

Encouraging the extended family to visit can be very supportive and reassuring to both the child and the parents, and can make the intensive care unit feel more like home. Brothers and sisters quickly accept the tubes and monitors, and can play a valuable part in helping to maintain normal family relationships. Siblings can feel neglected when their parents are spending much of their time at the hospital. By encouraging them to visit and play with their brother or sister, much can be achieved to help to prevent problems when the child returns home. With the use of extended ventilation tubing and /or hand-bagging circuits and a play mat, the child can happily and safely play on the floor. If a high chair is used for feeding at home, this can be brought to the unit and used during meal times. A baby walker can be used with the help of two people (one to support the tubing and the other to encourage the child to move around). By these methods, not only does their view of the unit become more varied, but they can begin to learn and discover motor and social skills. This is also an effective form of physiotherapy.

Parents should be encouraged to help and, with effective education and supervision, may be able to take over in these areas (Farrel, 1989). The toddler can be bathed in a baby bath and this can be an enjoyable experience. Parents who are involved in these everyday activities become more relaxed and hopeful for the future. One important concern for the parents of children in intensive care is that they can feel that the normal control they have over their child, with respect to simple care decisions, is often taken away from them. By allowing the parents gradually to take over their child's care, they will feel that this is given back to them and that they are again assuming their normal role. Routine is most important in a child's life and, by arranging a normal pattern of playing, sleeping and eating around routine nursing care, a sense of security is given to the child and the child is generally happy, content and secure. As soon as possible, the routine should match the child's normal routine at home with regards to meals, bedtimes and so on. These children must not be allowed to become isolated, but should feel needed, loved and encouraged.

Even children who are ventilated and unable to move their arms and legs can, with ingenuity, be helped to play and communicate with their family and nurses. Many different ways can be used and a certain amount of trial and error may be needed before a mode of communication that is effective and comfortable for the child is found. Careful assessment of the child's needs must be performed.

For the child over 4 or 5 years of age, the help of a school teacher can be sought. Being in hospital can seriously disrupt normal schooling, and many problems can arise in the future. The school teacher can be enormously helpful in maintaining some level of normality. This also gives the parents a chance to spend time at home, with other children, or simply away from the unit, as they will feel less guilty at leaving if the child is busy doing school work. Parents need to be able to continue their home life to some extent, especially when their child is in hospital for several months. A great strain is put on even the strongest marriages during these times.

By assessment of the child's needs and cooperation of the parents, nurses and technicians, appropriate aids can make the world of difference to the child (Mostyn, 1987). Children even with little or no computer experience can soon develop skills in working the equipment and may become angry if the nursing staff do not seem to be learning as fast. The medical equipment technician is often a useful person to contact. People are usually very willing to be of help in these circumstances. Obviously, access to a computer is required. A light-emitting wand attachment can be fixed to the side of the child's head or onto glasses if worn. Just by moving his or her head and directing the wand at the computer screen the child can draw on the screen, learn to read, play music and games, and many other things, which the school teacher will supervise. Suitable school programmes on television and videos can be used. However, it must be emphasized that the child may have a shorter concentration span than usual and that play is still important. Having stories read to them, watching favourite television programmes, listening to music and being appropriately involved in the unit are also important.

Swimming is another activity which with the help of an enthusiastic team of willing hands, becomes possible. Some hospitals do not have this facility but, if a pool is available, take advantge of it (Carter, 1988). Most children enjoy swimming and this is particularly beneficial for the paralysed child, both physically and mentally. Four people are needed for this exercise (an anaesthetist to hand-ventilate, a porter to help with the lifting in and out of the pool, a nurse and a physiotherapist) and parents are encouraged to assist if they wish. Swimming costumes are required for the child, the nurse and the physiotherapist. The anaesthetist and porter generally remain dry and clothed. As previously mentioned, the ventilator tubing can be lengthened; for a circuit long enough for use in the pool, elephant tubing can be used. This is white corrugated lightweight tubing cut to the required length. Extra care is needed to ensure that all connections are well fitting and that a portable suction machine and an oxygen supply are available. The resuscitation box discussed previously should also be taken. After the initial fear is overcome, great enjoyment is to be had by all, not only the patient. The child usually feels happy, relaxed and pleasantly tired and clean: a good combination rarely achieved with a bed bath. Plenty of dry towels and blankets need to be available to keep him warm and dry afterwards. The journey to and from the swimming pool can also help to break the monotony of the view from the bed space.

During warm sunny weather, if the intensive care unit has an exit leading directly outside either on the ground floor or on a balcony, sunbathing is a possibility. The child and the ventilator can be positioned near the open door or outside, depending on the availability of equipment such as extension plug boards, extensions to the ventilator tubing and so on. Being ventilated need not be a deterrent to getting a sun tan. However, plenty of suntan lotion must be used and exposure time must be sensibly limited to avoid sunburn. Fresh air and the everyday outside noises can brighten up a child's day, and getting ready to go outside can be part of the fun. Parents can be encouraged to bring in suitable clothing, sunhats and sunglasses.

There are a small group of children who spend long periods in the intensive care unit unconscious and unresponsive. The parents of these children live in a no-man's land where they have no idea if their child will ever wake up. Even if the child regains consciousness, there is no way of knowing to what extent he or she will be brain damaged. These parents will need extra help and care, as no honest assurance can be given when they ask many times whether the child will be alright. Many problems can arise within the family as each member tries to come to terms with the illness. Only constant support and encouragement to talk about their worries can be given by staff (Carnevale, 1990).

However, despite these difficulties, it is important to maintain the child's own personality. Parents can bring in the child's own clothes. Staff must continue to talk to the child when giving nursing care. Parents, if they wish, can be encouraged to take over most of the care. Special areas of care include nutrition and physiotherapy. The help of the dietitian can be sought to ensure that the child's nutritional needs are met. The physiotherapist will help to prevent chest complications by giving regular chest physiotherapy. Passive exercises to the arms and legs will help towards the prevention of muscle wasting and stiffness.

It must be remembered when encouraging parents to learn to care for their child that time at home is very important, as the continuation of normal life within the family must be maintained. By this means, staff can help to minimize the guilt that parents sometimes feel when trying to combine the running of a home and being with their child.

Although the paediatric intensive care unit is not an ideal environment for the growth and development of children, many things can be achieved. With plenty of help and an enthusiastic, motivated and committed team, including parents, grandparents, brothers, sisters and friends, the child's stay on the unit can be made relatively happy.

REFERENCES

Carnevale, F.A.. (1990) A description of stressors and coping strategies among parents of critically ill children – a preliminary study. *Intensive Care Nursing*, **6**, 4–11.
Carter, M.B. (1988) Simple pleasures. *Nursing Times*, **84**, (13), 38–9.
Farrell, M. (1989) Parents of critically ill children have their needs too! A literature review. *Intensive Care Nursing*, **5**, 123–8.
Mostyn, C. (1987) Educating Jamie. *Nursing Times*, **83** (41), 36–9.

Paediatric pharmacology

John Lockwood

Children always present special problems with regard to drug therapy, because the responses they show are both quantitively and qualitatively different from those of an adult. In the setting of the intensive care unit, these problems are compounded by the frequent need for multiple drug therapy and a need to maintain therapeutic drug concentrations for long periods of time, often via the intravenous route. In these circumstances an understanding of the pharmacology involved is an essential part of the care of the child. As always with children, the first problem is the calculation of the correct dose for the drug, or drugs, required.

CALCULATION OF DOSES

Whenever possible, specific dosage guidelines provided by manufacturers should be followed to ensure optimum drug therapy and to decrease the possibility of side-effects. Unfortunately, in many cases there are no guidelines available on the dosages of drugs for use in children. Even the choice of drug may be difficult because many manufacturers have disclaimers that their preparation should not be used in children. This may be due to real problems or, more often, to the absence of clinical trials of the particular drug in children. One is therefore often left with the need to calculate from basic principles suitable dosages for these drugs. This can often prove difficult because of the different way in which children react to drugs, and any dose calculated in this way should be administered with caution.

Although it is sometimes unwise to treat children as small adults, many of the methods of estimating paediatric doses are based on scaled-down adult doses as determined by age or body weight. Age is obviously not an accurate indicator as children may vary greatly in their weight within a given age range. Weight will provide more accurate results, and doses can be calculated using Clark's rule:

$$\text{children's dose} = \frac{\text{weight (kg)}}{70} \times \text{adult dose}$$

Probably more accurate is Clark's surface area rule, which relates the dose to the surface area of the child. This is thought to have the advantage that it corresponds better with renal function, cardiac output and fluid requirements in infancy and childhood. The surface area can be obtained from a knowledge of the height and weight of the child, and then by the use of a nomogram available in most paediatric text books or dosage guides. The formula is:

$$\text{children's dose} = \frac{\text{surface area of child (m}^2\text{)}}{1.8} \times \text{adult dose}$$

where 1.8 is taken to be the average surface area of an adult.

A useful rule of thumb for checking doses on a day-to-day basis is the percentage method, which is an extension of Clark's surface area rule. In this method, percentages of adult surface area for different ages of child are related to similar percentages of adult dose. This gives the results shown in Table 12.1.

Table 12.1 Children's dose as a percentage of adult dose

Age	Percentage of adult dose	Average weight (kg)
Newborn	12.5	3.5
4 months	20	6.5
1 year	25	10
3 years	33.3	15
7 years	50	23
12 years	75	39
16 years	90	58
Adult	100	68

A decision as to which method of dose calculation to use will depend primarily on the therapeutic index of the drug and the age of the child. For drugs with a high therapeutic index (i.e. drugs where the difference between the therapeutic dose and the dose where toxic effects become evident is large), the weight or even the age of the child may be used as the guideline. For drugs of a low therapeutic index, where adverse effects soon manifest themselves, the surface area method can be used. However, it is preferable with these drugs for the dose to be based on clinical experience or serum level measurements of the drug.

THE FATE OF DRUGS IN THE BODY

These dosage calculations use the adult as the basis; there are several physiological differences between children and adults, which can affect the way the drug is utilized. Children differ from adults in their ability to absorb, distribute, metabolize and eliminate drugs, and these differences alter with the age of the child. Some of the important considerations are as follows.

Absorption

Absorption is the rate at which a drug leaves its site of administration. Perhaps more important is the concept of bioavailability: the extent to which a drug reaches its site of action.

Oral absorption of drugs in children is different from that in adults owing to several factors. The two main differences are the changing pH of the stomach and the gastric emptying time.

The absorption of many drugs is dependent to some extent on the presence of adult values for gastrointestinal pH. At birth the gastric pH is approximately neutral, but within a few hours it falls to a value of about 2. After 2 weeks the pH has risen to about 5 and then falls gradually to adult levels around the age of 2. The effect of these differences is difficult to predict; some drugs may be more readily absorbed, and others will be less well absorbed than normal.

Gastric emptying time can also affect oral absorption, especially in neonates where it is prolonged. Adult values are not reached until 6–8 months of age. Peristalsis is also irregular and unpredictable, again particularly in neonates. All these effects prevent the rapid and regular absorption of some drugs by the oral route. For example, absorption of phenytoin has been shown to be slower in neonates than in older infants and phenobarbitone absorption is lower in the first 2 weeks of life than later.

Intramuscular absorption can be affected by decreases in local blood flow and a reduction in muscle mass. Absorption is likely to be unpredictable, and whenever possible the intramuscular route should be avoided, especially in neonates and in older children required to have long-term courses.

Caution should be exercised with the topical administration of drugs, because percutaneous absorption of many drugs is enhanced and may lead to unexpected systemic side-effects. These effects are due to a thin stratum corneum and better hydration of the skin. It should also be remembered that occlusive dressings will enhance these effects.

Distribution

In infants 75% of the body consists of water; this is gradually reduced to 60% at 1 year of age, and falls slowly over the years to reach an adult value of 55%. This can be important in the dosage of water-soluble drugs; for example, a drug such as gentamicin will achieve lower serum concentrations in the child than in the adult given the same dose per unit body weight.

This effect can be further compounded by the ease with which infants develop water retention with oedema, or water loss with dehydration, leading respectively to decreased or increased serum concentrations of the drug. For example, children being given phenobarbitone can rapidly show the effects of overdosage if they develop gastroenteritis and diarrhoea, leading to dehydration and a resultant rise in serum concentrations of the drug.

Metabolism

The liver is immature at birth and the various enzyme systems that metabolize drugs are not fully developed. Compounds that require metabolism to the active drug, e.g. pivampicillin, may therefore not be fully effective because of lower blood concentrations of the active metabolite and a consequent decrease in therapeutic benefit.

Other drugs require the liver's enzyme systems to be developed to produce non-toxic breakdown products. Absence of the enzyme can lead to toxicity owing to high plasma concentrations of the drug. For example, high chloramphenicol levels can lead to the grey baby syndrome (vomiting, hypotension, grey skin and shock, leading to death in 40% of cases).

After the first few months of life, and as the enzyme systems become fully effective, the relatively large liver can result in some cases in a more rapid metabolism of drugs. For example, diazepam, carbamazepine and phenobarbitone give lower blood concentrations and shorter duration of effects in children than might be expected.

Excretion

For most drugs, the principal route of excretion is via the kidneys. In the infant, tubular secretion and glomerular filtration rate only reach adult value at about 6 months of age. Drugs dependent on these processes for elimination (e.g. digoxin, gentamicin and penicillins) will therefore have longer half-lives than in the adult, and reduced dosages will be necessary. With drugs such as digoxin and gentamicin, in which the therapeutic level is close to the toxic level, such considerations are of considerable practical importance.

From the age of about 12 months, there may in some cases be faster elimination in infants than in adults. This can be for several reasons, including the more rapid metabolism at this age.

Summary

The way drugs are handled by the body in infants and children is affected by many factors, which may need to be taken into account. It is therefore often difficult to generalize on the response one may see. Caution is therefore always necessary, especially with drugs with which the doctor or nurse may be unfamiliar.

In the intensive care setting, other complicating factors may include the presence of liver or renal failure leading to uncertain metabolism and excretion of the drug.

Multiple drug therapy may alter the distribution and clearance of other drugs; for example, histamine H_2 receptor antagonists (especially cimetidine) decrease the clearance of a number of drugs (e.g. lignocaine, chlormethiazole, fentanyl and midazolam).

Side-effects due to these interactions may be difficult to recognize, and the monitoring of the plasma concentration may be necessary for drugs with a narrow therapeutic index.

ADMINISTRATION OF DRUGS

The administration of drugs to children gives rise to special problems which are not encountered in adults.

The oral route is the easiest and most convenient route to use when suitable preparations are available. Difficulties in measuring doses accurately can be overcome by using syringes, which should always be used for doses of less than 5 ml. Either normal syringes or specially manufactured oral syringes can be used; both allow a greater degree of accuracy than other methods and better control when giving the medicine.

When using a syringe the following procedure should be followed.

1. The child should be in a sitting position to reduce the possibility of choking.
2. The tip of the syringe should be placed in the inside of the cheek towards the back of the mouth.
3. The drug should be given slowly to avoid choking.

Giving drugs by the parenteral route produces more reliable blood levels and may be the only route considered in seriously ill patients. The intramuscular route should not be used if there are other alternatives because of the small muscle mass, particularly in neonates, and the poor vascular supply to the muscles. The intravenous route is to be preferred and, where frequent injections will be required, an intravenous catheter should be inserted.

A particular problem with injections is that most are available only in adult doses. This may mean the withdrawal of small volumes of the injection solution. Many antibiotic injections are supplied as powders for reasons of stability. Significant errors in dosage can result if the displacement value of the powder is not taken into account when calculating the volume to be given. The displacement value is the volume of diluent displaced by the powder. For example, 500 mg ceftazidime displaces 0.5 ml of diluent. To prepare a solution containing 500 mg in 2 ml, one must therefore add 1.5 ml of diluent, *not* 2 ml.

Pharmacy departments will normally be able to provide displacement values for the most common drugs, and these should be referred to before reconstituting the injection.

Intensive care problems in administration

Problems peculiar to intensive care are, as mentioned above, the need for multiple drug therapy and a reliance on the intravenous route for the administration of most if not all drugs.

Drugs to be given intravenously can be administered either as a bolus, or by intermittent or continuous infusion. The choice of method will depend largely on the stability of the drug and a useful guide to the preferred method for many drugs can be found as an appendix in the British National Formulary. Also important will be the therapeutic response required. For example, many drugs are required to be maintained at high concentrations for long periods of time, e.g. sedatives and analgesics for the control of intermittent positive pressure ventilation and pain relief. In these circumstances, the drug must be administered by continuous intravenous infusion.

If several drugs are required, the problem of venous access may become overwhelming. In these circumstances the use of multilumen catheters can be a great help. As well as providing a multiple access route, they also help prevent the problems of drug incompatibility on mixing, which frequently occurs.

DRUGS USED IN INTENSIVE CARE

Over a period of time, almost all the drugs available to the physician may be used on the intensive care unit. Included here are only the drugs and dosages used regularly in most hospitals. Doses have been expressed throughout in whole units to avoid confusion and errors; this is a practice to be wholly recommended when prescribing on treatment sheets.

The conversion between units is as follows:

$$
\begin{aligned}
1 \text{ kg} &= 1000 \text{ g} \\
1 \text{ g} &= 1000 \text{ mg} \\
1 \text{ mg} &= 1000 \text{ } \mu\text{g} \\
1 \text{ } \mu\text{g} &= 1000 \text{ ng}
\end{aligned}
$$

Ages are defined as follows:

1. Neonate: first 4 weeks of life
2. Infant: Up to 1 year of age
3. Child: 1–12 years of age
4. Adolescent: 13 and over

ADRENALINE

Action	α- and β- adrenergic receptor stimulator, inotropic vasoconstictor
Use	low cardiac output and low blood pressure
Dose	slow intravenous injection over 5 min, 10 μg/kg (0.1 ml/kg of 1 in 10 000): this may be repeated twice
Side-effects	tremor, tachycardia, arrhythmias, hypertension, peripheral vasoconstriction with reducing peripheral perfusion

AMIODARONE

Action	antiarrhythmic, lengthens refractive period of atrial and ventricular muscle
Use	refractory atrial or ventricular tachycardia
Dose	intravenous infusion 5 mg/kg over 20 min to 2 h
Side-effects	many, including phototoxicity, corneal microdeposits, skin discoloration, peripheral neuropathy; check thyroid and liver function
Caution	reduce dose of digoxin by 50%

ATRACURIUM
Action	non-depolarizing muscle relaxant
Use	long-term ventilation
Dose	300–600 μg/kg by intravenous injection, or 200–400 μg/kg per h diluted in normal saline for intravenous infusion
Side-effects	erythematous rash on the chest and neck related to histamine release

ATROPINE
Action	antiarrythmic, abolishes vagal tone
Use	bradycardia and cardiac arrest
Dose	intravenous 20 μg/kg, repeated if necessary
Side-effects	tachycardia, dry mouth, confusion

CALCIUM GLUCONATE
Use	cardiac arrest
Dose	0.2 ml/kg of a 10% solution, given slowly
Side-effects	bradycardia, arrythmias, irritation after intravenous injection
Caution	do not mix with sodium bicarbonate solutions

DOBUTAMINE
Action	positive inotrope and peripheral vasodilator
Use	low cardiac output and cardiogenic shock
Dose	2–2.5 μg/kg per min, increasing slowly to 10 μg/kg per min; dilute to 0.5–1 mg/ml before use
Side-effects	tachycardia and sudden increases in systolic blood pressure indicate overdosage

DOPAMINE
Action	positive inotrope and peripheral vasodilator
Use	low cardiac output, cardiogenic shock
Dose	intravenous 2–10 μg/kg per min to a maximum of 10 μg/kg per min
Side-effects	nausea and vomiting, peripheral vasoconstriction, hypotension

FENTANYL
Action	narcotic analgesic
Use	analgesia during operation, enhancement of anaesthesia, respiratory depressant in assisted ventilation

Dose   intravenous bolus 2–5 μg/kg; continuous infusion
                 1–3 μg/kg per h
Side-effects   respiratory depression, transient hypotension,
                 bradycardia, nausea and vomiting

FRUSEMIDE
Action   loop diuretic
Use   oedema, oliguria due to renal failure
Dose   0.5–1 mg/kg intravenous; if diuresis is not produced
                 within 2 h, a repeat single intramuscular dose of up
                 to 4 mg/kg may be tried
Side-effects   rashes
Caution   do not mix with adrenaline, dopamine or
                 dobutamine; do not dilute with glucose solution

HYDRALAZINE
Action   afterload reducing agent, peripheral arteriolar
                 dilator
Use   hypertension or hypertensive crisis
Dose   intravenous 1.5–3 mg/kg per day
Side-effects   tachycardia, fluid retention, postural hypotension,
                 nausea and vomiting, neutropenia, lupus-like
                 syndrome
Caution   start at lower dose because of problems with
                 hypotension and tachycardia; high doses (> 3 mg/kg
                 per day) can produce discoid lupus erythematosus-
                 like illness; over-rapid blood pressure reduction
                 occasionally results even with low doses

ISOPRENALINE
Action   antiarrhythmic, increases heart rate
Use   bradycardia, heart block
Dose   intravenous infusion 50 ng/kg per min, increasing to
                 a maximum of 500 ng/kg per min
Side-effects   tachycardia, arrhythmias, hypotension, sweating,
                 tremor
Caution   acidosis prevents isoprenaline, atropine and inotropes
                 from working

LIGNOCAINE
Action   membrane stabilizer, antiarrhythmic
Use   ventricular tachycardia and significant multifocal
                 ventricular extrasystoles

Dose   intravenous 1 mg/kg bolus over 1 min followed by
                    1 mg/kg per h infusion
Side-effects   confusion, convulsions

MANNITOL
Action   osmotic diuretic
Use   forced diuresis, cerebral oedema
Dose   intravenous 1 g/kg over at least 30 min
Side-effects   chills, fever

MIDAZOLAM
Action   sedative
Use   sedative during artificial ventilation
Dose   2 μg/kg per min as an intravenous infusion
                    increasing to a maximum of 6 μg/kg per min
Side-effects   hypersensitivity reactions, respiratory depression on
                    intravenous injection

PANCURONIUM
Action   non-depolarizing muscle relaxant of medium duration
Use   paralysis of ventilated patients
Dose   intravenous 100–200 μg/kg when required
Side-effects   caution where tachycardia could be dangerous
Comment   reduce dose in obesity and renal impairment

PHENOBARBITONE
Action   anticonvulsant
Use   seizure control
Dose   intravenous or oral up to 10 mg/kg per day, usually
                    in two doses (usually 6 mg/kg per day)
Side-effects   drowsiness, ataxia, allergic skin reactions,
                    hyperkinesia
Caution   impaired renal or hepatic function, severe respiratory
                    depression; avoid sudden withdrawal; prolonged
                    dosage may produce dependence

SODIUM NITROPRUSSIDE
Action   afterload reducing agent, peripheral vasodilator
                    (immediate action)
Use   hypertensive crisis, controlled hypotension in surgery
Dose   intravenous infusion 500 ng to 5 μg/kg per min

Side-effects   Nausea and vomiting, palpitations, retrosternal pain
                    (can be avoided by reducing the infusion rate)
Comment   has immediate action and immediate reversibility;
                    may result in thiocyanate or cyanide toxicity if used
                    in high doses or for prolonged periods of time

SODIUM BICARBONATE
Use   resuscitation, renal acidosis
Dose   for resuscitation, 1 ml/kg of 8.4% solution initially,
                    followed by 0.5 ml/kg if necessary every 10 min

VECURONIUM
Action   Non-depolarizing muscle relaxant
Use   muscle relaxant in ventilation
Dose   intravenous infusion 50–100 µg/kg per h
Side-effects   large doses may have a cumulative effect

REFERENCES

Timmins, J.G. (1985) Pharmaceutical problems in children. *British Journal of Pharmaceutical Practice*, 7(9), 242–7.
Insley, J. (1990) *A Paediatric Vade-Mecum*, 12th edn, Edward Arnold, London.
Alder Hey Book of Children's Doses, 5th edn, (1990)
Lewisham and North Southwark Health Authority (1990) *Paediatric Formulary*, 2nd edn.

Appendix A Support groups

Action for Sick Children
Argyle House
29–31 Euston Road
London
NW1 2SD   (071 833 2041)

Association for Children with Heart Disorders
35 Upper Bank End Road
Holmsfirth
Huddersfield
West Yorkshire
HD7 1EP   (0484 685431)

BODY
British Organ Donor Society
Balsham
Cambridge
CB1 6DL   (0223 893636)

British Epilepsy Association
Crowthorne House
New Wokingham Road
Wokingham
Berkshire
RG11 3AY

British Institute for Brain Injured Children
Knowle Hall
Knowle
Bridgewater
Somerset
TA7 8PJ   (0278 684060)

British Kidney Patients' Association
Bordon
Hampshire
DU35 9JP

Children's Head Injury Trust (CHIT)
National Headquarters
Atkinson Morley's Hospital
Copse Hill
London
SW20 0NE

Compassionate Friends
5 Lower Clifton Hill
Clifton
Bristol
BS8 1BT

Contact a Family (Pierre Robin type disorders)
16 Streaton Ground
London
SW1P 2MP

Courtney Foundation for the Welfare of Mothers and Babies (WOMB)
Trafalgar House
Grenville Place
Hale Lane
Mill Hill
London
NW7 3SA

Cruse
126 Sheen Road
Richmond
Surrey
TW9 1UR

Foundation for the Study of Infant Deaths
23 St Peter's Square
London
W6 9NW

Friends of the Foundation for the Study of Infant Deaths
15 Belgrave Square
London
SW1X 8PS

Guillain–Barré Support Group
45 Parkfield Road
Ruskington
Sleaford
Lincolnshire
NG34 9HT

Headway
7 King Edward Court
King Edward Street
Nottingham
NG1 1EW   (0602 240800)

MIND
22 Harley Street
London
W1N 2ED

National Advisory Service for Parents of Children with a Stoma
32 Suters Drive
Norwich
Norfolk
NR8 6UU

National Meningitis Trust
Fern House
Bath Road
Stroud
GL5 3TJ   (0453 755049)

National Reye's Syndrome Foundation of the UK
45 Parkfield Road
Ruskington
Sleaford
Lincolnshire
OX1 6JJ

National Society for Mentally Handicapped Children
117–123 Golden Lane
London
EC1Y 0RT

National Society for the Prevention of Accidents
Cannon House
The Priory
Queensway
Birmingham
B4 6BS

National Society for the Prevention of Cruelty to Children
1 Riding House Street
London W1

Research Trust for Metabolic Diseases in Children
53 Beam Street
Nantwich
Cheshire
CW5 5NF   (0270 629782)

Stillbirth and Neonatal Death Society (SANDS)
28 Portland Place
London
W1N 2ED

The Spastics Society
12 Park Crescent
London
W1N 4EQ

The Tracheostomy Society
Secretary Mrs F. Davis
Station House
Station Road
Market Bosworth
Nuneaton
Warwickshire
CV1 30PE

Index

Page numbers appearing in **bold** refer to figures and page numbers appearing in *italic* refer to tables